Malingering and illness deception

Malingering and illness deception

Edited by
Peter W. Halligan
School of Psychology
Cardiff University

Christopher Bass
Department of Psychological Medicine
John Radcliffe Hospital
Oxford

and

David A. Oakley
Department of Psychology
University College London

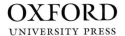
OXFORD
UNIVERSITY PRESS

OXFORD
UNIVERSITY PRESS

Great Clarendon Street, Oxford OX2 6DP

Oxford University Press is a department of the University of Oxford.
It furthers the University's objective of excellence in research, scholarship,
and education by publishing worldwide in

Oxford New York

Auckland Bangkok Buenos Aires Cape Town Chennai
Dar es Salaam Delhi Hong Kong Istanbul Karachi Kolkata
Kuala Lumpur Madrid Melbourne Mexico City Mumbai Nairobi
São Paulo Shanghai Taipei Tokyo Toronto

Oxford is a registered trade mark of Oxford University Press
in the UK and in certain other countries

Published in the United States
by Oxford University Press Inc., New York

A catalogue record for this title is available from the British library

Library of Congress Cataloging in Publication Data
(Data available)
ISBN 0 19 851554 5 (Pbk)

10 9 8 7 6 5 4 3 2 1

Typeset by Newgen Imaging Systems (P) Ltd., Chennai, India
Printed in Great Britain
on acid-free paper by
Biddles Ltd., Guildford and King's Lynn

Acknowledgements

The editors gratefully acknowledge the considerable assistance provided by Kath Little, Laura Morris, Sue Dentten and Lorraine Awcock. We would also like to thank all those contributors at the Woodstock meeting who provided constructive comments and feedback on the presentations: Mrs Diana Brahams, Professor Derick Wade, Dr Peter White, Professor John C. Marshall, Professor Gordon Waddell, and Professor Richard Lewis. We are grateful to Richard Marley, Carol Maxwell and Laura Johnstone at OUP for their editorial guidance and assistance. The meeting which formed the basis for this book would not have been possible had it not been for the enthusiastic support of Professor Mansel Aylward and funding from the Department for Work and Pensions.

Contents

Section 7 Disability analysis and insurance medicine

Section 8 Deception detection

List of Contributors

Mansel Aylward   Department for Work and Pensions, London, UK.

Charles Baron   Registered Specialist in Occupational Medicine, Mold, UK.

Christopher Bass   Department of Psychological Medicine, John Radcliffe Hospital, Oxford, UK.

Richard Byrne   Scottish Primate Research Group, School of Psychology, University of St Andrews, St Andrews, Fife, UK.

Kenneth D. Craig   Department of Psychology, University of British Columbia, Vancouver, B.C., Canada.

Tom Farrow   Academic Department of Psychiatry, University of Sheffield, Sheffield, UK.

David Faust   Department of Psychology, University of Rhode Island, Kingston, RI, USA.

Richard S. J. Frackowiak   Wellcome Department of Imaging Neuroscience, Institute of Neurology, London, UK.

Richard I. Frederick   Department of Psychology, US Medical Center for Federal Prisoners, Springfield, Missouri, USA.

Peter W. Halligan   School of Psychology, Cardiff University, Cardiff, UK.

Amy Herford   Academic Department of Psychiatry, University of Sheffield, Sheffield, UK.

Marilyn Hill   Department of Psychology, University of Western Ontario, Ontario, Canada.

Michael A. Jones   Liverpool Law School, University of Liverpool, Liverpool, UK.

Richard Kitchen   Department for Work and Pensions, Ladywood, Birmingham, UK.

David Leung   Academic Department of Psychiatry, University of Sheffield, Sheffield, UK.

Judith A. Libow   Department of Psychiatry, Children's Hospital and Research Center at Oakland, Oakland, CA, USA

John LoCascio   UNUM Provident Insurance Company, Portland, ME, USA.

Chris J. Main   Department of Behavioural Medicine, Hope Hospital, Salford Royal Hospital, NHS Trust, Salford, UK.

Bertram F. Malle   Institute of Cognitive and Decision Sciences and Department of Psychology, University of Oregon, Eugene, OR, USA.

Samantha Mann   Psychology Department, University of Portsmouth, Portsmouth, UK.

George Mendelson   Department of Psychological Medicine, Monash University, Australia.

Craig Neumann   Department of Psychology, University of North Texas, Denton, TX, USA.

David A. Oakley   Department of Psychology, University College London, London, UK.

Ian P. Palmer   Royal Centre for Defence Medicine TD, Fort Blockhouse, Gasport, Hants, UK.

Loren Pankratz   Department of Psychiatry, Oregon Health Sciences University, Portland, OR, USA.

Jon Poole   Dudley Priority Health NHS Trust, Health Centre, Dudley, UK.

Lindsay Prior   Cardiff School of Social Sciences, Cardiff University, Cardiff, UK.

Anna Rahman   Academic Department of Psychiatry, University of Sheffield, Sheffield, UK.

Adrian Raine   Department of Psychology, University of Southern California, Los Angeles, CA, USA.

Becky Reilly   Academic Department of Psychiatry, University of Sheffield, Sheffield, UK.

W. Peter Robinson   Department of Experimental Psychology, University of Bristol, Bristol, UK.

Richard Rogers   Department of Psychology, University of North Texas, Denton, TX, USA.

Samir Shah   Academic Department of Psychiatry, University of Sheffield, Sheffield, UK.

Michael Sharpe   Division of Psychiatry, School of Molecular and Clinical Medicine, University of Edinburgh, UK.

Sean Spence   Academic Department of Psychiatry, University of Sheffield, Sheffield, UK.

Alan Sprince   The Cayman Islands Law School, Grand Layman, B.W.I.

Emma Stokes   Scottish Primate Research Group, School of Psychology, University of St Andrews, St Andrews, Fife, UK.

Aldert Vrij   Psychology Department, University of Portsmouth, Portsmouth, UK.

Nicholas S. Ward   Wellcome Department of Imaging Neuroscience, Institute of Neurology, London, UK.

Simon Wessely   Department of Psychological Medicine, GKT School of Medicine and the Institute of Psychiatry, London, UK.

Fiona Wood   Cardiff School of Social Sciences, Cardiff University, Cardiff, UK.

Matthew K. Wynia   Institute for Ethics at the American Medical Association, Chicago, IL, USA.

Section 1

Introduction

1 Wilful deception as illness behaviour

Peter W. Halligan, Christopher Bass, and David A. Oakley

Deceiving others is an essential part of everyday social interaction

Aldert Vrij (2001)

You must believe in free will: there is no choice

Isaac Singer

Human freedom is real—as real as language, music, and money—so it can be studied objectively from a no-nonsense, scientific point of view. But like language, music, money, and other products of society, its persistence is affected by what we believe about it.

Daniel Dennett (2003)

Abstract

Sensitivities and confusion regarding the nature of illness deception continue to be a major feature of modern medicine and social security policy in most Western democracies. Although biomedical models continue to dominate current definitions of illness deception, neither of the standard psychiatric glossaries consider malingering—the intentional production of false or exaggerated symptoms motivated by external incentives—to be a valid diagnostic term. In this chapter, we argue that illness deception does not need to be medicalized in order to be understood as a coherent explanatory construct in its own right. The fact that health and non-health related deception is commonly practiced within society and that public attitudes towards fraud and deception are largely equivocal, suggests that it is reasonable to view illness behaviours from several conceptually non-medical perspectives. This is clinically and theoretically important, since disagreements both within and outside the medical community about the fundamental nature of illness deception are still largely framed in medical parameters given the absence of credible or acceptable non-medical accounts. Discussion of illness deception outside medicine is meaningless without an explicit recognition and acceptance that an individual's choice to feign or exaggerate symptoms is a legitimate explanation for some illness behaviours associated with personal or financial incentives.

Over the past 30 years, more generous benefits have became more widely available. It seems unlikely that medical factors alone can adequately explain the large uptake in work-related incapacity benefits in most countries since the 1970s, despite improvements on most objective measures of health. Significantly, most of the conditions associated with this increase are symptom-based illnesses which ultimately rely on the credibility of the subject's report. The key factor in any discussion of illness deception is the extent to which a person's reported symptoms can be considered a product of free will, 'psychopathology' or psychosocial influences beyond his/her volitional control or perhaps all. Distinguishing illness deception from psychiatric illness on the basis of a subject's assumed motives is not practical or always possible; there are no reliable or valid methods for objectively determining consciously motivated intention. Medical models of illness are rendered more congruent with existing sociolegal models of human nature, when they acknowledge and consider the capacity for patients (as human beings) to influence illness behaviour by choice and conscious intent.

Introduction

Malingering and illness deception are regarded by most in medicine and clinical psychology as pejorative terms best avoided in clinical practice. The 'M-word' is typically shrouded in negative and moralistic overtones aptly described by Rogers and Cavanaugh (1983) as 'deviousness and manipulativeness'. Labelling someone as a malingerer has far-reaching medicolegal, personal, and economic ramifications for both subject and accuser. In medicine, the imputation that symptoms are significantly exaggerated or feigned risks law suits (e.g. for defamation of character) and even personal danger (Hofling 1965). In Brisbane, in 1955, three of the four orthopaedic surgeons who labelled a patient as a malingerer were shot; two were killed (Parker 1979). Consequently, for much of the twentieth century, formal studies of malingering have been conspicuous by their absence and the subject has until recently been poorly researched (Rogers 1997) or couched under a variety of different medical and military euphemisms (see Palmer, Chapter 3). Even the courts are reluctant to entertain the label or to stigmatize individuals as malingerers (Miller and Cartlidge 1972; Knoll and Resnick 1999; see Jones, Chapter 16).

Despite general recognition that malingering is not a medical diagnosis '... it is clear from medical literature and the examination of law reports that many doctors consider detection of malingering as an integral part of the medical enterprise' (Mendelson 1995). With the increasing acceptance at the end of the twentieth century that symptoms alone may provide the basis for the diagnosis of discrete underlying mental diseases (Horwitz 2002) and the growing inclination to medicalize social deviance (Wakefield 1992), the traditional distinction between medical illness (or 'medical or psychological illness') and illness deception has become increasingly blurred.

Underlying attempts to medicalize illness deception is the assumption that one has to be ill to want to feign the sick role. The logic of this position was summarized by Menninger (1935) who wrote '... in the compulsive deception represented by the feigning of disease ... the malingerer does not himself believe that he is ill, but tries to persuade others that he is, and they discover, they think, that he is not ill. But the sum of all this, in the opinion of myself and my perverse minded colleagues, is precisely that he is ill, in spite of what others think. No healthy person, no healthy-minded person, would go to such extremes and take such devious and painful routes for minor gains that the invalid status brings to the malingerer'. The proposition that malingering was a mental illness became popular during the Second World War. 'It was believed that only a "crazy" or "sick" person would malinger ... Bleuler seems to have been the first to suggest that the simulation of insanity, irrespective of how conscious or unconscious the patient's motive, should be regarded as a manifestation of a mental illness' (Bash and Alpert 1980).

In this chapter, we question the prominent role that medicine and the biomedical model continues to play in shaping and defining current discussions of illness deception, despite the fact that neither of the established medical and psychiatric glossaries (the DSM-IV/ICD-10) (DSM 1994; WHO 2000) consider malingering to be a valid diagnostic term. The absence of credible or acceptable non-medical accounts, is clinically and theoretically important. Disagreements both within and outside the medical community about the fundamental nature of illness deception are still largely framed in medical parameters. The problem with this medical framing '... is that as soon as the language of "patient–treatment–disease" is used, . . . there is a merging of the language of medicine and the language of morality; if bad is sick, then sick is bad, and sane must be good. The more we treat someone as a patient, the more likely we are to give his sincerity the benefit of the doubt. We tend to ask "what makes him behave like that" instead of "is he telling the truth" and "could he behave differently if it was to his advantage?" ' (Mount 1984).

There is a need for a paradigm shift away from the implicit determinism of the biomedical model and a move towards the proposition that human beings, in most everyday situations (including many aspects of their illness) possess a sense of control and influence over their actions (as opposed to behaviour); that is, they can choose between different courses of action. This capacity is the necessary basis for morality, personal responsibility, democracy, and justice and is "concerned with things people sense themselves as doing, rather than with observed patterns of movement said to be caused by external events", (Shotter 1975). Considered as a volitional act, rather than a psychiatric disorder, illness deception (ranging from mild symptom magnification to frank and protracted feigning or malingering) is meaningfully conceptualized within a sociolegal or human model that recognises the capacity of free will and the potential for pursuing benefits associated with the sick role (see Prior and Wood, Chapter 9). This pervasive and deep-seated notion of free will and individual responsibility remains central to all democratic and legal conceptions of human nature, and provides a reasonable framework from which to explain and discuss illness behaviour not produced by disease, injury, or psychopathology. This emphasis on the non-medical aspects of illness behaviours is essential if we are to move the discussion away from the traditional reliance on medical or psychological 'causes' which discourages empirical investigation of the 'reasons' (together with psychosocial influences) and potential incentives which may explain why some individuals engage in socially deviant behaviours.

Another common belief about illness deception that has contributed to its neglect is the assumption that prevalence levels are small or relatively inconsequential. However, the absence of widely accepted validated measures, the difficulty in establishing reliable base rates and a general reluctance to research the topic suggests that it is too early to draw such definitive conclusions. Moreover, in the absence of convincing evidence regarding prevalence, there is no reason to believe that illness deception considered as one type of deception (extending from exaggeration of transient symptoms to protracted feigning of chronic illness) is any less common that other forms of deceptive behaviour (e.g. lying or fraud) commonly present in non-medical situations.

Finally, since illness deception is not recognised as a legitimate medical or psychiatric diagnosis—the role of doctors in determining illness deception remains unclear unless it can be shown that they are capable of distinguishing real from simulated illness. As suggested by Berney (1973) in dealing with malingering, the physician is caught 'between his duty to society and to his patient—a confusing problem which in the legal profession has been solved by separating the advocate from the judge. For the physician to try and use the term malingering without moral overtones is to change either the rules of the game, or the social meaning of malingering, or his own position within the game'.

Freed from the constraints and assumptions imposed by a biomedical model of illness behaviour, illness deception is best described and understood within a sociolegal framework that considers social responsibility and free will as paramount.

Illness without disease: the growth in 'symptom-based' diagnosis

The traditional medical model of illness assumes that an organ or bodily function is physically abnormal and that this provides the primary cause of the patient's complaint or presenting symptom(s). The diagnosis of illness assumes the presence of a disease that leads to conferment of disability, distress or handicap on the individual. In terms of a disease model, mental disorders are assumed to be a consequence of structural and functional changes occurring primarily in the brain (Horwitz 2002, p. 5). However, as Kendell and Jablensky (2003) point out, the term 'disease' has no generally agreed definition. In defining disease as an objectively and demonstrable departure from perceived adaptive biological functioning, Albert *et al.* (1988) 'emphasized that the clinical signs and symptoms do not constitute the disease and that it is not until causal mechanisms are clearly identified that "we can say we have "really" discovered the disease"'. Consequently, in the traditional biomedical model, establishing the disease or pathology thought to be responsible for a patient's illness presentation is a conceptually related but nevertheless independent aspect of diagnosis.

Whereas disease is dependent on demonstrable objective abnormalities of physical structure or function, illness describes the patient's experience and can be considered 'a social manifestation, a commentary, a role' (Taylor 1979) that can and increasingly does provide for diagnosis despite relying entirely upon the subjective reports of distress, suffering or disability reported by the subject.

Lacking evidence of objective disease, it is perhaps surprising how over the past two decades there has been a growing acceptance of 'medically unexplained symptoms' (an explanatory reference used mainly in psychiatry for symptoms that currently cannot be explained by disease or psychiatric disorder) and 'subjective health complaints' (a term used mainly within medical psychology and disability medicine—see Ursin 1997; Eriksen and Ihlebaek 2002) both of which ultimately depend on the patient's reports and the growing belief that relevant psychosocial factors play a contributing role in their presentation (Engel 1977; Waddell, 1998). Aylward and Locassio considered this acceptance of subjective health complaints to be a significant culture shift in medical practice. The same authors raised concerns regarding the 'creeping medicalization' that has particularly taken place in psychiatry (see Aylward 2002, Chapter 22). Since the first edition of the DSM-I, the total number of psychiatric conditions has more than tripled from 112 in 1952 to over 370 disorders in 1994 (DSM-IV).

Growing numbers of medical specialities are now confronted with increasing numbers of patients who present with disabling unexplained somatic and mental symptoms where no relevant pathology or known psychopathology can be established (Kroenke and Mangelsdorff 1989; Kroenke and Price 1993; Nimnuan *et al.*, 2001). Trends in social security in the United Kingdom also reveal a substantial increase in subjective health complaints during the past few years (Aylward 2002). This in turn has led to calls for a paradigm shift within medicine and a growing acceptance of illness-based conditions such as 'functional somatic symptoms/syndromes' particularly within psychiatry (where most of the mental disorders described by the DSM-IV remain medically unexplained by the same definition). Thus, the traditional requirement of an assumed relationship between symptom and demonstrable pathology has changed and become 'remedicalized around the notion of a functional disturbance of the nervous system' (Sharpe and Wessely 1997; Sharpe and Carson 2001).

Without evidence of a definitive neurobiological or physiological malfunction, calling a set of behaviours and symptoms a syndrome and treating it as such ultimately depends on the underlying beliefs of the patient, doctor, and society at large. In many cases however, 'diagnosis' operates along pragmatic rather than strictly definitional lines—some doctors believe they can recognize disease even if they cannot observe or explain the pathology. For example, none of the functional somatic syndromes are independently verifiable beyond what the patient says and how he or she behaves. Clinicians use the same features which define a disease to justify its status as a disease. For example, how do we know if someone has a factitious disorder? Because of the way they respond and behave. Why do they behave that way? Because they have a factitious disorder!

Notwithstanding issues of validity, it is generally recognized that 'medically unexplained symptoms' and their associated disability (alteration in or limitation of a subject's normal activity) are among the most common of health problems (Kroenke and Mangelsdorff 1989; Kroenke and Price 1993; Nimnuan *et al.* 2000). For example, Bass and Mayou (2002) reported that fewer than half of the patients referred to emergency departments and cardiac outpatient clinics with chest pain have any evidence of heart disease. Over two-thirds of these patients, however, continue to be disabled by their symptoms in the long term, and many remain understandably dissatisfied with their medical care.

In addition to their clinical importance and growing uptake of medical resources (Sharpe and Wessely 1997), subjective health complaints 'are very expensive and claim half or more of the funds available for sickness compensation' (Brosschot and Eriksen 2002, p. 99). In Norway, over 50 per cent of sick certification is currently based on subjective health complaints (Ursin 1997). In the United Kingdom, 'patients regularly seek and receive sick certificates for subjective health complaints' despite the fact that doctors and the general public are 'reluctant in principle to accept psychological and social problems as the basis for sick certification' (Waddell 2002, p. 10). These common, and often non-specific, subjective health complaints (e.g. back pain, musculoskeletal complaints, and stress) account for most of the rise in sickness absence and social security benefits (Waddell 2002, p. 10). In the United Kingdom, 70 per cent of recipients for incapacity benefit have health-related problems that are not sufficient to fully explain their incapacity in purely medical terms (Waddell *et al.* 2002, p. 21). Moreover, most of these current recipients 'and of the greater number on incapacity benefit compared with 20 years ago have less serious, musculoskeletal and mental health complaints' (Waddell 2002).

Although rightly accepted within an evolving and progressive biopsychosocial framework of illness behaviours, these subjective health complaints or medically unexplained symptoms can raise issues of authenticity when personal or financial benefits are involved (see Sharpe, Chapter 12). Thus, increasing reliance on uncorroborated health complaints has understandably raised 'issues of external consistency compared with objective findings and biomedical diagnosis; of internal consistency compared with previous medical history, current clinical history, medical attention and sickness absence record; of psychosocial issues; and ultimately of credibility.' (Waddell 2002, p. 11).

This is not to suggest that subjective health complaints or functional somatic symptoms are trivial or 'not real', but in the context where doctors are the sole diagnosticians and also gatekeepers for financial and related benefits, a symptom-based medical or psychiatric diagnosis alone is open to abuse and fraud given the elaborate bureaucratic social welfare and health-related insurance infrastructure that exists. Together with the growing perception of 'diagnostic creep' (Farah 2002), it is timely to confront the conceptual blurring that continues to impede meaningful discussion of illness behaviours that may stem from willful deception.

Defining issues and competing explanations

Illness deception has never been the exclusive preserve of medicine (see Palmer, Chapter 3). Under Article 115 of the US, Uniform Code of Military Justice (UCMJ) malingering (i.e. feigning illness, physical disablement, mental lapse, or derangement carried out in a hostile fire zone or in time of war) carries the penalties of a dishonourable discharge, forfeiture of all pay and allowances, and confinement for 3 years. Moreover, today, the term 'illness behaviour' is not reserved for exclusive medical use and has been employed to describe a protean range of non-medical conditions 'from unconscious symptom exaggeration to psychiatric disorders and malingering, characterised by mistaken beliefs, refusal to consider alternative explanations of symptoms, misattribution of symptoms, falsification of information, fabrication of complaints, manufactured disease and exaggeration for profit or revenge' (Ensalada 2000).

Illness deception, when encountered in the medicolegal context however, remains controversial, since the attribution describes a form of social deviance where the person is assumed to be using illness behaviours as a way of acquiring benefits of the sick role. Explanations of illness deception can be considered from at least three basic perspectives; medical, biopsychosocial, and non-medical. Disagreements among these different perspectives ultimately boil down to philosophical assumptions concerning the nature of humanity and the extent of personal responsibility. Although none of these accounts are mutually exclusive, it is meaningful to conceptually distinguish them for the purposes of examining their relative characteristics.

Biomedical explanations for illness behaviours

Within Western medicine, the biomedical account still remains the dominant paradigm for explaining most illness behaviours. Central to this account is the assumption that diseases are malfunctions of biological mechanisms and psychological disorders are disordered functioning of the brain, which can be corrected by psychotropic medication (see Aylward, Chapter 22).

Despite declarations by the established medical glossaries that malingering does not constitute a formal 'mental disorder'; in practice, malingering is often implicitly medicalized by contemporary clinical researchers (Miller and Cartlidge 1972; Gorman 1984; Overholser 1990; Hirsh 1998; Reynolds 1998) within a 'pathogenic model' (Rogers 1997), which considers illness deception to be the product of a mental disorder (Bordini *et al.* 2002, p. 94). More often than not and perhaps to avoid confronting the difficult sociolegal issues, many clinicians tacitly medicalize the term and employ it synonymously or equivalently with that of factitious, conversion or somatization disorders. This insidious inclusion within a medical framework is consistent with the view that the biomedical model largely ignores the fundamental notions of responsibility, free will, and the patient's capacity to choose (Wade and Halligan 2003). Horwitz (2002, p. 223) points out that the problem for diagnostic psychiatry 'is that its symptom-based logic makes no distinction between symptoms that are the products of internal dysfunctions and those that stem from chosen, although socially disvalued, activities'.

It is strange, therefore, that while many medical and psychological texts agree that malingering is not a mental or medical disorder, most cite the leading psychiatric nosological manual, the DSM-IV as the principal definition (Franzen and Iverson 1998; Gelder *et al.* 2000). Despite confirming that 'malingering' does not constitute a diagnosis (but, rather, a 'condition that may be a focus of clinical attention') the DSM-IV-TR (2000) nevertheless provides four operational criteria that are used to differentiate malingering from psychiatric conditions such as conversion hysteria and factitious disorders. These include the presence of a medicolegal context, complaints of illness that are far beyond objective findings, lack of cooperation in treatment and diagnosis and the presence of an antisocial personality disorder (APD). These criteria, however, are insufficient (Rogers 1997) and offer little guidance 'for determining consciousness of actions (voluntariness) or consciousness of motivation' (Ensalada 2000). Furthermore, the association with APD can be questioned given that most malingering research typically involves criminal forensic groups where such a diagnosis is not uncommon (Rogers 1997).

Many discussions of malingering continue to use the DSM-IV definition and its four 'diagnostic' criteria, despite the lack of specificity. This is understandable, however, when one considers the conceptual proximity between malingering and many current functional somatic and mental disorders. In what could be viewed as an effort to retain medical involvement in the growing number of unexplained illness-related disorders, ill-defined mental disorders such as 'compensation neurosis' and 'factitious disorders' were introduced into psychiatric nosologies at different times during the twentieth century. However, far from clarifying the distinction from malingering, the introduction of factitious disorders in particular have, if anything, had the opposite effect and closed the gap between an unprovable underlying (but as yet unspecified) disease process and a morally questionable but volitional choice to deceive others by feigning illness. The intentional production or feigning of illness behaviours is common to *both* factitious disorders and malingering. It seems incredible to many that the basis for this formal psychiatric distinction rests solely on the assumed motive thought to underly the individual's behaviour (see Bayliss 1984). The assumed goal in factitious illness is that of wanting to adopt the 'sick role', whereas for the malingerer it is seen as an external goal such as financial compensation, and the avoidance of unwanted social or legal requirements. Some of these shortcomings have been previously pointed out by Kalivar (1996) and Rogers, (Chapter 6).

Common to factitious disorders and malingering is the requirement of doctors or others to perform (often within the temporal confines of a clinical interview) the seemingly impossible task of inferring the level of conscious awareness, the degree of consciously mediated intention, and the motivations that accompany the symptoms presented by their patients! Moreover, the likelihood that more than one type of conscious intention or motivation could be concurrently involved in most forms of illness behaviour makes this distinction impractical and unrealistic. As pointed out by Miller (1961) the distinction between hysteria and malingering 'depends on nothing more infallible than one man's assessment of what is going on in another man's mind'.

The practical and significant impact of having a set of symptoms and behaviours explained in terms of a mental or medical disorder are, however, considerable. Converting an individual into a patient and by extension 'sick role' absolves them of moral responsibility and reclassifies them as the subject of a pathological process largely beyond his/her control (Parsons 1951). Although dependent on medical diagnosis, the 'sick role' can only be fully legitimized within a social context. For Parsons (see Prior and Wood, Chapter 9), this role had the positive benefits of exempting the individual from the usual obligations and attributing the incapacity to agencies other than themselves. If a biomedical account can be used to endorse illness deception then the proposition that malingering might one day be considered a formal mental disorder should come as no surprise. 'Many behavioural tendencies that the layman would consider "bad" but not medical illnesses have acquired diagnostic codes in the Diagnostic Statistical Manual of the American Psychiatric Association' (Farah 2002) and as a consequence of this, 'the "medical model" of condemnable behaviour has been criticised when used to excuse, not simply explain behaviour' (Farah 2002). This endorsement is to be avoided, since the medical model is about defining what is healthy and what is sick—but illness deception and malingering are not consistent with either of these.

Biopsychosocial explanations of illness behaviours

The traditional biomedical model is considered by many to be overly mechanistic, linear, and dated and best suited to demonstrable structural pathology (see Aylward, Chapter 22). It is now recognized that the patient–doctor relationship involves a spectrum of psychosocial factors that contribute to but extend beyond the conventional disease-based models. The biomedical model has been rightly criticised for failing to take account of the complex constitutional beliefs and experiences that individuals in their social context bring to any physical or psychological dysfunction. As pointed out by Nimnuan *et al.* (2000) '... many patients with medically unexplained physical symptoms do not have psychiatric disorders: they may instead be the result of minor pathological change, physiological perceptions and other factors including previous experience of illness'. In response to the perceived and growing need to consider these more complex, interactional and contextual paradigms, 'biopsychosocial models' applied to health sciences emerged in the late 1970s (Engel 1977). Symptom complexes and syndromes including somatization, fibromyalgia, conversion hysteria, irritable bowel syndrome (IBS), and factitious disorders have been included. These 'functional somatic symptoms' were often constructed to account for medically unexplained symptoms within the medical speciality to which the patient is first referred (Wessely *et al.* 1999). However, little is currently known about their aetiology and in the absence of a principled account, as to their pathophysiology it remains unclear what sets one group of descriptive but largely unexplained illness behaviours apart for medical consideration particularly as many, such as IBS, have a high incidence in the general population anyway. Furthermore, 'unfortunately, once a diagnostic concept . . . has come into general use, it tends to become reified. That is, people too easily assume that it is an entity of some kind that can be invoked to explain the patient's symptoms and whose validity need not be questioned' (Kendell and Jablensky 2003). In the case of medically unexplained symptoms, 'their definitive status in public consciousness and popular discourse contrasts markedly with their uncertain scientific and biomedical status' and unlike their predecessors in early twentieth century, patients who have these syndromes today are less 'relieved by negative findings on medical evaluation and less responsive to explanation, reassurance and palliative treatment' (Barsky and Borus 1999). Why should this be the case? Barsky and Borus suggest that 'the contemporary climate is marked by prominent political, legal, economic and regulary ramifications . . . the functional somatic syndromes form the basis for lawsuits and class actions seeking to attribute liability and fault . . .' and consequently remains a fertile source for disputes over health care insurance and the *validity* of current medical diagnosis.

Biopsychosocial models are still developing and one influential version developed by Waddell (1998) based on chronic back pain serves as a useful example of why such models are clearly relevant when explaining many symptom-based, or functional somatic, conditions. According to this model, acute and chronic symptoms that originate from benign or mild forms of physical or mental impairment are re-experienced as amplified perceptions with accompanying distress which, when filtered through the presenting patient's attitudes, beliefs, coping skills, and occupational or cultural social context, can affect patients' perceptions of their impairment and associated disability (Waddell 1998). Within such a model, behavioural symptoms and signs do not of themselves communicate indisputable information about the initial cause of the pain. Furthermore, the associated 'illness behaviours' (observable actions and conduct of the individual assumed to express and communicate the subject's own perception or interpretation of their 'disturbed health') are not considered a formal diagnosis nor should they be characterized along a continuum of pathology (pp. 168–9). Although psychosocial factors are held to be partly within the individual's control, the assumption for the most part is that 'Patients cannot help how they react to pain. Emotions are generally outside our conscious control and most illness behaviour is involuntary. Our professional role is not to sit in judgement, but to understand the problem with compassion and to provide the best possible management for each patient' (Waddell 1998, p. 176).

A related psychosocial account proposed by Rogers (1990) argues for a reconceptualization where feigning is considered an adaptive effort to deal with difficult life circumstances. This account claims the merit of providing the 'least pejorative explanation of malingering'. Using similar factors to those outlined in an 'economic model' of disability described by Waddell (2002), Rogers considers 'would-be malingerers' as engaging in a form of 'cost benefit analysis when confronted with an assessment they perceive as indifferent, if not inimical to their needs' (Rogers 1997, p. 8). The problem with these and other psychosocial accounts of illness deception is their failure to recognize and consider the potential role played by the subject's choice and personal values in deciding between options. Unfettered by such concerns, a psychosocial model could be used to explain all forms of illness deception; normal and deviant human behaviour. For example, Fallik (1972) suggested that 'laws of social welfare and work insurance were made mostly for law abiding people who really are in need. Therefore, it is not the individual who causes the problem of simulation and malingering but the society which created the legal framework for exploiting' (*Lancet* 20 May 1972, p. 1126). Emerging biopsychosocial models of illness are rendered more congruent with existing sociolegal models of human nature when they acknowledge and consider the capacity for patients (as human beings) to influence their illness behaviour.

Naturalistic sociolegal explanations of illness behaviours

Despite philosophical differences, most medical and biopsychosocial models share a common assumption: namely, that the person seeking help from a doctor is largely the victim of an endogenous biopsychosocial vulnerability or physical pathology which is beyond his/her control. Although biopsychosocial models permit medicine to successfully extend its powerful explanatory framework over new or emerging forms of illness behaviours, left unchecked the possibility exists that all forms of illness behaviours will be eventually explained within a medical or biopsychosocial framework. The case *against* such a mandatory medical/psychiatric monopoly for all illness behaviours however is compelling, particularly if crucial everyday human capacities such as intentionality, decision-making, and free choice are not to be surrendered to medical or psychiatric diagnosis. Together with the growing realization that subjective complaints can be influenced and modified by 'normal' beliefs, attitudes, and expectations—considerations of volition and value-laden choice provide an important additional non-medical framework for explaining illness behaviours. Adopting a medical reductionistic perspective in all cases is inappropriate, and removes the freedom of individuals to make decisions about their roles and actions in a society where they choose to deviate from its rules or values (a capacity not even denied to prisoners). Indeed, to suggest that malingering or illness deception is *not* the responsibility of the person with a conscious intention to commit an act is to deny them what is essential to our humanity—namely, our free will. As a form of deception, there is nothing particularly different or difficult about illness deception. Notwithstanding the social, ethical, and legal penalties surrounding malingering, the starting point has to be that while most of us are not motivated to do so, we are all nevertheless capable of exaggerating or feigning illness.

A human model is a reasonable and legitimate alternative to explain illness deception since it takes as its pivotal justification the potential exercise of 'free choice' and the fact that deception is an ubiquitous form of social behaviour (see Spence, Chapter 20 and Vrij, Chapter 27). A brief perusal of the daily news or reflection on our own everyday behaviours reveals that degrees of deception are a common practice in most sectors of society. In those cases, where the deception moves from the unethical to the fraudulent, the stakes and consequences are considerably greater than for many who choose to engage in illness behaviours.

Illustrative reminders of societal deception are not hard to find (see Robinson, Chapter 10) and include:

1. In 2002, senior executives at Worldcom, the second largest US long-distance phone company were found to have orchestrated one of the largest accounting frauds in history by misrepresenting profits of over US $9 billion. This followed the Enron scandal in 2001, where executives and directors, accountants, and law firms, engaged in massive insider trading while making false and misleading statements about the company's financial performance.
2. In 2001, UK credit card fraud amounted to losses of over £370 million.

A recent UK consumer survey (Mitchell and Chan 2002) showed that:

- More than 77 per cent of shoppers claim not to have owned up to getting too much change;
- 40 per cent of shoppers have walked out of shops without paying for goods;
- 77 per cent returned clothes after wearing them;
- 77 per cent lied about a child's age in order to get a reduced price.

Surveys of undergraduates in Australia found that 80 per cent admit to cheating including copying material from the Internet, textbooks, and sharing work with other students (*The Times Higher Education Supplement* (2003). According to estimates reported in the *Financial Times* (10 June, 1995) evasion rates for income tax in the United Kingdom were between 6 and 8 per cent of the GNP, whereas corresponding rates for other countries were: 15 per cent for Belgium, 25 per cent for Italy, and 100 per cent for Russia (Robinson 1996). In a recent national UK poll, almost one-third (30 per cent) of respondents admit to lying on their application form when applying for jobs (Mori Polls and Survey Archive, web page).

Findings from the British Social Attitudes Survey (Park *et al.* 2001), one of the largest and most authoritative indicators of contemporary British values, revealed that while 70 per cent considered value added tax (VAT) evasions for a home repair bill to be wrong (albeit to different degrees), 71 per cent were nevertheless themselves prepared to engage in the same evasion in a similar situation. In the United Kingdom, the Home Office and Serious Fraud Office estimated that the annual cost of fraud was £10.3 billion in 2000, an estimate that was not dissimilar from the £12 billion figure arrived at by the Association of British Insurers 2 years previously (Staple 2000).

Free will and illness deception

Central to the sociolegal account of illness deception as one form of illness behaviour remains the critical concept of 'free will', recognized and enshrined in The United Nations International Covenant on Civil and Political Rights (e.g. Articles 1 and 18—freedom to determine political status, economic, social cultural development, thought, conscience, and religion). Unlike bio-medical models, the human condition can be 'other than what it is' since all human actions can be regarded as value driven. Frankl (1963) called this our 'ultimate freedom' and refers to the potential freedom to choose one's attitude and thus one's actions in any given situation. This freedom to self determine, however, comes with the price that 'the individual is under responsibility to strive for the promotion and observance of the rights' of others. Without the explicit assumption of volitional choice and the known consequences that might follow its exercise in certain situations, any discussion of illness behaviour as deception is meaningless.

Not all deceptions are the same. Illness deception can involve the presentation of symptoms, which can be physical (e.g. weakness, paralysis, sensory loss) or mental (e.g. pain, memory loss), and can range from frank feigning (often used synonymously with the term malingering) to exaggeration of existing conditions or symptoms. Some consider malingering to lie along a continuum (Nies and Sweet, 1994) that varies according to the extent of conscious awareness; others distinguish categories of deception, all of which could apply to the same person. This fractionation of the term is useful given that malingering often means different things to different people. Lipman's (1964) typology included (1) *invention;* where a patient without actual symptoms claims that he has, (2) *perseveration;* genuine symptoms previously experienced are alleged to be present, (3) *exaggeration;*, symptoms or their associated effects (disabilities) are magnified or embellished, (4) *transference;* where genuine symptoms currently present are falsely attributed to previous or unrelated injuries. While all can be considered forms of malingering "there is general agreement that exaggeration of existing symptoms is more frequent than pure malingering of totally non-existent illness or injury" (Miller 1996, p. 7).

Furthermore, gain need not be confined exclusively to financial benefit (i.e. fraud) (Waddell and Norlund 2000) and can also include other incentives, such as:

- improved quality of life,
- avoidance of (stressful) work,
- avoidance of an uninteresting job,

- avoidance of criminal prosecution,
- obtaining drugs

together with some of the perceived social benefits of the sick (such as obtaining drugs) and of incapacity (e.g early retirement). Waddell (2002, p. 32) points out that for some, 'disability benefits are now seen as a right (earned by previous taxes paid) and it is socially acceptable to claim benefits and take early retirement provided it is "within the rules" and whatever the actual degree of (in) capacity for work'.

Any person who freely chooses *not* to participate in a given sociolegal system by engaging in deception might or should expect to be the subject of constraints from those systems they have chosen not to participate in. Even the DSM-IV recognizes this need to consider 'legal or other non-medical criteria' limitations when qualifying some of its more controversial diagnoses (e.g. pathological gambling and paedophilia). In these and related conditions the DSM recognizes that 'the clinical and scientific considerations involved in categorization of these conditions as mental disorders may not be wholly relevant to legal judgments, for example, that take into account such issues as individual responsibility, disability determination, and competency.' (DSM 1994, p. V).

Illness deception therefore stands apart from other illness behaviours *in not being* an illness or disease, although it can occur in patients with mental and other medical disorders (Ju and Varney 2000). It describes a conscious voluntary act or set of actions where the intention is to obtain personal advantage by securing benefits and/or lack of responsibilities that society and the legal system have bestowed upon the sick role. It is qualitatively no different from other forms of deception found in society save for the content and might never have been detached from its natural sociolegal context had it not been for the difficulty medical science had/has in establishing a definite diagnosis of illness behaviours in the absence of objective pathology. This theoretical reconceptualisation finds further support in the fact that malingering has its origins in the military and only became medicalized with the development of the welfare state and workmen's compensation schemes (Miller and Cartlidge 1972; see also Wessely, Chapter 2) at the beginning of the twentieth century.

Regarded as a non-medical explanation, it is not difficult to argue that people who engage in illness deception are not ill, nor are they mad—they simply lack the moral faculties that we assume most in society take for granted. To confound medical disorder with social deviance—by uncritically endorsing the medicalization of social deviance—serves neither medicine nor society and ends up denying one of the most fundamental characteristics of human nature. Indeed, it has been argued that, 'the whole fraudulent process is encouraged by the gradual redefinition of patterns of bad behaviour as bona fide illness. Even persistent lying about being ill has now been defined as an illness. In other words, you are sick if you think—or claim—that you are'. (Dalrymple 2001).

Viewed this way, malingering is not an illness in search of an underlying disease process but rather a form of social deviance—a manifestation of wilful choice for personal advantage. The absence of a reasonable non-medical alternative in which to locate the sociolegal and moral aspects of illness behaviours has, in the past, resulted in an uncomfortable rapprochement that varies precariously between forensic and psychiatric camps.

Although decisions to pursue the financial or personal incentives associated with the sick role provide one explanation for illness behaviours, we recognize that there are other 'psychological and psychosocial elements of illness behaviour, and interactions with health care, employers and the benefits system, over which the individual has little or no control' (Waddell 2000). While an emphasis on personal responsibility is central to the sociolegal account, if taken to extremes, it could result in wrongly attributing responsibility for illness behaviours that are not within an individual's control. The reality, however, is that illness behaviours can result from both exogenous and endogenous factors. In the context where potential external incentives are present or an outcome of the sick or disabled role, then in most cases other than those where psychiatric illness has been established, 'the decision that I am unfit for work, will go sick and apply for social security benefits' should be seen as "a conscious and rational decision, a free choice with full awareness and intent for which I must accept responsibility"' (Waddell 2002, p. 24).

Evidence of exaggeration or malingering is not, however, a reason for medicine to withdraw or abandon such patients. As Yudofsky (1991) points out, recognition of such behaviour is crucially important since it offers the opportunity, where possible, to 'help the patient and others affected by this behaviour' (Sheeley 1991). Freedom from the necessity to accommodate an implicit medical interpretation of some illness behaviours, however, ensures that future research can move beyond the questions of detection to the equally important issues of prevention and management of illness deception.

Distinguishing illness deception from medical or psychiatric illness

Given its origins in the military, in particular problems with motivating conscript armies faced with certain danger and possible death, it was understandable that soldiers might attempt to persuade medical officers and other colleagues that they had an illness which justified or sanctioned their removal from duty (Carroll 2001). Indeed as Palmer (Chapter 2) points out, illness deception in the armed forces both in peace time and war was not unusual, given the authoritative infrastructure and commitments required. The benefits, however, in the case of the military were not primarily financial but rather involved avoidance of criminal conviction or unwanted duty and the potential risks associated with it.

Although some of the prime motivations and benefits may have changed in the case of civilian medical health care systems, the role of the medical clinician as arbitrator has not for the most part. This requires doctors or other professionals to be able to identify illness behaviours that do not conform to known medical or psychiatric diagnoses in subjects with and without other co-existing medical disorders (see Sharpe, Chapter 12). In other words, the explicit remit for most doctors is not to 'diagnose' malingering but rather establish that the illness behaviour cannot be explained by established medical or psychiatric disorders (Hall and Pritchard 1996; Rogers 1997; Reynolds 1998). But given the growth of symptom-based conditions, is this assumed confidence in clinical and diagnostic skills well placed (see Chapter 8)? Are doctors capable of differentiating non-medical illness behaviours across a range of conditions where the doctors are unaware of the possibility of potential confederates?

To the best of our knowledge the relevant study has never been carried out, even with simulators or presumed malingers. The nearest and best-known study was that carried out by Rosenhan (1973) in America. This involved simulating psychosis and provides a compelling illustration of how relatively easy it was in the 1970s to obtain psychiatric diagnosis and gain admission to psychiatric hospitals. In his paper, aptly entitled, 'On being sane in insane places', Rosenhan (1973) and seven colleagues described how they posed as 'pseudopatients' (five men and three women) and gained admission to 12 different hospitals in five different states. In each case, other than giving a truthful normal history (save for their names) each of the pseudopatients complained of hearing voices which said 'empty', 'hollow', and 'thud'. All but one of the 12 were formally diagnosed with 'schizophrenia'. Not one of the pseudopatients was detected despite hospitalization lengths that ranged from 7 to 52 days (average 19 days). In response to criticisms of his study that the psychiatrists involved were unaware of the deception, Rosenhan subsequently secured partial

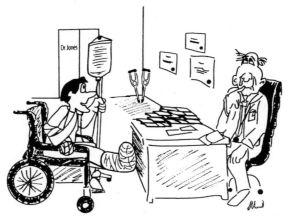

"Hi doc, I could be malingering, and then again I might
be the real article; I leave it up to you to decide"
(adapted from Faust, 1995)

Figure 1.1

confirmation of his original claims. After having said that he was intending to repeat the same study—but when in fact he did not—several individuals were subsequently identified as Rosenham pseudopatients in the months that followed (Faust 1995) (Fig. 1.1).

Furthermore, there is considerable circumstantial evidence to suggest that the traditional diagnostic skills and conceptual medical models adopted by doctors are unlikely to result in a reliable or positive diagnosis of the illness deception. Feigning illness is not as difficult or as obvious as some doctors appear to imagine, particularly since '. . . the possibility that an individual would ever feign illness runs contrary to the empathetic, trusting nature of the physician, the issue often never reaches the threshold of consideration' (Lande 1989). Moreover, the current sociolegal and medical predilection for avoiding the attribution of malingering, the attempts to medicalize social deviance and the difficulty in formally establishing the allegation makes feigning the sick role a relatively low-risk/high-gain form of deception for some.

Any physical or psychiatric disorder can be exaggerated, faked, or feigned. In 1971, Howard Barrow, working at the University of Southern California School of Medicine, showed that actors and non-actors ('simulated patients') could be trained to simulate histories and physical findings for all major features of neurological and psychiatric symptoms (Barrow 1971). His work showed that 'A wide range of psychiatric problems can be simulated, such as depression, agitation, psychosis, neurotic reactions and thought aberrations, with little problem'. The range was impressive 'In neurology, the simulated patients can show a variety: paralysis, sensory losses, reflex changes, extensor plantar responses, gait abnormalities, cranial nerve palsy, altered levels of consciousness, coma, seizures, hyperkinesias, and so forth . . . in other fields anything that features symptoms primarily with little physical findings (pain syndromes, angina, backache, dysmenorrhea, headache, fatigue) and so forth can be readily simulated'. Barrow's simulated patients could be trained, for example, to respond with the Babinski triad to stimulation of the lateral portion of the sole, and not the medial, and made convincing teaching aids for essential features of coma, seizures, paralysis sensory losses, reflex changes, and blindness, as well as many common neurologic diagnoses. Even after being warned that these 'benign' malingerers were among the examinees, experienced clinicians found it difficult to detect these simulated patients (see Oakley *et al.*, Chapter 21).

Prevalence of illness deception

Deception is clearly not peculiar to those who engage in malingering (see Robinson, Chapter 10 and Vris, Chapter 27). Humans apparently 'show considerable aptitude for deception . . . it appears that we all use and need deception in order to cope with social life' (Lewis and Saarni 1993, pp. v–vi). According to Vrij (2000), most on average lie about twice a day or in one quarter of interactions with others, and hence deception remains an 'essential part of everyday social inter-action'. Generally, people are rather good at lying but rather poor at detecting lies or liars (Faust 1995). This failure in detecting deception may be explained by the fact that many lies go undetected because the observer is not motivated or predisposed to the possibility (Vrij 2000). As Rogers (1997, p. 5) rightly points out: 'The problem is circular. If we never investigate dissimulation, then we may never find it.'

Many of the reasons why people engage in lying or deception are similar to those for illness deception (Vrij 2000). As long as humans are motivated by the prospect of personal (and not just financial) gain and perceived entitlements, then illness deception inevitably remains a real pos-sibility, no matter how difficult it is to establish or how morally disagreeable the prospect. Until recently, the most common and powerful argument levelled against the serious consideration of illness deception has been the charge that it occurs so infrequently that routine investigation is unwarranted (Rogers 1997, p. 4). However, infrequency is not to be equated with inconsequen-tiality (Rogers 1997) and in any case, prevalence rates for malingering are under-investigated (Rogers 1997). A major problem with all studies remains the difficulty of defining behaviour and identifying suitable subjects (with or without co-present mental disorders) who can be reliably assumed to be currently engaging in malingering. Consequently, much of the available research is inferential and has to be based on studies involving either paid simulators or those involving groups of patients 'assumed by health professionals' to be engaging in illness deception. The major weaknesses with both are obvious, given the absence of any independent validated criteria from which to justify the selection of subjects in the first place.

Moreover, there is little other than anecdotal evidence to support the clinical assumption that illness deception is rare (1 per cent, Keiser 1968; 5 per cent Waddell 2002): and in most cases; these estimates depend on a particular clinician's opinion of what they consider illness deception to be (Waddell et al. 2002, p. 61). Given the tendency to reserve terms such as malingering or feigning for those considered to be at the extreme end of the illness deception continuum, it is, however, not unreasonable to assume that frank illness deception (i.e. fabricating symptoms or conditions for the purpose of explicit health-related fraud) is less common than symptom exaggeration or other minor forms of illness deception (Miller 1996).

Boden (1996) estimated that at most 3 per cent of injured workers in the United States could be classified as engaging in fraudulent behaviour. Using the 'Composite Disability Malingering Index', Griffin et al. (1996) suggested that 19 per cent of disability claimants in the United States were malingering to some degree. Opinion-based surveys of forensic psychologists in the United States provide estimates of malingering that range from 17.4 per cent in forensic to 7.4 per cent in non forensic settings (Rogers et al. 1994). A recent study of 131 practising members of the American Board of Clinical Neuropsychology provided estimates of the prevalence of malingering and symptom exaggeration for a variety of different clinical conditions (Mittenberg et al. 2002). In this study, estimates of the base rate of malingering/symptom exaggeration were calculated using over 33 000 annual cases seen by a group of clinical neuropsychologists. The reported base rates (when statistically adjusted to remove for the influence of referral source) were 29 per cent for personal injury, 30 per cent in the case of disability or workers' compensation, 19 per cent in criminal cases, and 8 per cent in medical or psychiatric cases. The same rates broken down by diagnosis revealed 39 per cent in the case of mild head injury, 35 per cent in fibromyalgia and chronic fatigue, 31 per cent chronic pain, 15 per cent for depressive disorders, and 11 per cent in the case of dissociative disorders. In a separate review of 1363 compensation-seeking cases, Larrabee (2002) found similar figures for mild head injury (40 per cent).

The perception that illness deception is rare has its roots in the general belief that 'patients' seeking help from a doctor would *not* normally seek to deceive them (see Malleson 2002). Other reasons for this perception include a reluctance to entertain a non-medical account, since malingering is not a legitimate medical disorder and hence by definition not one that can easily return a positive diagnosis. Since most clinicians are not formally trained to actively consider or identify deception in their patients, it is reasonable to assume that many of the 'good' malingerers pass undetected and hence, perhaps, the minority (i.e. 'poor' malingers) of cases that give rise to suspicion provide for the low estimate.

Like other professionals, doctors presumably do not like to think of themselves as having been deceived. Indeed, Pilowsky (1985) coined the term 'malingerophobia'—to describe the 'irrational and maladaptive fear of being tricked into providing health care to individuals who masquerade as sick, but either have no illness at all, or have a much less severe one than they claim'. Coincidentally, it is interesting to note that the most popular course run by the American Psychiatric Association every year involves the detection of malingered mental illness (Wessely 1995).

If illness deception is not a medical disorder but rather a qualitatively distinct form of deception which in some circumstances can involve fraud, then it is useful to know about the extent of deception and fraud in other areas of health care and medicine. Documented reports of fraud and deception, together with the range of potential incentives and prevailing attitudes to fraud provide a relevant (albeit indirect) context from which to consider the extent of illness deception. It would seem somewhat incongruous if the prevalence of illness deception was significantly less than other forms of deception, particularly given:

- that most doctors are not explicitly engaged or trained in detecting deception;
- that clinical skills alone do not appear to be sufficient to identify feigned symptoms, particularly where these relate to mental health;
- the potential range of personal and/or financial benefits currently available.

It is also useful to remember that current rates of disability and incapacity benefits in most countries with welfare systems are generally higher than alternatives such as unemployment benefit and income support. Long-term incapacity is often higher than those on short-term sickness. Moreover, incapacity benefits often have less stringent conditions attached to them (Waddell *et al.* 2002, p. 316) in that they are:

- not means tested;
- not time limited;
- carry less social stigma;
- and carry comparatively less pressure to return to the work place.

Notwithstanding the fact that the vast majority of people not working are financially worse off on social security or workers compensation benefits, 25 per cent of incapacity benefits recipients in the United Kingdom are in the top 40 per cent of population income (Waddell 2002).

In exploring comparative levels of deception, there is clearly a need to be cautious about equating evidence of motivation (or incentive) with evidence of malingering (Rogers 1997) and drawing conclusions regarding the intentions and motivations of others (see Locascio, Chapter 23). However, as Malle (Chapter 6) points out, derivations of intentionality 'are well grounded in a systematic conceptual framework . . . that has evolved over our evolution and has been refined in everyday social practice'. Moreover, Malle points out that 'judging the intentions and goals of other people are made every day, by all social agents, and as such it is neither metaphysically impossible nor completely perfect'. Although motivations or intentions for behaviour can be multiply determined, the following section highlights situations where illness deception might reasonably be assumed to play a role in explaining some illness behaviours.

Examples of health-related deception

Health insurance fraud

The traditionally low estimates of illness deception maintained by same clinicians (see Malleson 2002) stand in marked contrast to the much larger estimates for general deception suggested by opinion polls and health related fraud documented by the insurance industry (see Locasio, Chapter 23). In the United States, the Coalition against Insurance Fraud (CAIF, a US association of consumers, government agencies and insurers) estimated that the total cost of insurance fraud in the United States to be in the region of $85 billion in 1985. The vast majority of this was due to health insurance fraud (LoPiccolo *et al.* 1999). The increase in false health insurance claims occurred at a time when claims fraud for other areas of insurance remained relatively stable. Interestingly, the CAIF tracked 249 significant fraud cases (i.e. those over $100 000) in 1997 and found that the largest group (32 per cent) identified for suspected fraudulent claims involved medical professionals themselves as claimants! They were twice as likely to be involved than that of the next largest group, insurance professionals (LoPiccolo *et al.* 1999).

Prescription fraud

In the United Kingdom, all medical prescriptions have to be paid for unless the patient is exempt or entitled to remission of charges. In 2000, almost 90 per cent of prescriptions claimed exemption. Sample checks showed that many of these were false. Prescription fraud was estimated to cost the National Health Service (NHS) at least £150 million per year (http://www.doh.gov.uk/dcfs/news dec98. htm).

Medical competency

Since the enactment in 1994 of the 'Three-Strikes' law in California, reports of malingering have become far more common during competency to stand trial evaluations, even for such minor crimes as petty theft following two serious prior convictions. Any new felony conviction for a person with two prior convictions (strikes) against them can result in a 25 years to life sentence (Jaffe and Sharma 1998).

Personal injuries compensation

The possible influence of compensation claims and litigation on medical outcome has always appeared to be an obvious target for those wanting to claim that large monetary sums were responsible, in part, for the high prevalence of illness deception in this group (Miller 1961). While obviously multi-determined, the motivation of financial compensation in these cases cannot be ignored, however powerful the case made for psychosocial factors (Wessely 1995; see Mendelson, Chapter 17).

Claims of persistent and disabling symptoms occurring after whiplash neck injury constitute up to 85 per cent of all motor accident personal injury claims in the United Kingdom, despite the fact that the condition is not associated with any specific type of psychiatric presentation not already found in other types of road traffic accident (Mayou and Bryant 2002). Explanations for persistent symptoms are thought to involve 'a subtle interplay between organic factors causing physical injury and functional factors such as personality type, pre-existing psychiatric disease or vulnerability, substance misuse, gender, employment status, legal framework, unrelated but coincidental life events and related life events such as ill health retirement, conscious and unconscious exaggeration' (Thomas 2002, p. 393). Although there is disagreement regarding the reported outcomes after accident-related compensation (e.g. Mendelson, Chapter 17; Kay and Morris-Jones 1998), the impact of financial incentives on disability, symptoms, and objective findings has been convincingly shown in several recent studies, including a systematic review of 13 cohort studies of whiplash injuries by Cote *et al.* (2001), a meta-analysis of 18 studies after closed-head injury by Binder and Rohling (1996) and another meta-analysis of 32 studies of patients receiving compensation for chronic pain by Rohling *et al.* (1995). A recent longitudinal study by Bryan Suter (2002) of 200 chronic back pain patients also adds support to this position. In this study, litigants scored higher on all measures of pain and disability in comparison with a matched non-litigating group. Moreover, litigants' scores on all measures dropped following settlement of litigation. Finally, a well-designed study of 202 unselected people involved in rear-end car collisions in Lithuania, where few drivers had personal injury insurance, showed clearly that the absence of a compensation infrastructure resulted in no significant difference between accident victims and uninjured controls with regard to head and neck symptoms (Schrader *et al.* 1996).

Previous differences in reported outcome in compensation cases may be due to several methodological factors, including what Thomas (2002) suggests are 'differences in mode of referral and orientation and attitude of the assessing specialist'. For example, he notes that most of the subjects assessed by Miller (1961) and Kay and Morris-Jones (1998), where the authors concluded that high levels of exaggeration were involved, were referred by the *defendant's* solicitors or insurance companies. By contrast, most of the litigants in the studies by Tarsh and Royston (1985) and Mendelson (1995) which reported persisting difficulties post-compensation, were seen on behalf of the *claimant's* solicitors.

There are several reasons why litigation and compensation outcome may be negatively affected. These include: (i) the adversarial administrative and legal systems that challenge the claimant to repeatedly prove he or she is permanently ill; and (ii) the fact that any improvement in the claimant's health condition may result in denial of disability status and potential reduction in compensation (Bellamy 1997). Psychosocial influences aside, it would be remiss in explaining such findings to ignore or neglect the important role that personal and financial incentives have in influencing illness presentation and motivating deception (Schmand *et al.* 1998). In this respect, it is worth remembering that many health professionals and social security employees derive 'much greater secondary gain from back pain than any patient ever did' (Waddell *et al.* 2002). Unless one claims that such patients are somehow bereft of volitional choice and decision-making capacity following their accident, then there is no reason to suppose that consideration of the financial circumstance, together with appropriating blame, may not be relevant factors in sustaining an illness presentation. Against a background of a large financial compensation and difficult social circumstances, few would argue that financial gain is not a major motivating force in our material society.

Medical collusion and attorney coaching

There is also evidence that some doctors collude with their patient's deception to help them obtain time off work and medical insurance cover that they are not entitled to (see Wynia, Chapter 15). In the United Kingdom, a qualitative study of the role of general practitioners (GPs) in sickness certification, (Hiscock and Richie 2001), showed that GPs admit to signing certificates when the medical evidence does not justify it. The findings of Wynia, where out of 700 physicians surveyed, 10 per cent admitted to fabricating signs or symptoms on behalf of patients and 54 per cent admitted to deception of insurance payers, confirms that patients are not alone in engaging in deception when the behaviour can be justified. A significant finding of this study was that 37 per cent of physicians reported that their patients 'sometimes, often or very often' *asked them to deceive health care payers*.

Concerns have also been raised in the US regarding attempts to overcome malingering measures using coaching or advice provided by legal attorneys. Youngjohn (1995) described the case of an attorney whose coaching of a 27-year-old man with mild head injury prior to neuropsychological testing provided him with literature regarding malingering measures and simulating injury. Lees-Haley (1997) provides further examples where attorneys were 'influencing data relied on by psychological experts in forensic cases'. The methods described included advising clients 'how to respond to psychological tests', 'making suggestions of what to tell the examining psychologist and what to emphasize' and, finally, leading clients 'not to disclose certain information important to psychologists'.

Sickness absence

In a qualitative study of absenteeism, 72 per cent of hospital workers who had just returned from a scheduled day off or an unscheduled day off that had been classified by the employer as due to sickness absence, admitted not being sick on their (sick) day off (Haccoun and Dupont 1987). According to the Institute of Personnel and Development (2000), of the 192 million sick days taken in 2000 (3.4 per cent of the total working time) more than one-third of these (estimated to cost in the region of £4 billion a year) were not related to ill health with the average worker taking three non-leave days off when they were not sick.

Incapacity benefits in the United Kingdom are replacement incomes provided to people of working age when they become sick or disabled. Incapacity benefits have risen in all developed countries over the past 20 years. Moreover, much of this rise is accounted for by non-specific and subjective health complaints (Waddell *et al.* 2002, p. 21). In November 2002, there were 2.7 million people of working age receiving incapacity benefit in the United Kingdom (Pathways to Work Green Paper 2002). These numbers are more than three times the level in the 1970s.

Estimates of Social Security fraud in the United Kingdom vary and details for health related fraud is difficult to estimate accurately. However, the 1998 Green Paper calculated the level of fraud throughout the social security system to be between £2 and £4 billion annually with a 'best estimate' of £3 billion—approximately 3 per cent of the total annual social security budget (Social Security Fraud Bill 2001-1 Research Paper 01/32, March 2001). To combat what the Public Accounts Committee considered to be unacceptably high levels of fraud, several measures were taken including:

- Establishing a new counter fraud unit and National Intelligence Unit.
- Setting up a benefit fraud telephone hotline.
- Passing the Social Security Fraud Act (2001).
- Introducing 'two strikes and you're out' for repeated benefit offences.
- Spending £1.5 million in TV advertising aimed at hardening public attitudes against benefit fraud.

According to a former Secretary of State in 1997, some 100 000 cases a year are pursued where the relevant department believe there are grounds for prosecution, but only 12 000 or so of these are ever taken to court (McKeever 1999). Many more are issued with benefit penalties or formal cautions. Suspicion of illness deception in claims for welfare related benefits was aroused in the United Kingdom and other countries by the fact that the expenditure on these benefits has tripled over the past 30 years despite improvements in many objective health measures such as life expectancy and morbidity rates over the same period. (Pathways to Work Green Paper 2002). Similarly, in the United States, concerns about malingering rose when 'workers' compensation outlays grew at an annual rate of 14% during the late 1980s and early 1990s outpacing the growth in general consumer spending' (Dembe 1998).

Suspicion regarding the increased up-take of work-related compensation benefits, however, go back to the very origins of the modern welfare state and in particular Germany's introduction of health-related insurance for workers in 1884 (Dembe 1998). Benefits first included 13 weeks of free medical care together with a cash payment equal to 50 per cent of the prevailing wage in the relevant occupation. The cash benefit began on the fourth day of an illness. After 1903, free medical care and cash payments were expanded to 26 weeks. In addition to the basic benefits, the compulsory-insurance funds often provided cash benefits equal to 75 per cent of the worker's pay depending upon family size. By the 1920s, these cash payments often started within one day after registration of the claim for illness (Ebeling 1994). Benefits paid out by the state insurance system always exceeded contributions received from member employees and employers and inevitably required government subsidization. Contributions from employers and employees in 1929 was 375 per cent larger than in 1913. By 1929 they were 406 per cent larger than in 1913 with the government subsidy increasing by some 270 per cent between 1924 and 1929 (Ebeling 1994). As compulsory workers's compensation grew '... the issues of fabricated back pain and malingering by industrial workers became a prominent concern of doctors, employers and insurance administrators' (Dembe 1996). Writing about this in his book, the *German Experience with Social Insurance*, Walter Sulzbach (1947) made the following points:

- Over a period of 50 years (1880–1930), and despite majors advancements in medical science and doctor access, it took the average patient under the compulsory health insurance scheme an increasing longer time to recover.
- In 1885, a year after socialized health insurance began, the average number of sick days each year was 14.1. In 1900, the average number had gone up to 17.6; in 1925, it had increased to 24.4 days; and by 1930, it was 29.9 days.

In the United States, the early studies involving work loss after illness tended to consider only medical factors. 'However, despite a strong desire on the part of the medical community to restrict disability to clinical criteria, medical conditions alone play[ed] a relatively minor role in the epidemiology of work loss' (Yelin 1986).

Early retirement due to ill health

A cross-sectional survey of ill health retirements in six UK organizations by Poole (1997) showed rates of ill health retirement that varied between 20 and 250 per 10 000. In four of the organizations studied, the mode rate of early retirement due to ill health coincided with enhancements in financial benefits and was interpreted as reflecting 'an understandable desire by retiring employees to secure the optimum pension possible' (see Baron and Poole, Chapter 19). It has been estimated that 75 per cent of men and 50 per cent of women now aged over 50 receive long-term incapacity benefit' which effectively forms a mechanism of financial support for early retirement (Waddell 2000, p. 32).

Public attitudes regarding insurance and welfare fraud

Findings from the British Social Attitudes Survey (19th Report) of 3500 adults living in Britain in 2001 (Park *et al.* 2003) confirmed that most people considered that fraud was commonplace in obtaining social security benefits. Seventy-nine per cent of respondents considered that large numbers of people were falsely claiming social welfare benefit. The level of respondents holding this view has never dropped below 70 per cent since 1994. Perhaps surprisingly, and more convincingly, 78 per cent of those who were either themselves (or their partner) currently receiving benefits also agreed that many people 'these days' were falsely claiming benefits. Moreover, the majority of respondents considered it unlikely that the level of false benefit claims was due to confusion rather than dishonesty. Finally, 54 per cent of respondents wanted the government to stop fraud more than facilitate those people entitled to claim benefits.

Public attitudes to fraud appear to be equivocal. In the United States, several public surveys have shown that many respondents considered fraud for insurance purposes as sometimes acceptable. A survey commissioned by the Pennsylvania Insurance Fraud Prevention Authority (IFPA) in 2002 found that while 90.6 per cent believed insurance fraud should be discouraged, 58 per cent (approximately 5.4 million Pennsylvanians) felt it would be appropriate for someone to commit some form of insurance fraud under certain circumstances (*IFPA Quarterly Newsletter* 2002). A similar survey ($N = 602$) by the CAIF showed that most respondents (69 per cent) to some extent endorse or could justify insurance fraud. The respondents could be divided into four distinct groups depending on their response. Some 31 per cent suggested that there was no excuse for insurance fraud and that perpetrators should be punished severely; however, 22 per cent expressed a low level of tolerance and considered that some behaviours involving fraud was justified in some circumstances. This group did not advocate strong punishment. Twenty-six per cent were fairly tolerant of insurance fraud largely because they believed that people did it and this made it more acceptable. These believed in more moderate forms of deterrent. Finally, 21 per cent were much more tolerant of insurance fraud and tended to blame the insurance industry for people's behaviour. Not surprisingly, this group did not hold with any form of punishment. Two-thirds of those asked to give the reasons why people might be motivated to commit insurance fraud indicated that the companies in question made undue profits or that they were entitled to commit fraud after paying high premiums (*The Rough Notes Magazine* 1998 web page).

In the United Kingdom, a similar survey carried out by the Association of British Insurers (ABI) found that 47 per cent of people considered making a fraudulent insurance claim and that 7 per cent admitted having already done so. The behaviour was perceived as being no different that stealing towels from a hotel bedroom (*The Daily Telegraph*, 12 Feb 2003).

Conclusions

Although there is now a number of source books on malingering and its clinical assessment (Rogers 1997; Hutchinson 2001, Reynolds 1998) there is certainly a wealth of information on 'malingering' and illness deception that still awaits investigation.

Sensitivity to issues surrounding the nature of illness deception continues to be a major feature of modern medicine and social security policy in most Western democracies, all of which has contributed to the paucity of published research on this subject. In the early part of the twentieth century, when their work took them out of hospital and into the work environment, many doctors were among the strongest advocates of illness deception as an explanation for unexplained illness behaviour (Dembe 1998). At the end of the twentieth century, a cultural shift within medicine occurred (Aylward and Locascio 1995) which resulted in the acceptance of growing number of symptom-based illnesses and a more tolerant attitude towards illness deception (Pilowsky 1985). By blurring this distinction between willful deception and medical disorder, illness behaviours could be explained in terms of an ever-expanding list of psychopathologies and the growing recognition of psychosocial disorders. However, a medical account alone has difficulty in explaining the three-fold increase in claims to incapacity benefits since 1970 in the United Kingdom and other countries despite improvements in most other indices of health (Dunnell 1995).

Aside from the question of reliable base rates and problems with assessment (Rogers 1997), the major problem for most non-medical accounts of illness deception has been the belief for many in medicine (and in society) that: (i) all illness behaviours have a medical cause; (ii) that all patients in describing their impairments and disabilities do so accurately; and (iii) that illness deception is not common. This 'medical bias' has effectively ensured that today most discussions and explanatory models are couched in psychiatric or psychological terms with little or no reference to the normal moral capacity of many of these persons to exercise choice and determine (at least to some extent) their actions.

Central to this debate on the nature of malingering and illness deception is the extent to which a subjects' illness presentation is considered a product of free will and hence social deviance or the result of psychopathology and or psychosocial influences beyond the volitional control of the subject. Although much theory and philosophy has been written about the illusionary nature of free will (Dennett 2003) the 'deep intuitive feeling of conscious will is something that no amount of philosophical argument or research about psychological mechanisms can possibly dispel . . . free will is the somatic marker of personal authorship, an emotion that authenticates the action's owner as the self' (Wegner 2002, pp. 325–7). Furthermore, considerable progress in cognitive neuroscience and functional imaging over the past decade (see Spence *et al.*, Chapter 20 and Oakley *et al.*, Chapter 21) are beginning to provide a conceptual and empirically based platform for developing a neuroscience of free will (Libet *et al.* 1999).

Significantly, a belief in the attenuation of free will undermines notions of moral and legal responsibility and encourages the acceptance of medical/psychiatric or other biological explanations for all illness behaviours. There are any number of reasons why otherwise normal individuals might choose to engage in activities that psychiatry might classify as illness behaviours. However, allowing medicine to classify all such activities as diseases or functional somatic syndromes carries with it by implication a deterministic diminution of personal responsibility and with it some of democratic society's deeply held values (Horwitz 2002, p. 224). Even in patients with established and well-recognized psychiatric and neurological conditions, the extent to which their illness behaviour is derived totally from their mental disorder or physical disorder is not always clear.

Given the levels of deception found in most areas of society, it remains unclear why deception in illness behaviour (and not just frank malingering) should be perceived as comparatively rare given some of the personal and financial benefits currently attached to the sick role and the low risk of detection. Much of the controversy surrounding malingering however, reflects the conflict between strongly held beliefs. Within the medical community there appears to be a large consensus that most people exhibiting illness behaviours are ill and hence cannot or do not consciously engage in illness deception. The evidence for this belief however is largely untested, since formal studies of illness deception are comparatively rare, difficult to carry out (see Oakley *et al.*, Chapter 21) and are often 'highly dependent on settings and referral questions' (Rogers 1997). While both volitional and non-volitional aspects are clearly relevant for any adequate explanation of illness behaviour, research into the nature and extent of deception have been constrained by the uncritical adoption of the medical model. This is not to argue that medical accounts do not have a role in differentiating unconscious or non voluntary deception, but rather to point out that conceptually it is not meaningful (at least in a non-psychiatric sense) to employ the term 'malingering' or illness deception when referring solely to unconscious deception or where the person is not considered to have control over their behaviour. Common sense requires acceptance that as human beings we all have the capacity to consciously and knowingly engage in subterfuge for the purpose of personal gain or avoidance of responsibility.

The unwillingness by some in medicine to consider the possibility that patients exaggerate or fabricate symptoms for reasons unrelated to their illness, often stems in part from a sense of misplaced compassion and inability (in many cases) to distinguish feigned from real illness behaviour. Another reason is the understandable attempt to minimise or avoid raising prejudicial overtones regarding the veracity of illness complaints. This reticence also finds support in the widespread belief that individuals, as patients, are somehow less likely to exploit or influence a medical situation for personal gain given the implications in terms of limited resources for those with genuine illness and disability. However, in neglecting non-medical explanations for illness behaviours modern medicine runs the risk of underestimating the capacity of individuals to influence and control their actions as they do successfully in many other non-medical areas of their life.

References

Albert, D. A., Munson, R., and Resnik, M. D. (1988). *Reasoning in Medicine*. Johns Hopkins University Press, Baltimore, MD.

Aylward, M. and Locascio, J.J. (1995). Problems in the assessment of psychosomatic conditions in social security benefits and related commercial schemes. *Journal of Psychosomatic Research*, **39**, 758–65.

Aylward, M. (2002). Health and welfare government initiatives and strategy: developing trends in incapacity related benefits. In *Trends in health, Chief Medical Officer's Report*. UNUM Provident, London.

Barrow, H. S. (1971). *Simulated patients*. Charles C. Thomas, Springfield, IL.

Barsky, A. J. and Borus, J. F. (1999). Functional somatic syndromes. *Annals of Internal Medicine*, **130**, 910–21.

Bash, I. Y. and Alpert, M. (1980). The determination of malingering. *Annals of the New York Academy of Sciences*, **347**, 86–99.

Bass, C. and Mayou, R. (2002). Chest pain. *British Medical Journal*, **325** (7364), 588–91.

Bayliss, R. (1984). The deceivers. *British Medical Journal*, **288**, 583–4.

Bellamy, R. (1997). Compensation neurosis: financial reward for illness as nocebo. *Clinical Orthopaedics*, **336**, 94–106.

Berney, T. P. (1973). A review of simulated illness. *South African Medical Journal*, **11**, 1429–34.

Binder, L. M. and Rohling, M. L. (1996). Money matters: a meta-analytic review of the effects of financial incentives on recovery after closed-head injury. *American Journal of Psychiatry*, **153**, 7–10.

Boden, L. I. (1996). Work disability in an economic context. In *Psychosocial aspects of muscoskeletal disorders in office work* (eds S. Moon and S. L. Sauter), pp. 287–94. Taylor and Francis, London.

Bordini, E. J., Chaknis, M. M., Ekman-Turner, R. M., and Perna, R. B. (2002). Advances and issues in the diagnostic differential of malingering versus brain injury. *NeuroRehabilitation*, **17**, 93–104.

Brosschot, J. F. and Eriksen, H. R. (2002). Editorial note. *Scandinavian Journal of Psychology*, **43**, 99–100.

Bryan Suter, P. (2002). Employment and litigation: improved by work, assisted by verdict. *Pain*, **100**, 249–57.

Carroll, M. F. (2001). Deceptions in military psychiatry. *American Journal of Forensic Medicine and Pathology*, **22**, 53–62.

Cote, P., Cassidy, J. D., Carroll, L., Frank, J. W., and Bombardier, C. (2001). A systematic review of the prognosis of acute whiplash and a new conceptual framework to synthesize the literature. *Spine*, **26**, 445–58.

Dalrymple, T. (2001) State fraud. *Spectator*, 21 July.

Dembe, A. E. (1998). The medical detection of simulated occupational injuries: a historical and social analysis. *International Journal of Health Services*, **28**, 227–39.

Dembe, A. E. (1996). *Occupation and disease: how social factors affect the conception of work related disorders*. Yale University Press, New Haven, CT.

Dennett, D. (2003). *Freedom evolves*. Viking Press, New York, NY.

Diagnostic and Statistical Manual of Mental Disorders (1994), 4th edn. American Psychiatric Association.

Diagnostic and Statistical Manual of Mental Disorders (2000). 4th edn. Text revision. American Psychiatric Association.

Dunnell, K. (1995). Population review (2): are we healthier? *Population Trends*, **82**, 12–18.

Ebeling, R. M. (1994). National health insurance and the welfare state (part 2). http://www.fff.org/freedom/0294b.asp.

Engel, G. L. (1977). The need for a new medical model: a challenge for biomedicine. *Science*, **196** (4286), 129–36.

Ensalada, L. H. (2000). The importance of illness behaviour in disability management. *Occupational Medicine*, **15**, 739–54.

Eriksen, H. R. and Ihlebaek, C. (2002). Subjective health complaints. *Scandinavian Journal of Psychology*, **43**, 101–3.

Fallik, A. (1972). Simulation and malingering after injuries to the brain and spinal cord. *Lancet*, **1** (7760), 1126.

Farah, M. J. (2002). Emerging ethical issues in neuroscience. *Nature Neuroscience*, **5**, 1123–9.

Faust, D. (1995). The detection of deception. In *Neurologic clinics: Malingering and conversion reactions*, vol. 13 (ed. M. Weintraub). W.B. Saunders, Philadelphia, PA.

Frankl, V. E. (1963). *Man's search for meaning*. Washington Square Press, Simon and Schuster, New York, NY.

Franzen, M. D. and Iverson, G. L. (1998). Detecting negative response bias and diagnosing malingering. In *Clinical Neuropsychology* (eds P. J. Snyder and P. D. Nussbaum) American Psychological Association, Washington, DC.

Gelder, M. G., Lopez-Ibor, J. J., and Anderson, N. C. (2000). *The New Oxford Textbook of Psychiatry*. Oxford University Press, Oxford.

Gorman, W. F. (1984). Neurological malingering. *Behavioral Sciences and the Law*, **2**, 67–73.

Griffin, G. A., Normington, J., May, R., and Glassmire, D. (1996). Assessing dissimulation among Social Security disability income claimants. *Journal of Consulting Clinical Psychology*, **64**, 1425–30.

Haccoun, R. and Dupont, S. (1987). Absence research: a critique of previous approaches and an example for a new direction, *Canadian Journal of Administrative Sciences*, 143–56.

Hall, H. V. and Pritchard, D. A. (1996). *Detecting malingering and deception: forensic distortion analysis*. St. Lucie Press, Delray Beach, FL.

Hirsh, H. L. (1998). Malingering. *Trauma*, **39**, 53–88.

Hiscock, J. and Richie, J. (2001). The role of GP's in sickness certification. Research Report No. 148. Department of Work and Pensions, London.

HMSO (2002). Pathways to Work: Helping People into Employment (CM 5690).

Hofling, C. K. (1965). Some psychologic aspects of malingering. *GP*, **31**, 115–21.

Horwitz, A. V. (2002). *Creating mental illness*. University of Chicago Press, Chicago, IL.

Hutchinson, G. (2001). Disorders of simulation: malingering, factitious disorders and compensation neurosis. International Universities Press/Psychosocial Press, Madison, CT.

Institute of Personnel and Development (2000). Cited in: Third of sick days taken by fit staff. *Institute of Personnel and Development*, May 15

Insurance Fraud Prevention Authority (IFPA) (2002). *Quarterly Newsletter*, **3** (2).

Jaffe, M. E. and Sharma, K. K. (1998). Malingering uncommon psychiatric symptoms among defendants charged under California's 'three strikes and you're out' law. *Journal of Forensic Science*, **43**, 549–55.

Ju, D., and Varney, N. R. (2000). Can head injury patients simulate malingering? *Applied Neuropsychology*, **7**, 201–7.

Kalivar, J. (1996). Malingering versus factitious disorder. *American Journal of Psychiatry*, **153**, 1108.

Kay, N. R. and Morris-Jones, H. (1998). Pain clinic management of medico-legal litigants. *Injury*, **29** (4), 305–8.

Keiser, L. (1968). *The Transgenic Neurosis*. J.B. Lippincott, Philadelphia, PA.

Kendell, R. and Jablensky, A. (2003). Distinguishing between the validity and utility of psychiatric diagnoses. *American Journal of Psychiatry*, **160**, 4–12.

Knoll, J. L. and Resnick, P. J. (1999). U. S. v. Greer: longer sentences for malingerers. *Journal of the American Academy of Psychiatry and Law*, **27**, 621–5.

Kroenke, K. and Mangelsdorff, A. (1989). Common symptoms in ambulatory care: incidence, evaluation, therapy and outcome. *American Journal of Medicine*, **86**, 262–6.

Kroenke, K. and Price, R. (1993). Symptoms in the community: prevalence, classification and psychiatric comorbidity. *Archives of Internal Medicine*, **153**, 2474–80.

Lande, R. G. (1989). Malingering. *Journal of the American Osteopath Association*, **89**, 483–8.

Larrabee, G. J. (2002). Detection of malingering using atypical perfomance patterns on standard neuropsychological tests. *The Clinical Neuropsychologist* (in press).

Lees-Haley, P. R. (1997). Attorneys influence expert evidence in forensic psychological and neuropsychological cases. *Assessment*, **4**, 321–4.

Lewis, M. and Saarni, C. (1993). *Lying and deception in everyday life*. The Guilford Press, New York, NY.

Libet, B., Freeman, A., and Sutherland, K. (1999). *The volitional brain: towards a neuroscience of free will*. Imprint Academic, Exeter.

LoPiccolo, C. J., Goodkin, K., and Baldewicz, T. T. (1999). Current issues in the diagnosis and management of malingering. *Annals of Medicine*, **31**, 166–74.

Malleson, A. (2002). *Whiplash and other useful illnesses*. McGill-Queen's University Press, Montreal.

Mayou, R. and Bryant, B. (2002). Psychiatry of whiplash neck injury. *British Journal of Psychiatry*, **180**, 441–8.

McKeever, G. (1999). Detecting, prosecuting and punishing benefit fraud: The Social Security Administration (Fraud). Act 1997. *The Modern Law Review*, **62**, 261–70.

Mendelson, G. (1995) 'Compensation Neurosis' revisited: outcome studies of the effects of litigation. *Journal of Psychosomatic Research*, **39**, 695–706.

Mendelson, G. (1995). The expert deposes, but the court disposes: the concept of malingering and the function of a medical expert witness in the forensic process. *International Journal of Law and Psychiatry*, **18**, 425–36.

Menninger, K. A. (1935). Psychology of a certain type of malingerer. *Archives of Neurology and Psychiatry*, **33**, 507–15

Miller, H. (1961). Accident neurosis. *British Medical Journal*, **1**, 919–25.

Miller, L. (1996) Malingering in mild head injury and postconcussion syndrome: clinical, neuropsychological and forensic consideration. *Journal of Cognitive Rehabilitation*, 14, 6–17

Miller, L. and Cartlidge, N. (1972). Simulation and malingering after injuries to the brain and spinal cord. *Lancet*, **1** (7750), 580–5.

Mitchell, V. W. and Chan, J. K. L. (2002). Investigating UK consumers' unethical attitudes and behaviours. *Journal of Marketing Management*, **18**, 5–26.

Mittenberg,W., Patton, C. Vanyock, E. M., and Condit, D. C. (2002). Base rates of malingering and symptom exaggeration. *Journal of Clinical and Experimental Neuropsychology*, **24**, 1094–102.

Mount, F. (1984). The flourishing art of lying. *The Times*, 30 April.

Nimnuan, C. *et al.* (2001). Medically unexplained symptoms: an epidemiological study in seven specialities. *Journal of Psychosomatic Research*, **51**, 361–7.

Nimnuan, C., Hotopf, M., and Wessely, S. (2000). Medically unexplained symptoms: how often and why are they missed? *Quarterly Journal of Medicine*, **93**, 21–8.

Overholser, J. C. (1990). Differenetial diagnosis of malingering and factitious disorder with physical symptoms. *Behavioural Sciences and the Law*, **8**, 55–65.

Park, A., Curtice, J., Thomson, K., Jarvis, L. and Bromley, C. (eds) (2001). *British Social Attitudes Survey*, 18th Report. Sage Publications, London.

Parker, N. (1979). Malingering: a dangerous diagnosis. *Medical Journal of Australia*, **1**, 568–9.

Parsons, T. (1951). *The social system*. Routledge & Kegan Paul, London.

Pilowsky, I. (1985). Malingerphobia. *Medical Journal of Australia*, **143**, 571–2.

Poole, C. J. (1997). Retirement on grounds of ill health: cross sectional survey in six organisations in United Kingdom. *British Medical Journal*, **314** (7085), 929–32.

Reynolds, C. R. (1998). *Detection of malingering during head injury litigation*. Plenum Publishing Corporation, New York, NY.

Robinson, W. P. (1996). *Deceit, delusion and detection*. Sage, Thousand Oaks, CA.

Rogers, R. (1990). Development of a new classificatory model of malingering. *Bulletin of the American Academy of Psychiatry and Law*, **18**, 323–33.

Rogers, R. (1997). Introduction. In *Clinical assessment of malingering and deception*, 2nd edn (ed. R. Rogers), pp. 1–19. Guilford Press, New York, NY.

Rogers, R. and Cavanaugh, J. L. (1983). 'Nothing but the Truth'. . . a re-examination of malingering. *Journal of Law and Psychiatry*, **11**, 443–60.

Rogers, R., Sewell, K. W., and Goldstein, A. (1994). Explanatory models of malingering: a prototypical analysis. *Law and Human Behavior*, **18**, 543–52.

Rohling, M. L., Binder, L. M., and Langhinrichsen-Rohling, J. (1995). Money matters: a meta-analytic review of the association between financial compensation and the experience and treatment of chronic pain. *Health Psychology*, **14**, 537–47.

Rosenhan, D. L. (1973). On being sane in insane places. *Science*, **179** (70), 250–8.

Schrader, H., Obelieniene, D., Bovim, G., Surkiene, D., Mickeviciene, D., Miseviciene, I., and Sand, T. (1996). Natural evolution of late whiplash syndrome outside the medicolegal context. *Lancet*, **347**, 1207–11.

Schmand, B., Lindeboom, J., Schagen, S., Heijt, R., Koene, T., and Hamburger, H. L. (1998). Cognitive complaints in patients after whiplash injury; the impact of malingering. *Journal of Neurology, Neurosurgery and Psychiatry*, **64**, 339–43.

Sharpe, M. and Carson, A. (2001). 'Unexplained' somatic symptoms, functional syndromes, and somatization: do we need a paradigm shift? *Annals of Internal Medicine*, **134**, 926–30.

Sharpe, M. and Wessely, S. (1997). Non-specific ill health; a mind–body approach to functional somatic symptoms. In *Mind–body medicine* (ed. A. Watkins). Churchill Livingstone, New York, NY.

Sheeley, W. F. (1991). Malingering. *Journal of Clinical Psychiatry*, **32**, 281.

Shotter, J. (1975). *Images of man in psychological research*. Clancer Press. Suffolk.

Staple, G. (2000). *The Daily Telegraph*, 20 July.

Sulzbach, W. (1947). *German experience with social insurance*. National Industrial Conference Board, New York, NY.

Tarsh, M. J. and Royston, C. (1985). A follow-up study of accident neurosis. *British Journal of Psychiatry*, **146**, 18–25, January.

The Times Higher Educational Supplement (2003). 24 January, p. 17.

Taylor, D. C. (1979). The components of sickness: diseases, illnesses, and predicaments. *Lancet*, **2** (8150), 1008–10.

Thomas, C. S. (2002). Psychological consequences of traumatic injury. *British Journal of Psychiatry*, **180**, 392–3.

Thomson, K., Park, A., Bromley, C., Curtice, J., and Jarvis, L. (2003). *British Social Attitudes: 19th Report*. Sage Publications, London.

Ursin, H. (1997). Sensitization, somatization, and subjective health complaints: a review. *International Journal of Behavioural Medicine*, **4**, 105–16.

Vrij, A. (2000). *Detecting lies and deceit*. John Wiley & Sons Ltd, Chichester.

Wade, D. T. and Halligan, P. (2003). New wine in old bottles: the WHO ICF as an explanatory model of human behaviour. *Clinical Rehabilitation* **17**, 349–54.

Waddell, G. (1998). *The back pain revolution*. Churchill Livingstone, London.

Waddell, G. (2002). *Models of disability: using low back pain as an example*. Royal Society of Medicine Press Ltd, London.

Waddell, G., Aylward, M., and Sawney, P. (2002). *Back pain, incapacity for work and social security benefits: an international literature review and analysis*. Royal Society of Medicine Press Ltd, London.

Waddell, G. and Norlund, A. (2000). A review of social security systems. In *Neck and back pain: A scientific evidence of causes, diagnosis and treatment* (eds A. Nachemson and E. Johnson), pp. 427–71. Lippincott, Williams and Wilkins, Philadelphia, PA.

Wakefield, J. C. (1992). The concept of a mental disorder: on the boundary between biological facts and social values. *American Psychologist*, **47**, 373–88.

Wegner, D. (2002). *The illusion of conscious will*. Bradford Books, MIT Press, Cambridge, MA.

Wessely, S. (1995). Liability for psychiatric illness. *Journal of Psychosomatic Research*, **39**, 659–9.

Wessely, S., Nimnuan, C., and Sharpe, M. (1999). Functional somatic syndromes: one or many? *Lancet*, **354**, 936–9.

World Health Organization (2000). *Manual of the international statistical classification of diseases and related health problems*, 10th revision. WHO, Geneva.

Yelin, E. (1986). The myth of malingering: why individuals withdraw from work in the presence of illness. *The Millbank Quarterly*, **64**, 622–49.

Yudofsky, S.C. (1991). Malingering. *Journal of Clinical Psychiatry*, **32**, 281–2.

Youngjohn, J. R. (1995). Confirmed attorney coaching prior to neuropsychological evaluation. *Assessment* **2**, 279–83.

Section 2

Historical, military, and evolutionary origins

2 Malingering: historical perspectives

Simon Wessely

Abstract

The practice of deliberate deception by feigning illness would appear to be long standing, with numerous examples from the biblical and classical world. The setting was usually either political or military. However, in this contribution I will outline how malingering moved from being a judicial or disciplinary problem to one that was brought within the sphere of medical expertise. I will argue that the key stimulus was the introduction of progressive social legislation in Bismarckian Germany between 1880 and 1890, with the Workmen's Compensation Act of 1908 and the National Insurance Act of 1911 playing a similar role in the United Kingdom. This legislation appeared, to the medical profession at least, to allow financial rewards to malingering, as opposed to simply escaping onerous duties such as military service. The conservative medical profession saw itself as a gatekeeper for the State against such temptations. The sceptical attitudes shown by much of the profession and authorities towards war-induced psychiatric injury that became an epidemic during the First World War owes much to the spectre of 'compensation neurosis' that was already a contentious issue in the decade before the War. However, one result was that the malingering debate now entered the psychological as well as the physical realm.

Introduction

It seems reasonable to assume that the simulation of illness is as old as humankind, and whenever people gather together in societies with duties and obligations some will use illness to avoid those obligations, or otherwise alter social relations. As writers on malingering never tire of telling us, examples abound in the biblical and classical literature, involving characters from Ulysees to King David, suggesting that such behaviour was recognized and well understood. For example, in Suetonius is the story of a Roman knight who amputated the thumbs of his two sons so they could escape military service—they did not, and the Emperor Augustus confiscated the property of the father. Likewise, as Kinney has entertainingly described, the phenomenon of beggars and assorted vagabonds feigning disease to extract money from the populace was a familiar one (Kinney 1990). In general, such behaviours were seen within the political and military field, and their detection and punishment was a matter for the political or military authorities.

In this chapter I wish to address only one period in the history of malingering. It is the period at the end of the nineteenth and beginning of the twentieth century, when I will argue that malingering moved from the political to the medical sphere—when it in effect became medicalized. That malingering moved into the medical sphere during this period is not in doubt. Before about 1880 there are the occasional texts on malingering, but these are few and far between (e.g. Gavin 1836). After 1880, a steady stream of articles in the learned journals and books devoted to the subject appear in all the industrialised countries. The stimulus to this increased interest was clear at the time—it was the beginnings of the welfare state, and in particular the rise of workmen's compensation schemes in the post industrial revolution societies of North America and Western Europe (Mendelson and Mendelson 1993; Dembe 1996).

The beginnings of the welfare state

The impetus came from Imperial Germany. For some this will come as a surprise, given the predominance of reactionary and conservative politics in Wilhelmine Germany, which might appear to have been the least likely state to implement socially progressive legislation, and indeed the Imperial Chancellor Bismarck was a convinced enemy of the growing influence of socialism and social democracy. His policy to remove working class support was a classic example of 'stick and carrot'. The stick was the 1878 Socialist Law, which outlawed a vast range of political activity. But the carrot was a series of progressive legislation designed to wrong foot the social democrats, and indeed did so successfully. Thus socially progressive legislation represented a way to undermine the labour movement and at the same time to buttress the political and economic elites (Eghigian 2000). The methods were the 1883 Sickness Insurance Act, The Accident Insurance Law of 1884, and the Old Age and Disability Insurance Act of 1889 (Craig 1978).

Britain was less affected by a direct contest between labour and the authoritarian/militaristic state that was being played out in Germany, but nevertheless, the growth of Trade Unionism and its political expression in the Labour Party necessitated similar legislative proposals, culminating in the famous Lloyd George National Insurance Act of 1911.

A link between the new legislative actions and medical interest in malingering was perfectly clear to contemporaries. In the introduction to Jones and Llewellyn (1917) the authors write explicitly that the 'sudden access' of interest by the civil (as opposed to military) practitioner, was the result of the 'social changes initiated during the last twenty-five years—the amalgamation of small industries into huge combines, the establishment of the Employers' Liability and Workmen's Compensation Acts, and the installation of State Insurance.' The pages of that key reference book return regularly to the iniquitous consequences of the recent legislation, the encouragement of 'skulking', the 'benefits trap', and the related phenomenon of 'over insurance' rewarding idleness and at the expense of work.

Social insurance legislation had placed the doctor in a key role—that of gate keeper to the new system, and it was a role which many doctors accepted with alacrity. The reasons why doctors were so keen to accept this new role were not that they accepted or agreed with the aims of the new social insurance schemes—rather the opposite.

The physician and the status quo

It was inevitable that the coming of the welfare state would provoke considerable disquiet and indeed a backlash amongst those traditionally aligned with conservative social policies, which definitely included the medical profession in Britain and Germany. Three years later, in an oration published in full in the *British Medical Journal*, one medical mandarin referred back to the dispute saying that all his audience would no doubt remember the 'very keen debates' in which the attitude of the profession was one of conflict with the Government . . . and he continued 'I advise you to regard the Chancellor of the Exchequer [Lloyd George] as one of the cosmic forces.' But the

Chancellor was to be pitied, for he 'merely expressed social tendencies', and hence his audience was advised to remember this and avoid being 'swept away' in spite of our 'impotent splutterings'.

And impotent splutterings there were. It was a moral issue. The physicians clearly believed that the malign influence of the social insurance legislation was '*a loosening of the grip of men on the principles of justice and equity*' (italics in original) (Jones and Llewellyn 1917). Said another 'a highly developed and conscientious principle of right and wrong is not a characteristic feature of a large number of working men...' (Dewar 1912).

Between 1880 and 1900, doctors in all the industrialized countries that had followed the German lead were united in raising the spectre of the opening of the floodgates to the new armies of malingerers. It would take at least two decades before such fears began to decline—in the period 1880 and 1900 German neurologists tended to classify about one-third of cases of so-called functional nervous disease as due to malingering, but in the next two decades the proportions fell dramatically. By 1917, in their standard text Jones and Llewellyn saw fit to issue a warning against 'wild and extravagant statements as to the increase of malingering under the influence of recent legislation are but too common'—suggesting that such fears remained widespread, even if no longer endorsed by the 'opinion leaders'.

Many physicians viewed the increase in claims under the new schemes as proof of the inequities of the new system. Collie (1917) noted the rise in claims since the introduction of the Compensation Acts in 1906—and as work was not getting more dangerous he concluded that 'malingering and dishonesty must have had an influence in raising the figures to their present abnormal height.' He later adds some statistical data to the effect that fatal accidents were increasing but only by 7 per cent over the 6 year period (being around 3500–4000 per year—which should be contrasted to the current rate of between 200 and 300 per year), but non-fatal accidents were increasing from 323 000 in 1880 to 469 000 in 1913—he concludes that non-fatal accidents were increasing at six times the rate of fatal accidents. That claims were increasing is of course not the issue—what is missing from all of the contemporary literature is any understanding of why such claims might be rising. We should remember that during the period in question the balance of power between worker and employer was completely towards the latter—no matter how dreadful the working conditions or negligent the employer, personal injury litigation against an employer was almost impossible—workman's compensation was the only avenue open to a person who felt they had been harmed by their employment.

'If the case were difficult before the passing of the Workmen's Compensation Act, it is doubly so now, for the injured workman has an Act of Parliament at his back which makes it worth his while to magnify his troubles. Without casting any unjust aspersion on the honest workman, we must be alive to the possibility of simulation especially with regard to injuries of the nervous system. It is wonderful how the malingerer learns the symptoms he has to simulate, and the only pity from his point of view is that he usually overdoes them, and thus betrays himself' (Barnett 1909).

Collie's reactions to the problem of chronic back pain was explicitly set in terms of a conservative social agenda in which he clearly felt some of the profession were acting as class traitors—'it is abundantly apparent to those who have much to do with working-men that there are certain persons who deliberately set class against class, who by day breed discontent, who prolong the period of incapacity caused by illness, and debase honest working men... as long as medical men who attend the working classes are dependent on the working man for their position, so long will gross exaggeration and malingering be rampant' (Collie 1917).

For the physicians, the new climate represented an affront to their values and principles. Wedded as most were to principles of social Darwinism, they could see no reason why the working classes would not use the new mechanisms to avoid their social obligations, namely to work. Old-fashioned virtues such as thrift, hard work, duty, and obligation were now penalized—but what would be rewarded was fecklessness, idleness, and sloth. It was the physician's duty to stem the flood of idleness and deceit unleashed by the new legislation. The detection of malingering was thus a semi class war, with the workman assumed to be trying to outwit the physician to gain money, and the physician standing to uphold the rights and resources of the state against this deception.

The culture of industrialism was exceptionally sensitive to the perceived threat posed by malingerers (Eghigian 2000). They represented an ever present threat to the viability of insurance. The only response was ever constant vigilance, with the medical profession acting as the gate keepers.

Doctors, patients, and the spectre of malingering

Reading the accounts of the period gives a vivid impression of the drama being played out between doctor and patient in the consulting room. On the one hand was the doctor, determined to uphold old-fashioned virtues, and to use his skills to trap the patient into giving proof of the attempted deception. For this purpose, the physician had a repertoire of clinical tricks, signs, and traps, listed in the texts of this period. The doctor had indeed become detective, and in their writings many made conscious analogies to the new literature of detective fiction.

In this period of the medicalization of malingering, exemplified by Collie and Llewelyn and Jones, it is the physician who plays detective, armed with intuition and a series of clinical tricks and traps. Many contemporaries themselves drew the analogy between the clinical skills needed to detect malingering and the skills of a detective—one army surgeon quoted by Bourke when asked if he was a doctor replied 'no, I am a detective' (Bourke 1996). Even with the psycho-logization of illness, and indeed malingering, this process did not stop. Indeed, the Freudian method itself owes perhaps more than we care to admit to the Conan Doyle tradition (Shepherd 1985).

Doctors were now doctors exhibiting what Pilowski has called 'malingerophobia'—the fear of missing malingering, which remains unchanged in certain insurance and medico-legal contexts ever since (Yelin 1986) (see LoCascio, Chapter 23). For the doctor it was a game, and a very one-sided game. For the doctor the rewards could be fame and fortune, exemplified by the career of the most eminent authority on malingering, Sir John Collie, who indeed dedicated his book to 'My friend The British Workman, to whom I owe so much' (Collie 1917).

Meanwhile, the patient was of course all too aware of the doctor's agenda. For the patient the game was in earnest. If the game was lost, and they were branded a malingerer, the consequences were dire. Not only would they be denied their entitlement, but they would also join, either literally or metaphorically, the under class, the beggars, itinerants, paupers, and so on. It was therefore crucial that the patient be seen as of 'good character'. As Eghigian has shown in his analyses of German social insurance claims before the First World War, the result was the frequent repetition of such stereotypic phases as 'I have never avoided work,' and the frequent claims of willingness to work, and good character (Eghigian 2000).

Just as one consequence of the doctor adopting the role of gate keeper for the new systems was that the doctor became convinced that he was the only defence against a legion of claimants out to deceive and defraud, for the patient came the opposite perspective—of a doctor who did not believe you whatever you said or did. 'If it was true, as employers seemed to think, that self interest and self-aggrandizement were the engines of society and the individual, then how could the testimony of claimants be believed?' (Eghigian 2000). And they were not.

The result was that the profession began to be held in contempt. 'Sensitivity to disbelief also helps explain the particular contempt in which workers held the certifying physicians of accident insurance boards. Insured workers saw these doctors as little more than "hired guns" of employers, intent only on finding a way to release insurers from their obligations' (Eghigian 2000). In the unequal struggle between patient and doctor, the only weapon left for the patient was dislike and contempt, a legacy which certainly continues to the present. One might say that every psychiatrist or physician who has been insulted or harried by patients with symptoms or syndromes such as chronic back pain or chronic fatigue is reaping the legacy of the insurance doctors.

Did the floodgates open?

By 1917, some of the worst fears were recognized as spurious. Looking back, Llewellyn and Jones were able to say that the 'moral debacle among the industrial classes' that the Workmen's Compensation Acts were expected to trigger had not happened to the extent foretold, not least in Germany where the concerns were the greatest. In the United Kingdom, said Jones and Llewellyn in 1917, the 'same gloomy forebodings were indulged in, to be, if anything, accentuated when State Insurance followed in their wake,' but again, overall had not been realized (Jones and Llewellyn 1917).

But nostalgia for the past remained. It perhaps puts our current preoccupation (and one which I must plead guilty to endorsing) with the alleged new culture of compensation (Furedi 1997) into some form of perspective to read a similar lament for the good old days; 'the morale of the Fife miner, which prior to the passing of the Compensation Act was of a high order, has since markedly deteriorated, and that traumatic neurasthenia is now a common topic of conversation among the miners' (Collie 1917). That it may have lead to a reduction in morale among the mine owners is plausible, but it seems hard to ascribe a similar deterioration to the miners' themselves, whose living and working conditions in the Scottish coal fields are hard for us now to comprehend.

Malingering and the First World War

The First World War brought a new dimension to the professionalization of malingering. Whereas Sir John Collie famously, and indeed now notoriously, dedicated his book to 'My friend The British Workman, to whom I owe so much' (Collie 1917), Llewellyn and Jones dedicated their volume to Lloyd George—the year was 1917. Lloyd George was the war premier (although of course had also been the architect of social insurance), and the results of three years fighting culminating in the Somme battlefields had led to a manpower crisis. Detecting malingering was now part of the war effort. Collee's own textbook was reissued in 1917—the second edition was nearly twice as long.

As Palmer's contribution (Chapter 3) shows, malingering and the military have always been closely linked. As a recent account of the psychiatry of the US Civil War demonstrates, the Army authorities in that conflict took it for granted that soldiers would attempt to avoid military service, and assumed that all symptoms or disability not associated with obvious physical injury were malingering until proven otherwise—'every means should be adopted to ascertain positively the reality of the deception' (Keen *et al.* 1864).

But what was different about the First World War was its scale. The coming of total war and the mass mobilization of civilian armies placed unprecedented strains on manpower in all the combatant nations. The deliberate avoidance of war service, if true, was a threat to the war effort and the survival of the Nation itself. Its detection was now not just a moral and economic duty, it was a patriotic one as well.

I have already stated my belief that what the turn of the century witnessed was the medicalization of malingering, and its shift from military to civilian settings. The First World War itself, given its scale, size and ferocity, saw the emergence of 'total war' with the mass mobilization of civilian armies. That the mobilization of such human resources was accompanied by the determined efforts of some to escape those duties comes as no surprise to us, nor of course to the medical and military authorities at the time. As Bourke (1996) has shown, some men went to great lengths of bodily mutilation to escape the War. This ranged from deliberately exposing limbs over the top of the trench so as to attract enemy fire and those that wished for 'Blighty' wound, to direct self-mutilation with weapons, or the simulation of disease by a variety of ingenious, and sometimes dangerous, methods. Soldiers would go to considerable, and dangerous, lengths to feign diseases, and, for a fee, there were a variety of orderlies, chemists, or other people to assist with inducing septic joints and simulated appendicitis. Those with genuine illnesses could sell specimens to others less 'fortunate'—there was a trade in genuine tubercle infected sputum (Bourke 1996). And yet, given our present knowledge of the conditions on the Western Front, and the final scale of the casualty lists (something of course that could not be known at the time), what is surprising is not the scale of such behaviour, but why it was not more common.

Medicine, of course, had to devise new methods of detecting malingering—the intuition of the doctor no longer being sufficient. New technologies were brought into play—chemical analyses were used to detect turpentine-induced abscesses, egg albumin in urine, and jaundice secondary to picric acid ingestion (Cooter 1998). X-rays were increasingly used—one of the reasons Sir John Collie undertook to revise his textbook between 1913 and 1917 was because of the increased used of the X-ray in determining the presence or absence of disease pathology.

The attitude of the soldiers themselves towards shirkers and malingerers was unclear. According to Bourke it was regarded as 'part of the game', putting one over on the system, a common practice that was far from being censured, and regarded as acceptable practice. She may well be correct when referring to what Palmer calls 'skrimshanking', the day to day minor games played between officers and men in the attempts of the latter to avoid onerous duties, but she is probably wrong when it comes to overt malingering, which far from being an accepted part of military culture, as Palmer argues for skrimshanking, was a threat to that culture. Those who managed to successfully evade their military duties were abandoning those who for whatever reason remained behind. In what I regard to be the finest fictional account of the war, Frederic Manning speaking via his main character makes it clear that there was little sympathy for those who consciously avoided their duties (Manning 1999). It is hard for us now, with our knowledge of the cost of the First World War, now an inescapable part of our own culture and imagination (Fussell 1975; Hynes 1990), to grasp just how popular was the War, and how deep rooted were the Edwardian values of service, patriotism, and duty.

But Bourke's evidence, whilst intriguing and certainly glossed over by both contemporary and later commentators, did not represent a fundamental shift in the nature of contemporary views of malingering, just its scale. In contrast, Cooter (1998) has argued that the increasing involvement of the medical profession in the psychological consequences of warfare, was indeed a radical departure and extension of medical authority into the domain of the psychological, and in doing so brought about the 'Psychologization of malingering' (Cooter 1998).

The scale of war medicine was unexpected, but not its scope, with the possible exception of the medical consequences of poison gas. The effects of bullets and explosives on the human body posed challenges of scale, but were not entirely unexpected. However, it was the effect of war on men's minds that provided the greatest challenge to medical thinking. The story of 'shell shock' has become well known through the work of the war poets, and latterly their central position in literary culture both on their own merits and as the subject of the fictional work of others, such as Pat Barker's Regeneration Trilogy. At the same time, a rich and varied historical scholarship has emerged looking at the phenomenon of war related psychiatric injury from numerous perspectives (see Leed 1979; Stone 1985; Showalter 1987; Bogacz 1989; Eckart 2000; Micale and Lerner 2001).

By the beginning of 1915, it was clear that something unprecedented was occurring, as doctors were faced with increasing numbers of soldiers with inexplicable symptoms and signs that could not be explained by conventional injury (Myers 1916). Was this still a manifestation of occult brain injury caused by the exploding shell? Was it a psychological reaction to the stressors and strains of modern conflict, stressors on a scale beyond previous experience or imagination? Was it fear, to be controlled? Was it an unconscious desire to escape from the fighting and dangers? Or was it a conscious attempt to avoid one's duties by simulation—in other words, malingering?

And just as the physicians had been subverted, and not unwillingly, into acting as gatekeepers of the insurance system, detecting malingering with varying degrees of enthusiasm, now the same happened to the RMOs, neurologists, nerve specialists, psychologists, and even the occasional psychiatrist, who were called in to assess the apparently psychiatrically damaged servicemen. Just like the physicians and surgeons had willingly policed the insurance system, these doctors were equally 'determined not to become their patients' allies, their actions were designed instead to identify "malingerers" and "moral weaklings" ' (Eckart 2000). The arguments were even more intense because of the invisibility of the presumed injury—the nosological status of psychiatric injury remained very much in dispute, and for many of the doctors the possibility that these conditions simply did not exist was a very real one.

The fate of one doctor, the German neurologist Herman Oppenheim, encapsulates the arguments that raged in all the major combatant nations, and has been brilliantly analysed by Lerner (2001). Oppenheim was a neurologist, arguably the most influential and brilliant of the period, with an international reputation as author of the most famous neurological textbook. He was also Jewish, which may have accounted for the fact that despite his reputation, he had failed to be appointed to the prestigious Chair of Neurology at Berlin. Long before the war, Oppenheim had been identified with the concept of traumatic neurosis—that illness could be caused by trauma. Oppenheim's explanations were a blend of the physical and psychological—he certainly did not espouse what we would call a modern psychological model of trauma—but he did believe that trauma caused illness. In the context of the compensation and insurance legislation discussed above, this was more than controversial, since Oppenheim was in opposition to those who saw that if someone became ill after an accident it was really the result of their predisposition of personality and hereditary. Oppenheim was at the centre of the 'pension wars' (Rentenkampfneurosen) that had divided German medicine before the First World War (Fischer-Homberger 1975; Eghigian 2000).

Now the same issues reappeared, but the stakes were much higher. The German medical establishment, like the British and the French, had thrown themselves whole heartedly into the war effort, and allied themselves completely with the military and national objectives. But what should they do? Should they be treating these people who had developed illnesses, whether physical or psychological, attributable to the stressors of war? Or alternatively should they be agents of military discipline, driving out, shaming and punishing shirkers and malingerers? Oppenheim was identified with the former view, but many of his colleagues were in the opposing camp.

Matters came to a head at the so-called 'War Congress' of the German Association for Psychiatry and the German Neurological Society, which began in Munich on 21 September 1916. The timing was important. The war was in its third year, and the German Army was still engaged in the battles of the Somme and Verdun. Falkenhayn's strategy of 'bleeding the French white' at Verdun had failed, instead it was the German Army that was suffering massive casualties. All were aware of the manpower situation, and the conference took place in an atmosphere of crisis. It was indeed a gathering of the German and Hapsburg neurological and psychiatric establishment.

The arguments raged for 3 days. Oppenheim lost, and lost heavily. He could not explain the oft-repeated observation that prisoners of war (POWs) showed no evidence of psychopathology—which was taken as strong evidence against his position, it being argued as proof that at best war neurosis was little more than fear, and at worst a conscious effort to avoid military duty. Oppenheim's detractors argued that POWs had no need of neurosis, since for them 'the war was over'.[1] His organic explanations were ridiculed. He accused his colleagues of failing to understand the enormous psychic strain imposed by the war, but his was a lost cause. All the old arguments from the pension wars resurfaced. For some, these conditions simply did not exist—what was being witnessed was the interaction between malingering soldiers and gullible doctors. However, the wider view was that Oppenheim and his supporters had misunderstood the nature of war neurosis, which was not conscious deception, but an unconscious desire to evade responsibility and duty. Either formulation, however, was both repugnant and damaging to the war effort.

Once again, doctors were the gatekeepers—but this time they were defending not only the moral order, nor the exchequer, which even if Germany won the war would be bankrupt by the war pensions bill if Oppenheim's arguments prevailed; his opponents were also defending the war effort itself. Oppenheim lost, resigned all his positions, and died the following year, by all accounts a broken man. War neurosis was definitely now a hysteria, and possibly little more than malingering. German (and of course British) treatments for the war neuroses became increasingly punitive.

Of course, it would be grave mistake to assume that either British or German medicine ended the War convinced that all the war neuroses were merely malingering. But despite the new psychological insights, the problem, real or perceived, of wartime malingering, was never far from the surface of war and post war policy. The possibility that the victim of war neurosis was in reality malingering was a British preoccupation as well, and constantly surfaced in the deliberations of the Southborough Committee, established after the end of the war to enquire into the problem of shell shock (Bogacz 1989). The many ambiguities and uncertainties of the final report reflected the absence of any satisfactory resolution of the problem—the distinction between neurosis and malingering, and between courage and cowardice was never satisfactorily resolved. And the prevailing attitude towards psychological injury was best encapsulated by the re-emergence of the foremost pre war expert on malingering, Sir John Collie, as the man in charge of determining war pensions for psychological injury.

After the War

The story of malingering, or more properly our preoccupation with malingering, continues after the First World War, and begins to merge directly with many of the contributions in this book. Several themes can be discerned.

First, the continuing saga of the attempts of doctors to detect deception, whether present or not. As the scope of occupational and compensatable conditions increased, and continues to increase, the same arguments reappeared again and again. For example, there is direct lineage between 'railway spine' and the epidemic of back pain, which began after the First World War and is covered in more detail by Main (Chapter 13). That argument raged during the 1920s and 1930s, but as that

---

[1] The apparent lack of nervous illness in POWs was a commonplace observation of the period, and presents us with some problems. It was shared by many authorities in all the belligerent nations–for example, Thomas Salmon, the man usually credited with inventing US military psychiatry and developing the doctrine of forward psychiatry, held the same view. Albert Glass, perhaps the most impressive military psychiatrist of the century, active during the Second World War and Korean War, also made the same observations. Yet modern follow up studies suggest exactly the opposite—that POWs are more, not less, at risk of long-term psychiatric disorder. I am not able to explain this discrepancy. It may reflect prejudices of the observers, or shame and unwillingness to admit to psychological distress in those who perceive themselves to have 'failed' in their military duties. As far as I know, no scholar has addressed this curious anomaly.

debate subsided the same issues resurfaced with the legitimisation of workmen's compensation for noise induced hearing loss in the 1950s (Dembe 1996). This had been a long-standing preoccupation during the 1920s and 1930s, but gained in strength with the widening scope of compensation. As late as 1967, we find a noted British ENT specialist writing that 'cases of malingering are encountered mostly in connection with pensions or compensation claimed as due to deafness resulting from employment. Such allegations are not only the by product of discontent, but also of social mal-integration. A sense of responsibility is lacking toward any but the subject, and a preoccupation with "getting", at a minimal expenditure of effort, is characteristic' (Mawson 1967).

One result of the continuing efforts at detecting deception was the continuing search for new technologies to detect it. Collie, Llewellyn, and their contemporaries relied on clinical intuition and some bedside tricks in their efforts to unmask the fraudulent. However, this reliance on intuition became increasingly unsatisfactory as we move away from the age of the consultant as King, whose word would be accepted as unquestionable by the Courts. In its place, and parallel to the psychologization of malingering, came a presumed understanding of human nature based on something more than intuition—the coming of age of the science of psychology. Now, to replace the Sherlock Holmesian deductive reasoning and intuition, comes the quasi-scientific certainty of the test—which, by substituting numbers for clues, seemed to promise a scientific certainty to what had previously been a matter of detection. We had entered the world of psychometrics, of the detection of deception by means of quantitative testing (see contribution by Frederick, Chapter 25).

Second, the attempt to obtain a psychoanalytic or psychological understanding of malingering. Physicians and surgeons had, as I have shown, enthusiastically embraced the cause of first medicalizing malingering by which I mean accepting that its detection and hence control was a medical rather than juridicial duty. The experiences of the First World War brought psychiatrists into the same role. And after the war, with psychoanalysis rampant, came attempts to use psychological understanding not to detect fraud, but to explain it. This had begun before the war—Dewar, for example, writing in the *British Medical Journal* uses the prevailing notions of degeneration to suggest that the malinger was not simply to be condemned, but 'There will always be a certain amount of sympathy with malingerers because from a psychological point of view they are not altogether to be blamed for being the possessors of a weak mental stamina, often the fault of heredity' (Dewar 1912).

After the War, the idea that malingering was itself a psychopathology to be understood was a frequent comment, coming close to becoming the dominant paradigm during the inter-war years, and indeed is considered by several of the contributions in this book. By the 1920s, it 'had become almost impossible to conceive of malingering outside a psychological or psychopathological framework' (Cooter 1998).

Third, continuing work on the sociological perspective on malingering (see contribution by Robinson, Chapter 10). During the 1950s, and following the seminal work of Talcott Parsons, came a similar perspective on malingering by the irresistibly named Dr Twaddle.

The apotheosis of the sociological perspective came with the work of Thomas Szasz, who first used his considerable oratorical talents in his assault on the psychologization of malingering. 'Malingering is considered in every textbook of psychiatry, and in psychoanalytic writings, as if it were a scientific concept designating a distinct mode of behaviour or a psychopathological syndrome' (Szasz 1956). But, for Szasz, malingering was not a diagnosis, but more a form of moral condemnation by the physicians, and reflected the identification of physicians with the prevailing values of the social group in which the physician operates. Szasz almost certainly had not read Collie, but he might have done. His arguments were convincing, but less so when he went on to apply them to what most of us accept as legitimate disorders such as depression or schizophrenia.

Conclusion

I have outlined what I take to be the principle reasons for the sudden increase in medical interest in the question of malingering at the beginning of the twentieth century. At its heart was the general reaction felt by those more privileged in society against the perceived decline in the pre-war moral codes that had governed society. Malingering seemed to be another sign of the general decline in social responsibility and social control, the questioning of previously accepted values and status (Bogacz 1989). Few could deny the growing power of Labour, and the consequent eclipse of the Liberal Party in the UK. These fears were exacerbated by the challenge of the First World War. In other countries, particularly those that had lost the war, these fears and resentments were even more dramatic, the 'stab in the back' by the profiteers, the conscientious objectors, and of course, the malingerers.

Finally, throughout the story of malingering one theme emerges time and time again. For those physicians and surgeons who took on the new task of determining eligibility for social welfare, there was never any doubt. Malingering was lying—it was, as Llewllyn and Jones put it 'a species of deceit'. That generation of doctors also believed that the medical man was best placed to detect this deceit. What has happened since is largely the story of how the latter, rather than the former, view has become challenged. True, there were many attempts by the early psychiatrists to lay claim to special expertise in detecting malingering, and in classifying malingering as a psychiatric disorder, but this has proved unconvincing. It was such efforts that prompted a barrister to note in 1938 that 'Malingering is not a disease but a species of fraud, and it might well be considered that a medical man as such has no special qualifications to decide whether his patient is guilty of fraud' (Norris 1938), a view echoed in this book by Mendelson (Chapter 17).

References

Barnett, C. (1909). *Accidental injuries to workmen with reference to Workmen's Compensation Act of 1906*. Rebman, London.

Bogacz, T. (1989). War neurosis and cultural change in England, 1914–1922: the work of the war office committee of enquiry into shellshock. *Journal of Contemporary History*, **24**, 227–56.

Bourke, J. (1996). *Dismembering the male: men's bodies, Britain and the Great War*. Reaktion Books, London.

Collie, J. (1917). *Malingering and feigned sickness*. Edward Arnold, London.

Cooter, R. (1998). Malingering in modernity: psychological scripts and adversial encounters during the First World War. In *War, medicine and modernity* (eds R. Cooter, M. Harrison, and S. Sturdy), pp. 125–48. Sutton Publishing, Stroud.

Craig, G. (1978). *Germany 1866–1945*. Oxford University Press, Oxford.

Dembe, A. (1996). *Occupation and disease: how social factors affect the conception of work-related disorders*. Yale University Press, Newhaven, CT.

Dewar, M. (1912). Medical training for the detection of malingering. *British Medical Journal*, **ii**, 223–5.

Eckart, W. (2000). War, emotional stress, and German medicine. In *Great War, Total War: combat and mobilization on the Western Front, 1914–1918* (eds R. Chickering and S. Förster), pp. 133–49. Cambridge University Press, Cambridge.

Eghigian, G. (2000). *Making security social: disability, insurance and the birth of the social entitlement state in Germany*. University of Michigan Press, Ann Arbor, MI.

Fischer-Homberger, E. (1975). *Die traumatische Neurose: vom somatischen zum sozialen Leiden*. Hans Huber, Bern.

Furedi, F. (1997). *Culture of fear: risk-taking and the morality of low expectation*. Cassell, London.

Fussell, P. (1975). *The Great War and modern memory*. Oxford University Press, London.

Gavin, H. (1836). *On feigned and factitious diseases*. Edinburgh University Press, Edinburgh.

Hynes, S. (1990). *A war imagined: the First World War and English culture*. Bodley Head, London.

Jones, A. B. and Llewellyn, L. (1917). *Malingering or the simulation of disease*. Heinemann, London.

Keen, W. M., Mitchell, S.W., and Morehouse, G. (1864). On malingering, especially in regard to simulation of diseases of the nervous system. *American Journal of Medical Science*, **48**, 367–74.

Kinney, A. (1990). *Vagabonds and sturdy beggars*. University of Massachussetts Press, Boston, MA.

Leed, E. (1979). *No man's land: combat and identity in World War One*. Cambridge University Press, Cambridge.

Lerner, P. (2001). From traumatic memory to male hysteria: the decline and fall of Hermann Oppenheim, 1889–1919. In *Traumatic pasts: history, psychiatry and trauma in the modern age, 1860–1930* (eds P. Lerner and M. Micale), pp. 140–71. Cambridge University Press, Cambridge.

Manning, F. (1999). *Her privates we*. Serpent's Tail, London.

Mawson (1967). *Diseases of the ear*. Edward Arnold, London.

Mendelson, G. and Mendelson, D. (1993). Legal and psychiatric aspects of malingering. *Journal of Law and Medicine*, **1**, 28–34.

Micale, M. and Lerner, P. (eds) (2001). *Traumatic pasts: history, psychiatry and trauma in the modern age, 1860–1930*. Cambridge University Press, Cambridge.

Myers, C. S. (1916). Contribution to the study of shell shock. *Lancet*, **1**, 65–9.

Norris, D. (1938). Malingering. In *British encylopedia of medical practice* (ed. H. Rolleston), p. 363. Butterworth, London.

Shepherd, M. (1985). *Sherlock Holmes and the case of Dr Freud*. Tavistock Publications, London.

Showalter, E. (1987). *The female malady: women, madness and English culture, 1830–1980*. Virago, London.

Stone, M. (1985). Shellshock and the psychologists. In *The anatomy of madness* (eds W. Bynum, R. Porter, and M. Shepherd), pp. 242–71. Tavistock, London.

Szasz, T. (1956). Malingering: diagnosis of social condemnation. *Archvies of Neurology and Psychiatry*, **76**, 432–43.

Yelin, E. (1986). The myth of malingering: why individuals withdraw from work in the presence of illness. *Milbank Memorial Fund Quarterly*, **64**, 622–49.

3 Malingering, shirking, and self-inflicted injuries in the military

Ian P. Palmer

'Sure there's a catch,' Doc. Daneeka replied. 'Catch-22. Anyone who wants to get out of combat duty isn't really crazy.'

Heller (1962)

Abstract

Soldiers of all nations have indulged in malingering and shirking to avoid duty since time immemorial; indeed the term originates with the military. Malingering is the simulation of injury or illness and may be understood as a way soldiers and sailors attempt to 'control' their environment; the results may be positive or negative. Avoidance of military duty is viewed seriously within British Military Forces given its potential to undermine group cohesion, discipline, morale, military culture, and ethos. Malingering therefore remains a concept extant within the minds of military commanders even today. It may be wittingly or unwittingly aided by gullible doctors; more importantly, however, it may reflect poor leadership, group dysfunction, learning difficulties, mental illness, or personality vulnerabilities or disorder. The greatest care is therefore required before the possibility of malingering is contemplated and all cases must be examined on their individual merits with an open mind.

Introduction

Feigning illness is behaviour indulged in by soldiers of all nations. It is one way of trying to control their environment and the results may be positive or negative for the individual or the group. As the role of military medical services is to maintain fighting strength, there is a potential conflict of interests from the outset; in combat the needs of the group are always more important than those of the individual.

Etymology

Malingering derives from the French [*malinger—sickly, weakly, prob. from mal, ill + OF heingre, haingre—thin, lean, infirm from L. aeger*] and describes a soldier who feigns himself as sick, or who induces or protracts an illness, in order to avoid doing his duty; hence, in general, one who shirks duty by pretending illness or inability (Webster 1890). Within the military, such behaviour is seen as malign as the individual puts his own interests before those of the group [malignus— *of an evil nature or disposition, ill-disposed, wicked, mischievous, malicious, spiteful, envious, malignant, malign*] (Lewis and Short 1844).

History

In order to escape the Trojan War, Ulysses feigned insanity by yoking a bull and a horse together, ploughing the seashore, and sowing salt instead of grain. Palamedes detected this deception by placing the infant son of the King of Ithica in the line of the furrow and observing the pretended lunatic turn the plough aside, an act of discretion that was considered sufficient proof that his madness was not real (Glueck 1915).

Self-inflicted injury was recognized by the Anglo-Saxons and "shoot-finger" was the term that described the mutilation of the index finger so vital in archery, and latterly in small arms. This action was always a 'most punishable offence', for which the laws of King Alfred inflicted a penalty of fifteen shillings' (Smyth 1867). In 1403, the Earl of Northumberland 'lay crafty sick' to avoid in the Battle of Shrewsbury, and in 1813 some 3000 soldiers apparently shot their trigger fingers off during the battles of Lutzen and Bautzen (Brussel and Hitch 1943).

During the American Civil War, psychiatric symptoms were seldom feigned (Carroll 2001) and any man seeking discharge for physical or psychological disability was felt to be a malingerer (Dean 1977). To fail as a soldier in the First World War carried a terrible stigma and officers went to great lengths to keep men fighting. Without any understanding or training in psychiatric matters, Medical Officers (MOs) found it difficult to disentangle malingering from shellshock, hysteria, and authentic amnesia (O'Connell 1960). Differing usages and definitions of the term malingering led to confusion and differing conclusions (Myers 1940, p. 33). The variation of symptoms reported were due to the personalities of the observers, the places of observation, and the variability of material; minor casualties never reached base hospital, for example, and gross disorders often developed only in the safety of hospital (Ritchie 1986, p. 255). The 1922 Shellshock Committee identified three types of malingering: true, partial, and quasi-malingering (HMSO 1922).

Whilst malingering and self-inflicted injuries were common in the Indian Army before the First World War, they took on epidemic proportions in Europe. Many sepoys were exhorted by their comrades to 'swing the lead' and even advised on various subterfuges; shellshock was apparently particularly easy to ape (Harrison 1999). Mental breakdown and malingering in the Wehrmacht were seen as cowardice and decidedly 'non-Aryan'; yet as Germany approached defeat officers and soldiers were increasingly felt to be 'delaying' their recoveries (Schneider 1987, p. 96). 'Disciplinary' management included the denial of gain and the summary execution of 15 000–30 000 soldiers (Shephard 1999).

There was less enthusiasm in British forces to fight and less intolerance of malingering in 1939. Many younger officers were reluctant to retain unenthusiastic men and attempted to get rid of them, through psychiatric channels if possible (Shephard 1999). Mental disorders comprised 35–41 per cent of all medical discharges (MDs) between 1943 and 1945 (Mellor 1972). In the Nigeria–Biafra War, 1967–70, malingering was a 'formidable' problem involving forcibly returning men to duty (Kalunta 1987). As recently as 1996, cases of mental disorder, personality disorder, and learning disabilities in ultra-orthodox Jewish men were labelled by psychiatrists as malingering (Witztum 1996).

Classification of malingering

Military malingering may be triggered by fear or desire (Trimble 1981) and is different in peace and war. It occurs for personal gain and equals manipulation, deceit and dishonour to military authorities. During the First World War, over 300 000 offences relating to shirking and malingering resulted in a conviction rate of 90 per cent (Bourke 1996, p. 77; War Office, 1922). Malingering to avoid punishment undermines military discipline and can lead to conflict between medical and disciplinary commands. Gain includes avoidance of conscription, duty, prosecution, danger; respite from danger; optimal job placement; retention in service; monetary, educational, and other welfare benefits; and enlistment with a disqualifying pre-existing medical condition.

Behaviours

Physical
- Self-mutilation—cutting, gunshot wounds, crushing, burns, etc.;
- Exaggeration/prolongation of current/past symptoms;
- Medically unexplained symptoms—fatigue, muscle and joint pains, sweats, memory difficulties (see Table 3.1).

Psychological
- Suicidal threat;
- Post-traumatic stress disorder (PTSD).

Self-inflicted injury (SII)

The risks of self-inflicted injury (SII) in war are great and may be fatal. They range from shooting, crushing, and burning through wilful infliction of frostbite and sexually transmitted diseases to eating cordite (Flicker, 1942). The incidence is not known as many will not be recognized as such by medics. Less than 1 per cent of injuries seen by surgeons in the First World War were thought to be SII (Bourke 1996, p. 37). One First World War study of 3000 soldiers revealed that 105 had attempted suicide, 3 of whom were successful (Stanford Read 1920, p. 152). Interestingly, the vast majority of British soldiers used a razor to cut their throats whereas gunshot wounds were the preferred method of suicide in the US Army, this method increasing from 38.4 per cent in 1907 to 55 per cent in 1910. Occurring against a reported 'increase' in suicides among schoolchildren, 1117 child suicides in Prussia were studied in 1907 (Stanford Read 1920, p. 154). Deliberate self-harm (DSH) and threatened suicide are now common ways of manipulating situations in armed forces (*The Times*, 2000). In nearly all cases they relate to distress and job dissatisfaction and few have a psychiatric disorder. Such individuals are rapidly removed from duties and sent for psychiatric assessment (Carroll 2001).

In military law, many 'crimes' would not be considered as such in civilian society. It is easy therefore for individuals to acquire a 'criminal' record and for some to even be labelled as personality disorders; this is a deception if they are subsequently medically discharged (MD) for they will receive a pension, often for the rest of their lives for a condition they may not have. Medical discharge obviates dishonourable discharge and may at times ensure that a commander's leadership skills are not called to account (Carroll 2001).

Learning disabilities (LDs)

During the First and Second World Wars, learning disabilities (LDs) were commonly seen in unselected recruits who often ran into disciplinary problems as they failed to understand the

Table 3.1 Methods of illness simulation employed in World War II

Gastric disorder
Oil and tobacco +/− ipecac (either tachycardia or jaundice)
Diarrhoea
Mix stools, urine, and water; Add fat pork and bits of raw meat
Tapeworm
Carriers supply others
Jaundice
Smoke mixture of antipyrin and tobacco; Drink tocacco juice; Inject picric acid
Haemoptysis
Irritation of throat surfaces with a needle
Albuminuria
Eat kitchen salt to excess in a bowl of milk; Oedema and albumin disappear on surveillance; Albumin injected into bladder
Incontinence
Difficult to prove fraudulent. True incontinence in middle of night—simulated, just before waking
Skin diseases
Eruptions: mercury, arsenic, iodine, bromide
Eczema: rubbing skin with slightly warmed thapsia. Rubbing excoriated skin with acids, Croton oil, bark of garou, sulphur, oil of cade, mercurial pomade
Erythema: astringent herbs
Herpes: Euphorbiacae
Oedema: constriction
Recurrent wounds
Cover with wax sealed bandages
Abscesses
Induction of septic material. Thread soiled with Tatar from teeth is drawn through the skin—characteristic odour of resulting abscess
Phlegmons
Subcutaneous petrol or turpentine
Sprain
A stopper put under heel; compress the leg with bandages to stop circulation and knock below repeatedly and forcibly—oedema and ecchymoses follow
Conjunctivitis
Ipecac, pepper, septic, or faecal material. Belladonna
Ears
Otitis externa—urine or chemical product in EAM
Emaciation and pallor
Ingestion of large amount of vinegar; Abuse of strong tobacco
Muscular weakness
Arsenous acid in eggs. Voluntary mecurial and lead poisoning
Intra-abdominal projectiles
Swallowing a bullet
Diabetes
Phloridzin or oxalate of ammonia. Glucose added to urine

Source: Southard (1919, p. 642).

nature of regulations and the reason for them. In the Second World War, the US Army calculated that about 0.75 per cent of servicemen were Mentally Defective, a figure less than the general population. However, in military prisons, the rate was about 20 per cent, a figure twice the general population (Piotrowski and Hobbs 1945). The incidence of veneral disease (VD), scabies, pediculosis, and the general sickness rate were appreciably greater amongst this group (Ahrenfeldt 1958, p. 78) as was mental instability, breakdown, and malingering (although such a pejorative concept could be debated within this group).

The military malingerer

All military malingerers require the ability to mimic disease or infirmity, take risks and have clearly defined goals. They may be 'outsiders' from the outset and some will have disciplinary records.

Some individuals receive grudging respect for their tenacity and ability to endure discomfort and even risk death in pursuit of their aims (Anon 1905). All authors, however, agree that where doubt arises as to the 'genuineness' of the illness, the soldier should be given the benefit of the doubt to avoid unjustly punishing one innocent man (Pollock 1911). Commanders *should* know their charges well enough to spot the malingerer but whilst peer groups will know who is malingering this information is seldom available if unit morale is poor and 'informers' are universally detested.

What is military malingering?

Civilians have views about soldiers and their behaviours (Hall 1999). Lepine, for example, stated that even in peacetime the (French) Army was a school for malingering (Lepine 1919, p. 144). To best understand soldiers, an exploration and understanding of military culture is essential; for example, soldiers have feigned health to *return* to the front line and possibly even going AWOL from hospital! (RMAS 2001).

Malingering has been defined in many ways: as wilful fraud (Lumsden 1916); an evasion of duty to the state and comrades (Bourke 1996, p. 77); a slur on the nation/race (Ossipov 1943; Schneider 1987, p. 89); lack of social conscience (Williams 1921); delinquent behaviour (Ross 1941); part of a 'process' of learnt behaviour (Lepine 1919, p. 149; Williams 1921); a result of inappropriate medicalization of behaviours (Culpin 1920); or a question of morality (Stanford Read 1920, p.150; HMSO 1923).

The current definition and sentencing policy for UK Armed Forces is broadly the same and contained in the various Naval, Army, and Royal Air Force Acts.

Army Act 1955. Part 2 42. Malingering

(1) Any person subject to military law who
   - (a) falsely pretends to be suffering from sickness or disability, or
   - (b) injures himself with intent thereby to render himself unfit for service, or causes himself to be injured by any person with that intent, or
   - (c) injures another person subject to service law, at the instance of that person, with intent thereby to render that person unfit for service, or
   - (d) with intent to render or keep himself unfit for service, does or fails to do anything (whether at the time of the act or omission he is in hospital or not) whereby he produces, or prolongs or aggravates, any sickness or disability, shall be guilty of malingering and shall, on conviction by court-martial, be liable to imprisonment for a term not exceeding two years or any less punishment provided by this Act.

(2) In this section the expression 'unfit' includes temporarily unfit.

In the US Armed Forces, malingering is a prosecutable offence under the *Uniformed Code of Military Justice (UCMJ) Article 115*. In practice, charges of malingering are difficult to substantiate and many commands seek to handle this type of behaviour through other disciplinary or administrative means (US Marine Corps 2002).

Not all men are equal in their propensity to malinger (Cheyne 1827; Bourke 1996, p. 92) and whilst the military hierarchy believed that the incidence of malingering was inversely proportional to the 'quality' of recruits (Young 1995, p. 57), it was subsequently revealed that the quality of leadership was equally, if not more, important in its genesis and a vicious circle could be created within units (Stanford Read 1920, p. 150).

In wartime, 'selfish' acts can endanger the lives of other men, and as soldiers live in a mutually interdependent world built on trust, malingering runs counter to the honesty and truth required for the efficient functioning of the military community (Wallace 1916; Bourke 1996, p. 111). Therefore, the establishment of special treatment centres encourages evasion and invalidism and results in wastage of manpower (Ahrenfeldt 1958, p. 5).

Maleness and the military family

The concept of maleness is important in understanding perhaps why more soldiers do not malinger. Men strive for pride, honour, and identity and whilst they may identify with what is evil, they seldom identify with what is shameful. Military culture, like many others, seeks to strengthen masculinity with culturally imposed qualities or 'initiation rites' that the male is expected to master, or face humiliation (Blimes 1992). These tasks include aspects of the *physical*—e.g. acts of endurance; the *moral*—displays of courage and loyalty; or the *social*—e.g. achieving success.

Culture fosters and shapes maleness through the use of shame sanctions. Failure and loss of control are humiliating yet there is a 'need' for men to 'prove' themselves with other men despite fearing their derision and humiliation. The expression of emotions and feelings for example makes many men feel 'unmanly'. Psychological defences against feeling shame include: concealment; attack and destruction of those before whom one has been ashamed; compliance and conforming in order not to stand out and (heroic) achievement (Miller 2000).

Shirking versus malingering

The motivation for malingering may not always be clear to an outside observer. Malingering is a dance that requires at least one partner. The key players are of course the individual and the medical officer. The first lesson for new MOs on joining a unit is 'trial by sick parade' where soldiers shirk to 'test them out' to see whether they are strict or lenient. Given that most are fresh out of medical school, they may easily be manipulated, seldom to their amusement (Hunt 1946).

Shirking has many names such as: scrimshanking, swinging the lead, goldbricking, working your ticket, etc. It is a timeless, perhaps a common human response to unwanted situations, real or imagined (Cooter 1998). It occurs in normal individuals when encouraged by the social situation and is not carried to extremes involving severe social consequences for the malingerer. Management is easy as such an individual is accessible to social pressure.

The malingerer occurs in 'abnormal' individuals without encouragement from the social environment. If carried to extremes it will have serious medical or disciplinary consequences. But when does scrimshanking become malingering? One metaphor is the familial nature of the Army as an institution (Rees 1945; Trustram 1984). Within this model, other ranks are perpetual children (or adolescents), and service reflects *rites de passage* between childhood and manhood. In terms of the 'sick role', scrimshanking is a 'normal' testing of boundaries whereas malingering is a more goal-directed and individual activity. Discovery may lead to either benign or disciplinary management dependent on the 'parent' dealing with the situation. Such management will depend on a mixture of 'child and parent' personality, temperament, and current mental state. Most families adopt a fairly flexible approach to the behaviour and in the same way medical officers come to learn what approach to use with each individual (Myers 1940, p. 50).

Good malingering

There are times when malingering is considered 'a good thing'. The first is in order to fulfil the soldierly duty of trying to escape the enemy. Feigning illness has worked for numerous POWs and if there are language difficulties, it is one of the times when feigning mental illness is easier to get away with (Stanford Read 1920, p. 664; Russell and Hersov 1983, p. 239). Second, psychological operations (Psych Ops) have always dropped leaflets advising enemy soldiers how to feign illness and escape fighting and the inevitable death which will face them should they stay and fight.

Soldiers and civilians

Soldiers have always been set apart from society and to a degree stigmatized (Hall 1999). There was, and remains, a class dimension to the military. In the nineteenth century, army officers were drawn from the upper classes and the ranks from the lower echelons of working classes—two disparate groups with strong and long-standing associations with low morals and debauchery (aristocratic vice and lower class immorality). Latterly, terrorist threats have led to an invisibility of soldiers within society as they seldom wear their uniforms off duty.

Disciplinary (behavioural) management

Soldier's behaviour is open to differing interpretations and, given the strictures of military law, commanders are frequently presented with 'misbehaviour' and the question of whether the individual is responsible for his/her actions. If they are (and guilty!) they are bad, if not they are mad! Such behaviour reflects badly on the reputation of a regiment which, in the First World War at least, 'had' to be 'protected' at all costs (Bourke 1996, p. 98).

Malingering is most likely to appear at times of great social upheaval when punishments for crimes are very severe or when the situation is such that one's life is threatened (Ossipov 1943). At such times, preservation of the group is of the utmost importance and any threats to the group from within are more feared and hated and produce more violent reaction than does external threat. The 'aberrant' individual may be regarded with revulsion and fierce hatred and no penalty is considered too severe for him (Flicker 1947).

Management of malingerers was and remains disciplinary. According to General Haig, punishment had to inflict physical discomfort and shame. Imprisonment was inappropriate during wartime as prison compares favourably with combat and, despite a lack of opportunities of spending money and working to the limits of their endurance, the commonest punishments were extra work and the forfeiture of pay. Coercive measures such as denying separation allowance to widows, wives, and mothers could be implemented; pay was forfeited by men in hospitals accused of inflicting their own injuries. Individuals could also be removed from military service without pensions and imprisonment could even be suspended until after the war (Bourke 1996, p. 102). But coercive punishments risk creating mistrust and discontent and may lead to a situation where shirking or malingering is tolerated, encouraged, supported, and even admired (Bourke 1996, p. 109).

Medical officers (MO)

If an individual's complaints have no physical basis, doctors tend to oscillate uneasily between two alternative attitudes: either there is nothing wrong with him, or he is psychiatrically ill (Russell and Hersov 1983). An organic label may allow collusion between MO and soldier and exculpate the MO's guilt or dislike of their role of identifying a malingerer.

Malingering has always presented military doctors with a dilemma which was succinctly enunciated in 1827 by Cheyne, '... to force a soldier who is unfit for the hardships of military life to continue in service, would be undoubtedly an act of great oppression, as well as a source of frequent disappointment to the commanding officer. While, on the other hand, every instance in which fictitious or fabricated disease escapes detection and punishment, becomes not merely a reward granted to fraud, but a premium held out to future imposition' (Cheyne 1827). He recognized the link between malingering and the morale of a unit and his observations are as valid today as 1827.

The Commanding Officer often regards doctors as encouraging soldiers to seek their discharge through delinquency and avoiding responsibility for their actions (Ahrenfeldt 1958, p. 103). One famous US general criticized doctors for 'aiding' or encouraging malingering by their 'shameful use of "battle fatigue" as an excuse for cowardice' (Patton 1947).

In the First World War, MOs were novices, unused to military life and unprepared for trench warfare with no psychological training. Civilian experience was poor preparation for military work and many of the conditions they saw were new to them (Harrison 1999; Whitehead 1999). Attempts to 'explain' malingering and other behaviours (shellshock, etc.) were felt to reflect the tendency of alienists to find everyone abnormal which, if carried to its logical conclusion would lead to an end of social responsibility. MOs became the moral arbiters of military misbehaviour and medicalization of malingering was seen as a method of increasing demand for war pensions (Ritchie 1986, p. 58; Cooter 1998). MOs may, on the one hand, not recognize or 'choose' to identify malingering as a function of inexperience or naivety, or on the other collude by over- or under-identification with the soldier (Binneveld 1997).

The MO's dilemma is whether to be on the one hand too lenient and flooded with cases that will diminish force levels and strength and lose them the confidence and respect of officers and senior NCOs; or on the other to be too strict and thereby lose the confidence of their soldiers which will affect morale. In either case their standing, abilities, motivation, professionalism and judgement will be called into question.

The identification of malingering continues to remain difficult. The touchstone is to catch the soldier *in flagrante delicto*. Failing that, a good knowledge of the individual coupled with close observation and common sense offers the best chance of success.

All MOs owe allegiance to the codes of practice and ethics of both military and medical professions. How they discharge these duties and obligations will relate to the degree to which they manage their identification with both cultures and will be different in different operational scenarios. There has, and always will be, a conflict between the requirements of the service and medical recommendations, particularly in time of war. MOs must recognize this and work

Table 3.2 A differential diagnosis for malingering

	Hysteria	Neurasthenia	Malingering	Shock (not shellshock)
Cause	Heredity; emotional upset female; sex repressed (usually sexual desires)	Heredity; worry; overwork; debilitating diseases; masturbation	Dislike of work; desire for money; ease or sympathy not earned	Accident; injury (physical/psychological); operation; haemorrhage
Onset	Sudden; variable	Gradual; even	Varies	Sudden or gradual
Symptoms	Emotional; mercurial temperament; quick active mind; protean symptoms involuntary all may malinger, too; globus, spasms, fits, faints, etc.; 'subconscious malingering'	Weak for action, but hypersensitive; memory weak; mind and body easily tired; introspective; dyspeptic; depressed and irritable	Any which are easily feigned; pains in back; giddiness; lost senses—sight etc.; corresponding with the gain sought for; voluntary and conscious	Collapse; cold sweat; dilated pupils; weak pulse of low tension; pallor
Cure	Marriage; full and pleasing occupation; suggestion	Sleep, rest, and food build up Ergogen; exercise	Detection, or if it ceases to pay well	Stimulants, fluids, alkalis, rest, food
Pathology	Motives beyond conscious control; 'auto-suggestion'; 'buried complex'	Brain cells run down; bankrupt of ergogen	Conscious and fraudulent, ''a moral cell disease''	Falling blood pressure, brain cells ill supplied with blood

Source: Lumsden (1916).

within its constraints, which may at times present them with moral, philosophical, and ethical challenges.

Feigning psychiatric symptoms

Before shellshock, soldiers were very unlikely to attempt to feign mental illness as they might run the risk of ending their days in an asylum as a consequence of the Lunacy Laws. In addition, early observers noted the inability of malingerers to feign true mental illness—they simply feign their belief of what a lunatic is (Gunn and Taylor 1993a). A 1955 study of American soldiers in military prison revealed 50 cases of the Ganser Syndrome out of the study population of 8000 (Werner and Braiman 1955; Gunn and Taylor 1993b).

Shellshock caused major problems in the First World War as it did not fit the distinctions between real and feigned illness, and added little to the debate about physical versus psychological aetiologies of mental diseases (see Table 3.2). Previously, constructs of psychological illness were considered either organic/social; mad/bad; guilty/not guilty; and honest/deceitful (Bourke 1996).

With advances in medical science, it is more difficult to feign physical conditions. Although individuals no longer shoot themselves in the foot, they are more likely to present with vague multi-system, non-specific subjective symptoms. In addition, there is less stigma attached to mental illness, hence the tendency to feign psychiatric disorders. In the US Veterans Administration system, malingering of PTSD is now extremely common (Carroll 2001 and see Pankratz, Chapter 14).

Conclusion

Malingering may be encouraged by doctors and is more likely to occur in those with learning difficulties and psychopathy. It may reflect poor leadership and has a number of consequences which include undermining unit cohesion, discipline, and authority. In extreme cases it may lead to sedition, which could be exploited by the enemy. Shirking is ubiquitous and occurs in normals, particularly when facilitated by the social situation. Malingering, however, is a more extreme form of illness behaviour which is more likely to occur in conscript armies at times of great danger. Shirking and malingering threaten to diminish the capacity to fight and put other soldiers at risk and, as such, military authorities will always regard them negatively.

References

Ahrenfeldt, R. H. (1958). *Psychiatry in the British Army in the Second World War*, pp. 5, 78, 103. Routledge & Kegan Paul, London.

Anon (1905). Malingery. *Lancet*, 45–7.

Binneveld, H. (1997). *From shellshock to combat stress. A comparative history of military psychiatry*, p. 134. Amsterdam University Press, Amsterdam.

Blimes, M. (1992). Macho and shame. *International Forum of Psychoanalysis*, **1**, 163–8

Bourke, J. (1996). *Dismembering the male. Men's bodies, Britain and the Great War*, pp. 37, 77, 92, 94, 98, 102, 109, 111. Reaktion Books, London.

Brussel, J. A. and Hitch, K. S. (1943). The military malingerer. *Military Surgeon*, **93**, 33–44,

Carroll, M. F. (2001). Deceptions in military psychiatry. *American Journal of Forensic Psychiatry*, **22**(1), 53–62.

Cheyne, J. (1827). Medical Report on the Feigned Diseases of Soldiers, in a letter addressed to George Renny, Director General of Military Hospitals in Ireland. *Dublin Hospital Reports and Communications in Medicine and Surgery*, **4**, 127–8.

Cooter, R. (1998). Malingering and modernity: psychological scripts and adversarial encounters during the First World War. In *War, medicine & modernity* (eds R. Cooter, M. Harrison, and S. Sturdy), Chap. 7, pp. 125–48. Sutton Publishing, Stroud.

Culpin, M. (1920). *Psychoneuroses of war and peace*. Cambridge University Press, Cambridge.

Dean, E. T., Jr. (1977). *Shook over Hell. Post-traumatic stress, Vietnam and the Civil War*. Harvard University Press, Cambridge, MA.

Flicker, D. J. (1947) Sedition: a case report. *Psychiatric Quarterly Supplement*, **22** (2), 187–99.

Flicker, M. D. (1942). The self-inflicted injury—a case report. *American Journal of Psychiatry*, **99**, 168–73.

Glueck, B. (1915). The malingerer: a clinical study. *International Clinics*, **3**, 200–51.

Gunn, J. and Taylor, P. J. (1993a). *Forensic psychiatry. Clinical, legal and ethical issues*. Butterworth-Heinemann, Oxford.

Gunn, J. and Taylor, P. J. (1993b). *Forensic psychiatry. Clinical, legal and ethical issues*, pp. 44–6. Butterworth-Heinemann, Oxford.

Hall, L. A. (1999). War always brings it on: war, STDs, the military, and the civilian population in Britain, 1850–1950. In *Medicine and Modern Warfare* (eds R. Cooter, M. Harrison, and S. Sturdy), Chap. 8, pp. 205–23. Volume Clio Medica 55, Editions Rodopi B.V.

Harrison, M. (1999). Disease, discipline and dissent: the Indian Army in France and England, 1914–1915. In *Medicine and Modern Warfare* (eds R. Cooter, M. Harrison, and S. Sturdy), Chap. 7, pp. 185–203. Volume Clio Medica 55, Editions Rodopi B.V.

Heller, J. (1962). *Catch-22*. Jonathan Cape, London.

HMSO. (1922). Report of the War Office Committee of Enquiry into 'Shellshock,' p. 141. HMSO, London.

HMSO. (1923). *History of the Great War: medical services—diseases of the War. (Neurasthenia and War Neuroses)*, pp. 1–67. HMSO, London.

Hunt, W. A. (1946). The detection of malingering: a further study. *US Navy Medical Bulletin*, **46** 249–54.

Kalunta, A. (1987). Experience of a non-military psychiatrist during the 1966–1970 Nigerian Civil War in the area of 'Biafra'. In *Contemporary studies in combat psychiatry* (ed. G. Belenky) Chap. 9, pp. 133–41. Greenwood Press, New York, NY.

Lepine, J. (1919). In *Mental disorders of war* (ed. C. A. Mercier), pp. 144, 149. University of London Press, London.

Lewis, C. T. and Short, C. (1844). *A Latin Dictionary*. Clarendon Press, Oxford.

Lumsden, T. (1916). Malingering in peace and war. *Lancet*, 862.

Mellor, W. F. (1972). *Statistics of the Great War*. HMSO, London.

Miller, W. I. (2000). *The mystery of courage*. Harvard University Press, Cambridge, MA.

Myers, C. S. (1940). *Shellshock in France*, pp. 33, 50. Cambridge University Press, Cambridge.

O'Connell B. A. (1960). Amnesia and homicide. *British Journal of Delinquency*, **10**, 262–76.

Ossipov, V. P. (1943). Malingering; the simulation of psychosis. *Neuropathologica I Psychiatrica* **12**, 3–10. (Translated for the *Menninger Clinic Bulletin* (1944) **8** (2), 39–42.)

Patton, G. S. (1947). *War as I knew it*, pp. 381–2. Houghton Mifflin, Boston, MA.

Piotrowski, Z. A. and Hobbs, J. M. (1945). Mental deficiency and military offence. *Psychiatric Quarterly Supplement*, **19**, 5–10 (Part 1).

Pollock, C. E. (1911). Malingering. *Journal of the Royal Army Medical Corps*, **16**, 50.

Rees, J. R. (1945). *The shaping of psychiatry by war*, pp. 16–29; 43–5. W.W. Norton & Co., New York, NY.

Ritchie, R. D. (1986). *One history of shellshock*, pp. 58, 255. PhD Dissertation, University of California, San Diego, CA.

RMAS. (2001). Department of War Studies, Royal Military Academy Sandhurst, Personal communication.

Ross, T. A. (1941). *Lectures on the war neuroses*. Butler & Tanner Ltd, London.

Russell, G. F. M. and Hersov, L. A. (eds) (1983). *Handbook of psychiatry*, Vol. 4, p. 239. Cambridge University Press, Cambridge.

Schneider, R. J. (1987). Stress breakdown in the Wehrmacht: implications for today's army. In *Contemporary studies in combat psychiatry* (ed. G. Belenky), Chap. 6, pp. 89, 96. Greenwood Press, New York, NY.

Shephard, B. (1999). Pitiless psychology: the role of deterrence in British military psychiatry in the Second World War. *History of Psychiatry*, **X**, 491–524.

Smyth, W. H. (1867). The sailor's wordbook. Referenced in Kacrik, J. (1997). *Forgotten English*. Quill Press, New York, NY.

Southard, E. E. (1919). *Shell-shock and other neurospsychiatric problems presented in 589 case histories from the War Literature* 1914–1918. W. M. Leonard, Boston, MA. (Reprinted ARNO Press 1973.)

Stanford Read, C. (1920). *Military psychiatry in peace and war*, pp. 150, 152, 154, 664. H.K. Lewis and Co. Ltd., London.

The Times Newspaper. (2000). Jail for soldier who shot himself. 1 November, p. 3.

Trimble, M. R. (1981). *Post-traumatic neurosis. From railway spine to the whiplash*, Chap. 4, pp. 57–73. John Wiley & Sons, Chichester.

Trustram, M. (1984). *Women of the regiment: marriage and the Victorian Army*. Cambridge University Press, Cambridge.

US Marine Corps. (2002). Available online at www.usmc.mil.

War Office. (1922). *Statistics of the military effort of the British Empire during the Great War*, p. 643. HMSO, London.

Webster, N. (1890). *International dictionary of the english language*. Revised and enlarged by N. Porter. George Bell & Son, London.

Werner, B. A. and Braiman, A. (1955). The Ganser syndrome. *The American Journal of Psychiatry*. **111**, 767–74.

Whitehead, I. R. (1999). The British Medical Officer on the Western Front: the training of doctors for war. In *Medicine and modern warfare* (eds R. Cooter, M. Harrison, and S. Sturdy), Chap. 6, pp. 163–84. Volume Clio Medica 55, Editions Rodopi B.V.

Williams, T. A. (1921). Malingering and simulation of disease in warfare. *Military Surgeon*, **48**, 520–33.

Witztum, E. (1996). The erroneous diagnosis of malingering in a military setting. *Military Medicine* **161**(4), 225–9.

Young, A. (1995). *The harmony of illusions. Inventing post-traumatic stress disorder*, pp. 56–9. Princeton University Press, Princeton, NJ.

4 Can monkeys malinger?

Richard W. Byrne and Emma Stokes

Abstract

It is often helpful, when examining a subtle or vexed issue, to take an outside perspective. The non-human primates present opportunities for doing just this, with respect to malingering. Monkeys and apes live in long-lasting and often complex social milieus, in which there are profits to be made by malingering—and indeed, malingering has been found in many species, and of a rich panoply of types, limited more by opportunity than cognitive flexibility. Yet most of these animals are believed, with reason, not to understand the intentional states of others; only the great apes may properly intend to malinger. Perhaps much more malingering in humans is 'unintentional' than is commonly thought? Disablement in chimpanzees and gorillas, a result of snare injury, allows us to see how well they can compensate for loss of capacities, uncontaminated by the help of others since help is not offered in ape society. Nevertheless, remarkable compensation is possible, by means of low-level flexibility rather than reorganization of technique, sometimes enabling severely maimed apes not only to survive but thrive. Considerable overlap in apparent efficiency levels was found between disabled and able-bodied apes, even though there could be no profit from malingering. This raises the question of whether measures of overt efficiency can ever be reliable in assessment of human malingering, where there may be real motivation to conceal capacities for gain.

Introduction

A number of ingredients are needed for successful malingering.[1] Any would-be malingerer evidently must have a *problem* to which malingering might be a solution, or there would be no point; he/she must have an *audience* which has the power to offer help, but his/her audience may be another individual(s) or an organization; he/she must have the *means to affect* this audience by feigning or exaggerating pain, sickness, or injury, usually engaging their sympathy and getting help or resources; and he/she must have the *cognitive capacity* to organize his/her behaviour in the appropriate way at the right time to achieve this effect.

Notice that we have not mentioned that our malingerer must have the *intention of creating a false belief* in his/her audience in order to gain the necessary sympathy. Instead, the malingerer may only intend, by simulating illness or suffering, to get the (undeserved) reward or avoid the (richly deserved) punishment. It might be thought that this is a hair-splitting distinction, the sort of logic-chopping that only a heinous malingerer would go in for, most likely to avoid his/her just

---

[1] The sense of malingering used here is that of the *Concise Oxford English Dictionary* (5th Edition, 1964), 'Pretend, produce, or protract illness in order to escape duty'. In some of the clinical conditions examined elsewhere in this volume, it may be difficult to discern to what problem, if any, the sickness deception is addressed.

retribution when caught! When we begin to ask questions about the evolutionary underpinnings of human malingering, however, we must look towards non-human species for answers. It cannot be assumed *a priori* that individuals of species other than human are able to comprehend the mental states of others, or to make attributions about their intentions. Nevertheless, it does not seem impossible that non-humans might still malinger, if a definition of malingering were accepted that did not include full understanding of the mental processes involved. Moreover, it may be very difficult in some human cases to be sure that behaviour that functions as malingering is fully comprehended by the perpetrator. In this chapter, we will examine some real cases, where the behaviour of non-human primates functions to allow malingering. We hope that this will serve a heuristic purpose, in illuminating some of the 'grey areas' in the human domain—where a deliberate intention, to create false beliefs about the self's physical status and thereby profit unfairly, is hard to prove or unlikely to be the correct ascription.

We will begin by focusing on cases of deception in non-human primates (hereafter, primates) that involve misleading others about pain, health status, or personal risk. This will illuminate the restricted opportunities that primates have for malingering, while showing that such deception does indeed occur. When the circumstances give primates an audience whose emotions can be affected in the necessary direction, functional malingering sometimes does occur. Evidently, then, primates have the cognitive capacity to deceive in this way: but what is this capacity based upon? To begin to answer this, we use the same corpus of data on deception; but now we remove the restriction that the means should involve feigned pain or sickness, since the focus is now on the underlying cognition rather than the precise rewards and costs. This analysis in the main will indicate that effective deception in primates does *not* depend on understanding of the situation by modelling it in the mind. Perhaps, then, the same may often be true in humans? There is, however, some evidence that a few species of primate (the great apes) may intend to create false beliefs. It may therefore be that the intentionality necessary for deliberate, planned malingering is more ancient than is often thought, dating from an ancient time when humans and apes shared common ancestry. Finally, we turn the question around, and ask, how do primates cope if they are *genuinely* disabled, yet—as is so often the case—no other individual will help them. Can they survive, and how do they manage?

Functional malingering in primates

Consider our earlier check-list of ingredients for successful malingering, and how it might apply to primates. These animals certainly have plenty of *problems* in their lives, which other individuals could help them with if they so wished. Living in the wild, they must obtain adequate nutrition, under often harsh conditions; they must avoid predation, heat-stress, dehydration, and exhaustion; and they must breed successfully. But what audience is liable to be manipulated into providing help? Evolutionary theory makes it clear that only in restricted circumstances can any behaviour evolve that is not purely for an individual's own direct benefit, and by far the most probable circumstance is close genetic relatedness (Hamilton 1964). Evolution of altruistic traits that confer benefit indirectly, via genes shared with relatives, is known as 'kin selection'. In most circumstances, kin selection depends on the ability to recognize and remember other individuals as such, and can only operate in situations when certainty of genetical relatedness is ensured. For these reasons, in all mammals the most obvious place to look for altruism is the mother–offspring relationship. Mother and offspring share 50 per cent of their genes by direct descent, and they need have no uncertainty about identity or relatedness. We can also predict the direction of the malingering. The mother is usually larger and more powerful than its offspring and often able to control or give effective aid, so we should expect occasional malingering by the offspring, since it would certainly pay. This is surely not so different from the human case: most children begin their malingering with their mother as the target audience.

Like many species of mammal, in primates there may be a considerable period of conflict at weaning, between the mother—who benefits from efficient, early weaning of her offspring, since she can that way maximize her life-time reproductive output—and the infant, who benefits from every last bit of care it can obtain from its mother (Trivers 1974). Probably, infants often exaggerate their distress at this time. One primatologist, David Chivers, was convinced this was the case in the siamang (*Hylobates syndactylus*), a monogamous species of gibbon in which the father often carries the infant: 'During the second year of life, once the male has taken over carriage of the infant when it is weaned from the female, the male progressively encourages the infant to travel after him. Often the infant protests at this, with squeals, calls used to signal distress. It is deception to the extent that the infant is not really in distress, but is hoping for the easy way out—for the male to retrieve and carry him' (record #150 in Byrne and Whiten 1990, from which all numbered citations are taken). Unfortunately, it is very hard to be certain of *precisely* how much distress a member of another species is feeling, so this sort of exaggeration is always problematic as evidence.

However, sometimes infants go further, into outright temper tantrums. Fernando Colmenares describes this in baboons, 'the infant exhibits temper tantrum behaviours, including throwing itself about and jumping into the air, geckering, screaming and mewing. When this happens it may elicit two sorts of response: care-giving behaviour by other group members, and tension among group members that sometimes leads to the mother being threatened by the leader male. The ultimate consequence of this is that the infant will reach its goal, which is to regain physical or nipple-contact with the mother' (record #99). Throwing temper tantrums evidently 'works', but one might wonder whether the effects are coincidental: perhaps the infant is simply out of control? However, Jane Goodall's knowledge of chimpanzees (*Pan troglodytes*) makes her suspect that this would be an oversimplification: 'The temper tantrum seems to be an uncontrolled, uninhibited, and highly emotional response to frustration. . . . It is observed most frequently in youngsters who are going through the peak of weaning, after they have begged, whimpered, and cajoled their mothers for an opportunity to suckle, but to no avail. In some ways it seems absurd to think that such a spontaneous outbreak could be a deliberate strategy for achieving a goal. Yet Yerkes (1943, p. 30) wrote, "I have seen a youngster, in the midst of a tantrum, glance furtively at its mother . . . as if to discover whether its action was attracting attention." And de Waal (1982, p. 108) says, "It is surprising (and suspicious) how abruptly {chimpanzee} children snap out of their tantrums if their mothers give in." At Gombe {where Goodall's chimpanzee studies took place, in Tanzania} a mother almost always does give in. The tantrum seems to make her tense and even nervous. She hastens to embrace the screaming child—who, of course, begins instantly to suckle. As he does so, the mother often gives a soft bark of threat. Her behavior, roughly translated, might read "Anything for peace!" ' (Goodall 1986, p. 576, record #227). If temper tantrums usually do result in favourable consequences, considerable scepticism is justified towards accounts that portray them as uncontrolled: infants are certainly capable of instrumental learning, and the use of temper tantrums may even be planned as a deliberate strategy.

Other tactics are used for the same purpose. Instead of merely appearing to be in distress, an infant may actually incite some real risk, and thereby gain the necessary reaction from its mother. Robin Dunbar describes an example of this in the gelada (*Theropithecus gelada*), a relative of the baboon, 'A yearling was geckering and mewing at its mother after failing to gain access to the female's nipples while she was feeding. It then moved across to the harem male who was grooming with another female nearby and geckered and mewed at them; they ignored it. The infant hit out at the male's back, then pulled his cape; the male ignored it. After holding onto his cape for a few seconds, the infant pulled it again. This time the male turned round and hit out at the infant. The infant then ran across to its mother, who had looked up at the commotion. When the infant approached, the mother allowed it to go on nipple at once, and then she moved off carrying the infant away from the male' (record #114). Another infant gelada 'ran across to the adult male sitting about 1.5 m away and threw itself at the male, bouncing off the male's back (the male was facing the other way). The male whipped round in surprise. The mother at once looked up, ran across to the infant and picked it up, allowed it to go on the nipple and began to groom it assiduously. The male returned to his feeding' (record #117). The gelada infant's use of another individual as a social tool can be applied to other targets, and for other purposes. Dunbar gives the example of a 2-month old infant who, when left to walk a few metres by its mother, 'jumped onto the dorsum of a 2-year old juvenile of the neighbouring reproductive unit who was feeding nearby. The mother at once ran back to retrieve the infant and pulled it onto her ventrum. The 2-year old ignored the whole thing, but the infant's older sibling, a 2-year old male, rushed across and began to threaten the juvenile female' (record #116). The primary social unit of geladas is the harem, and no doubt infants run little risk from their harem male who is normally their father; to involve an unrelated juvenile of another harem seems more risky, but a 2-year old is a small animal compared to the infant's own mother.

An even safer tactic would simply be to behave *as if* some risk or pain has been incurred, and this also happens in primates. The innocent primatologist may be the fall-guy in such deception, as Guy Norton describes in yellow baboons (*Papio cynocephalus*), 'an 8 month male infant was attempting to suckle and being repeatedly rebuffed by his mother who was feeding on the ground. After repeated attempts and a prolonged weaning geek and tantrum he walked calmly to where I was sitting and sat within 5 m—an unusually close distance for an infant. He then proceeded to scan alternatively between his mother and me and then quite suddenly flopped to his back wriggling in apparent agony and make distress calls. His mother scanned me and her infant, turned her back and continued to feed' (record #108). With any single anecdote, interpretation is tricky. Here, could it just have been a coincidence that the infant was near Norton when its tantrum occurred? In a more elaborate example reported by Toshisada Nishida, this becomes less probable. Here, the tactic was used twice, but on different 'victims'. A 5-year old male chimpanzee, Katabi, was being weaned by his mother Chausiku, who often rejected suckling attempts and on 27 November 1979 had done so repeatedly while she was consorting with the only adult male of the group, Kamemanfu. Nishida then describes how, 'Katabi came towards me, and began to scream loudly, reaching his hand towards me, as if pointing. Then, he went round me, repeatedly screaming loudly while still reaching a hand to me. Chausiku and her consort Kamemanfu at once glanced at me, with hair erect. I retreated a little bit away from Katabi, to avoid possible attack from Chausiku or Kamemanfu or both. Undoubtedly both Kamemanfu and Chausiku misinterpreted that Katabi had been attacked or teased by me. In fact I did nothing to him.' If this had been the end of it, we would be wondering the same as in the baboon case: was the primatologist really being deliberately involved by Katabi, or was it only a lucky coincidence for him. But 6 months later, the juvenile did the same thing, this time with a chimpanzee as the victim. 'Katabi . . . approached an older adolescent male Masisa, who was sitting alone, away from Chausiku, Katabi and Kamemanfu. Katabi displayed the same temper tantrums, reaching a hand to Masisa, who appeared embarrassed. As soon as Kamemanfu and Chausiku looked at Masisa he stood and pant-grunted {a submission call} to Kamemanfu. He then left Katabi, going away from the side where Chausiku and Kamemanfu were sitting. This was the same reaction as I did, although of course I did not pant-grunt; thus it appeared that Masisa understood the dangerous situation which he was driven into by Katabi. Katabi was finally allowed to suck 3 minutes after the second episode' (record #251).

There need not even be a plausible 'danger' for this sort of tactic to be found useful. Jane Goodall describes following the chimpanzee Fifi and her 4-year old son, Frodo, when the latter was being weaned, 'After he had twice tried to climb onto his mother's back and twice been rejected, he followed slowly with soft hoo-whimpers. Suddenly he stopped, stared at the side of the trail, and uttered loud and urgent-sounding screams, as though suddenly terrified. Fifi, galvanized into instant action, rushed back and with a wide grin of fear gathered up her child and set off—carrying him. I was unable to see what had caused his fear response. Three days later, as I followed the same mother–infant pair, the entire sequence was repeated. And, a year later, I saw the same behavior in a different infant, Kristal, who was also being weaned' (Goodall 1986, p. 582, reprinted as #247).

The tactical device of behaving as if some attack or threat has been experienced, when none has, is used among primates in a much wider range of contexts than merely weaning conflict. In some cases, the mother or other relatives of the apparent victim are induced to give support. As with weaning, this may simply be a matter of exaggerating need, as noted by Julie Johnson, who comments that baboons seem 'to learn to use—or exaggerate—screams, not to express pain but as a cry for help.' After describing a particular case in which the older brother interceded on behalf of a young female baboon, Johnston noted that 'her reaction was out of proportion to either any pain she felt or any perceived threat . . . the bipedal stance and orientation to the thicket differed from "real" screaming' (record #106). But deception is clearer when the observer can be certain that no threat at all has been received. A series of instances, in which the same young chacma baboon (*Papio ursinus*) manipulated adults to his advantage, shows that his actions were tactical not lucky chance. For instance, on 16 September 1983, 'Adult female Mel is digging, probably to obtain a deep growing corn. Young juvenile Paul approaches to 2 m and looks at her, then scans around; no other baboons are in view. Paul looks back at Mel and screams. Adult female Spats runs into view towards them, then chases Mel over a slight cliff and out of view. Spats, who is Paul's mother, normally defends him from attack. When both females are out of sight Paul walks forward and continues digging in Mel's hole' (Byrne and Whiten 1985, and record #104; see Byrne 1997, for detailed consideration of how this tactic may have been learned). On other occasions, Paul used the same tactic of an unwarranted scream to manipulate his father to displace adult females, and once it was his own mother that was the victim! (records #103, 105; this baboon group was a single-male unit, so paternity is certain.)

Innocent humans may also sometimes be targeted. Bertrand Deputte records a white-cheeked gibbon (*Hylobates concolor*) group, in which, 'Suddenly without any previous warning the juvenile male, partly hand-reared and very tame, gave a call I've previously never heard despite working at that time on vocal repertoire of this species; this call sounded like a scream. The three other gibbons immediately and simultaneously lunged to my head, mouths opened, but fortunately soon retreated' (record #152). Gibbons are monogamous, so the other gibbons would include the parents and sibling of the caller. Deputte notes, 'I have many times observed a young animal giving a scream without apparently being threatened, and also apparently aware, at least the second or third time, that a partner (e.g. the mother) will jump on the "opponent".'

As in the weaning context, note that in all these cases it is *genetic relatives* who have been manipulated to give sympathy, reassurance, or support. For some captive primates, humans can quite easily be recruited into the same role. A Guinea baboon (*Papio papio*), that became an expedition pet and was brought back to Holland, showed remarkable innovation in her tactic of deception to avoid walking to a feared area, as R. Pfeiffer describes, 'Bandi resisted heavily by seizing anything she passed, but eventually gave up and followed me slowly. About half-way, when I looked back, I saw her foot was bleeding. Apparently she had stepped on a piece of glass on the muddy path. I therefore decided to go home with her. After healing, next week, I decided to try again. This time I watched out for glass on the path. However, after 100 m her foot again was bleeding—and we returned. Another week later, in a new try, I stealthily watched her. Then, when she thought I didn't look, in a lightening fast movement she bit her foot and was bleeding again.

So it seemed she had deceived me all three times because in earlier events she had learned that we would go home when she had wounded a foot' (record #80). A bonobo (*Pan paniscus*) involved in an 'ape language' project had easier means available to elicit sympathy and thereby use one human to manipulate another, as noted by Sue Savage-Rumbaugh, 'A common strategy was to send me out of the room on an errand, then while I was gone she would grab hold of something that was in someone else's hands and scream as though she were being attacked. When I rushed back in, she would look at me with a pleading expression on her face and make threatening sounds at the other party. She acted as though they had taken something from her or hurt her, and solicited my support in attacking them. Had they not been able to explain that they did nothing to her in my absence, I would have tended to side with Matata and support her as she always managed to appear to have been grievously wronged' (record #249). For these captive primates, kept in close proximity to benevolent humans, their carers readily take on many of the roles of relatives and the animals can evidently discover this fact. Living in human homes, there were presumably many opportunities for these animals to learn how to manipulate their carers' behaviour.

More puzzling for biologists, there are also a few reported cases in which primate individuals, who are not known (or sometimes, known not) to have any genetic affinity to the malingerer, are induced to respond. Jane Goodall observed a male chimpanzee, Mr Worzle, who 'after begging persistently and unsuccessfully for a share of meat, threw a tantrum so violent that he almost fell out of his tree. Goliath, the higher-ranking possessor of the carcass, immediately tore the prey apart and gave half to his screaming companion' (Goodall 1986, p. 576; record #229). In a captive chimpanzee group, Frans de Waal describes how the researchers were themselves convinced that one chimpanzee, 'Yeroen, was injured after a fight with another male, Nikkie, until a student noticed that Yeroen only limped when his former adversary was present. de Waal went to check, and records, 'Yeroen walks past the sitting Nikkie from a point in front of him to a point behind him and the whole time Yeroen is in Nikkie's field of vision he hobbles pitifully, but once he has passed Nikkie his behaviour changes and he walks normally again. For nearly a week Yeroen's movement is affected in this way whenever he knows Nikkie can see him' (de Waal 1982, record #238).

Both these cases, in which a primate non-relative shows apparent sympathy, are in the same species, the chimpanzee. It may therefore be that our closest primate relative shows compassion beyond the behaviour expected on the basis of kind selection (see de Waal and van Roosmalen 1979; de Waal 1996). However, note also that the manipulated individual and the manipulator are both *males*. This is significant, since chimpanzees are a patrilocal species in which females transfer between communities. Males of a natural community are therefore genetically closer relatives than would be expected in a random population; their average genetic distance has been estimated at the equivalent of half-brothers, and so some altruism among them might be expected by kin selection.

Primate cognitive capacities for malingering

In any lasting social group, deception is necessarily rather infrequent (or it is likely to be ineffective). Records are therefore rare, and recorded on an *ad libitum* basis rather than collected systematically. If we wish to study primate deception, there is little choice but to make the best of this less-than-ideal situation. The approach taken by Whiten and Byrne was to survey a wide range of primatologists, with the help of the main international academic societies in the field (Byrne and Whiten 1988b; Whiten and Byrne 1988). This led to the creation of a large corpus of records (Byrne and Whiten 1990), from which this chapter's accounts of functional malingering in primates are taken. The criteria used to define deception were purely functional: the sequence of behaviour should reflect tactical use (not coincidental conjunctions of events), potentially benefit the agent to some other(s)' disadvantage, and rely on some individual being deceived. No requirement was made that the agent *meant* to deceive, or that any primate individuals *understood* the mechanism of what happened. The records were all submitted by experienced primatologists who were familiar with the scientific method and the need for objective evidence; they are not, therefore, 'anecdotes' in the pejorative sense of casual incidents, unreliable, and often badly remembered.

All the major groups of primates were represented in the corpus, although not at equal frequency: baboons and chimpanzees were distinctly over-represented (Byrne and Whiten 1990). However, these particular species have been the focus of much more study in the wild than most primates, so the opportunities for primatologists to detect deception were greater. Perhaps all variation in frequency can be explained by observer effort, as would be expected by theorists who assert that animals do not differ in intelligence (Macphail 1985). Yet, when the true frequency of deception was compared with that predicted from the number of long-running field studies on that species, there was significant difference (Byrne and Whiten 1992). Evidently, there is more than observer effort behind the distribution. Among the primates, the neocortex varies more than other brain parts (Stephan *et al.* 1981; Barton and Harvey 2000) and the neocortex is often credited with higher cognitive functions in humans. Byrne (1993, 1996*b*) therefore created an index of deception frequency, corrected for observer effort by taking account of the number of long-running field studies on each species, and compared this to a measure of neocortical enlargement, the ratio of neocortex to the rest of the brain in mass. The correlation was both significant and high, accounting for 60 per cent of the variance in deception frequency. This strongly supports theories that suggest that the enlarged brains of the primate order, and those of simian primates in particular, reflect intragroup selection on brain areas that underlie abilities at social manipulation (Humphrey 1976; Byrne and Whiten 1988a; Brothers 1990; Byrne 1996*a*).

The question remains, do the primates *understand* their malingering, or their deceit in general? And the problem is, a learning-theory account that does not involve intention can usually be given. As cognitive psychologists are still uneasily aware, the radical behaviourists seriously argued that all human behaviour could be described without giving any causal role to intentions or any mental states (Skinner 1953, 1981). Many of the major thinkers within psychology were for many years comfortable with this position, which treats all human action as a product of simple learning principles, so it is not surprising that it is often possible to account for even complex aspects of animal behaviour by learning alone. In the case of primate deception, this can certainly be done (Byrne and Whiten 1991). However, the plausibility of such an account varies across records. Byrne and Whiten (1990, 1992) rated all the 253 records according to whether it was possible to construct a reasonably plausible reinforcement history. That is, they judged whether the series of past events that would have to be imagined, in order to give rise to the behaviour in each record, were understandable in the context of what was known of the behavioural ecology of the species. In the vast majority of cases, this was indeed so. Only in 18 cases did Byrne and Whiten consider that the simplest 'imaginary history' was bizarre or highly improbable, either because it involved a complex conjunction of rare events, or assumptions about the animal's behaviour that did not fit with anything previously recorded. In each of these cases, they considered it less implausible to accept that the primate agents had an intentional understanding of what they were doing than to write off their actions as a product of reinforcement learning. If they were wrong, and these records simply represent the sort of flotsam that emerges from a wide trawl of non-systematic data, we should expect the records to roughly match the frequencies of deception reported as a whole, but they do not. Instead, records of apparently intentional deception are tightly clustered in a single, closely related group of primates, the great apes (i.e. chimpanzee, bonobo, gorilla, orangutan). This is consistent with other, independent assessments of primate cognition (Parker *et al.* 1994;

Russon *et al.* 1996; Byrne 1998, 2000). Since humans are also great apes, it may be concluded that the level of intentional understanding necessary to intend to deceive or malinger most probably originated in the ancestors we share with the other living great apes, perhaps 12 million years ago.

Surviving disablement

Surveying the range of primate deceptive tactics that involve feigned injury and sickness, it becomes apparent that the stakes are not usually high. Youngsters exaggerate the distress of weaning, they get into minor scrapes that encourage maternal comfort, or they simulate fear and distress and gain occasional food rewards from maternal intervention on their behalf. Adult primates feign minor injury and gain respite from harassment, or recruit supporters by showing fear of non-existent attack. The potential gains from successful malingering in these circumstances do not appear to be matters of life and death. Although ill-gotten gains might become cumulatively significant for survival if the tactics were repeated sufficiently often, the fact is that primate deception is relatively rare, so accumulated benefits are unlikely to be great. The reason would appear to lie not in primates' lack of cognitive capacity to deceive—as we have seen, this is not in doubt—but in the limited scope that their victims give for valuable manipulation. Big profits are not on offer.

The restricted nature of help available within primate societies is most clearly illustrated in response to severe disability. This was well illustrated during an outbreak of polio at Gombe, Tanzania, in which 15 chimpanzees were afflicted: several died, and others became permanently paralysed in some way. How did unaffected chimpanzees react to a paralysed member of the community? 'Initially, almost certainly, they were frightened by the strangeness of his condition. . . . the group of chimps already in camp stared for a moment and then, with wide grins of fear, rushed for reassurance to embrace and pat one another, still staring at the unfortunate cripple. . . . Eventually the others calmed down, but, though they continued to stare at him from time to time, none of them went near him—and presently he shuffled off, once more on his own' (Goodall 1971, p. 201). This pattern was typical throughout the polio outbreak. Only one male, thought to be the brother of a very severely afflicted individual, showed any affinitive reaction, and this went no further than remaining near to the sick animal until it eventually died. At no point was help offered. For instance, each night a chimpanzee constructs a bed to sleep in the branches of a tree, and without help the polio victims could not do this and were forced to sleep on the ground. Nor was any food shared, although the chimpanzee, unusually among simian primates, does show food-sharing in other contexts (de Waal 1989). It is not that such aid would not have been beneficial: both food and mechanical help were in fact offered by human observers, and was evidently gratefully received by a dying chimpanzee. The chimpanzee community simply avoided the victims.

Avoidance of victims of any mystery sickness has clear survival value: it is the reaction of humans to their sick fellows that is remarkable, and even that has its limits, as shown by the history of the Great Plague. Simple physical injury is in a different category, and when primates are injured others do not seem to avoid them. Quiatt and Reynolds (1994) found injured chimpanzees at Budongo to be well integrated spatially with able bodied ones. But nor do primates help their injured fellows. Closest to helping behaviour is an incident described by Boesch (1991), where a chimpanzee was seriously injured by a leopard, and, following the attack, conspecifics surrounded him and began to lick the wound clean, removing blood and particles of dirt.

The most frequent context for recording primate reactions to injury, sadly, is occasioned by the wire and plastic snares set to catch animals for local consumption or the bush-meat trade. Primates are often not the intended victims, but as infants and juveniles they are curious and investigative so are put greatly at risk. Moreover, the 'right' approach to getting out of a snare is counter-intuitive: pulling only makes a noose tighten further. This makes particularly remarkable the report of Dian Fossey at Karisoke, Rwanda, that the silverback gorilla 'Beethoven, possibly because of numerous past experiences with snares, had once managed to release 4-year old Puck from a wire noose' (Fossey 1983, p. 91). This observation remains unique, although snares continue to be a common cause of injury of gorillas at Karisoke and of chimpanzees at several sites, so it may be that Beethoven was just lucky. Nevertheless, this particular gorilla demonstrated understanding of snares in a more routine way, clearly distinguishing *set* snares, in which a 5-m stem of living bamboo is bent in a taut arc to power the noose, from *sprung* ones, where the bamboo is released and the wire hangs down from it. Beethoven often herded young gorillas away from set snares, but allowed them to examine and play with a large snare and the antelope caught within it (personal observation). If his protective actions were often effective, it may be that he only once confronted the difficult task of releasing an entrapped gorilla. Whatever the explanation, by far the more normal result is injury or death for the ape, and yet there seems to be no published record of help offered to a disabled individual by any of its associates (Stokes *et al.* 1999). Disabled primates are on their own.

Remarkably, in at least two species, the chimpanzee and the gorilla, severe disablement does not necessarily spell death in the wild. Individuals of both species have been known frequently to survive with missing feet, but hand injuries are potentially even more serious because of the need for skilled manual food processing for survival (Byrne 1999). Many individuals may indeed have died for lack of the necessary survival skills, but the success stories are striking. For instance, the female gorilla Pandora was first seen as an adult in August 1976, when it was noted that 'she had only a thumb on her right hand (in 1989 only the proximal phalange of the thumb was present, personal observation; see Figure 4.1), which ended in a stump. Her left was claw-shaped, with atrophied and twisted fingers. The backs of both hands bore old scars and suggested that past wounds, rather than birth defects, were responsible for her deformities. Undoubtedly, Pandora had been a poacher's trap victim' (Fossey 1983, p. 233). Nevertheless, Pandora was alive in February 2002 when she must be at least 36 years old, and she is the mother of several healthy offspring. About 16 per cent of the Karisoke gorilla population show permanent, disabling injuries to the hands, though none more severe than Pandora's. In some chimpanzee populations, more than 20 per cent of the population display severe injuries to the hands (Quiatt 1996).

We compared the gorilla Pandora with two severely injured adult chimpanzees (Byrne and Stokes 2002). Tinka retained some function only in the thumb of the left hand (see Fig. 4.1), apparently because most of the muscles of his left wrist were paralysed and when relaxed the wrist was hooked and weakened, while his right hand showed even greater deformity, with complete paralysis of the wrist and no voluntary movement possible. Muga, lacked a right hand. His amputation was distal to the wrist, and the wrist joint appeared to function normally. For the chimpanzees and the gorilla, we examined leaf-processing tasks that demand multistage techniques involving the use of both hands in complementary, coordinated roles. Nettles *Laportea alatipes* have abundant painful stings on the stem, petiole and leaf-edges. Gorillas accumulate multiple whorls of leaves by stripping up a growing stem with half-closed hand, detaching the petioles by tearing or twisting them off with the other hand, removing inedible debris, and then carefully folding the bundle of leaf-blades so that the parcel is wrapped in a single leaf-underside— the least stinging part of the plant—before ingestion by popping through open lips (Byrne and Byrne 1993). This minimizes the number of stings that contact the palm, fingers and lips. Bedstraw *Galium ruwensoriense* has tiny hooks which are most numerous on stem- and leaf-edges. An able-bodied gorilla selects multiple green stems from a large mass which usually also contains dead matter, folds the hank of trailing stems, concertina style, until it is grasped firmly in one hand, removes any remaining inedible debris, rolls the bundle against chin or hard-palate until it is tightly

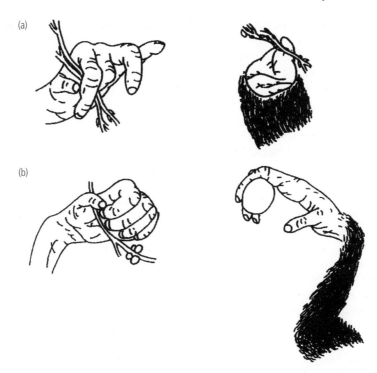

Figure 4.1 Snare injuries to the hands of wild great apes. (a) left and right hands of gorilla Pandora; (b) left and right hands of chimpanzee Tinka. In each case, the best grip the hand can exert is indicated by the material held in the hand.

rolled, then eats it with shearing bites. This technique compacts the troublesome hooks into the mass of other plant material. In both techniques, one or more stages may be iterated to build up larger amounts of food, which involves separate motor control of individual digits since the partly processed food is retained in the hand as more is dealt with (Byrne *et al.* 2001), and hierarchical organization of the overall process, since parts of the process are treated as subroutines (Byrne and Russon 1998). Budongo chimpanzees eat young leaves of paper mulberry *Broussonettia papyrifera*, an exotic species introduced for paper production in the 1950s. The leaves have large fleshy blades with a rough hairy surface. The leaf petioles are tough, and chimpanzees remove them before eating the leaves. In order to process the leaves, chimpanzees use a variety of related techniques, each stage of which requires a distinct set of actions, involving bimanual coordination and delicate manipulation. The majority of these techniques involve stripping up a stem to form a roll of leaves in the palm with leaf blades aligned parallel. In this way, the chimpanzee can remove petioles in one action. The direction in which the leaves are stripped further determines the sequence of actions required and hence the particular technique used. Leaves can be stripped towards the individual, in which case leaf blades are first consumed and petioles discarded at the end of the handful, or leaves can be stripped away from the individual, in which case petioles must first be discarded before the leaf blades can be eaten.

Processing speed gives a first approximation to feeding efficiency, provided the size of handful does not vary. Pandora tended to process handfuls of similar size to those of able-bodied gorillas, so for gorillas we were able to use the mean time to process a handful to measure efficiency. Since we were concerned that the injured chimpanzees might be systematically unable to process handfuls as large as their intact counterparts, we calculated the mean number of leaves processed in a single handful for each individual. Then, from processing rates we calculated the average time to process a single leaf and used it to measure the individual's feeding efficiency. For each plant species, we calculated a mean value and 95% confidence intervals for feeding efficiency in the able-bodied members of the ape populations. The chimpanzee Muga's feeding efficiency for paper mulberry, and the gorilla Pandora's feeding efficiency for nettles, both fell within the normal ranges. When eating bedstraw, Pandora's feeding rate fell below the lower 95 per cent interval for able-bodied individuals, and slowing was even more striking in the case of Tinka feeding on paper mulberry, where he ate at half the rate as an average able-bodied chimpanzee. Nevertheless, considerable compensation must be occurring in these individuals, all three of whom have dramatic injuries.

We found that severely injured gorillas and chimpanzees use the same techniques as able-bodied individuals, and compensate primarily at the level of detailed elements of action. They do not innovate wholly novel techniques more suited to their remaining capacities. Changes to technique are essentially a matter of omission or frequency: for example, Tinka never used the technique of able-bodied chimpanzees for making a tight roll of leaves, and both he and one-handed Muga relied on techniques used only occasionally by the able-bodied. When only one technique is used by able-bodied individuals, it is retained: Pandora used the same technique to process nettles and bedstraw as able-bodied gorillas. All three injured individuals had developed a set of novel actions to achieve the necessary intermediate operations in the complete processes, and were thus able to use the same approaches to the problems as those of uninjured peers. The compensations included holding with a thumb, or chin, or foot, instead of a power grip by the non-preferred hand; stripping leaves unimanually, when no other hand was available as a counter-force; and repeating a less efficient, unimanual operation, when a bimanually coordinated one was impossible.

Low-level flexibility therefore underlies compensation to injury in great apes, and imparts the hallmarks of each particular injury. This finding strongly suggests that, at the level of individual elements of action, each individual is learning from their own experiences. In contrast, the basic organization of techniques is found in individuals regardless of injury type, a finding which is most consistent with its acquisition by imitation of (able-bodied) adults, most likely the mother. In this way, disabled chimpanzees and gorillas obtain adequate nutrition from the more difficult-to-process plants by working around their impairments in such a way that they can employ the same techniques as the able-bodied population. The ability to accommodate flexibly to rather extreme disablement evidently buffers populations from the effects of snare injury.

More comprehensive analysis of five chimpanzees at Budongo with permanent and debilitating manual injuries confirmed these findings (Stokes and Byrne 2001). Mean time taken to process a single leaf of *Brousonnettia papyrifera* was taken as a measure of feeding efficiency. Only two of the five chimpanzees had processing rates outside the 95% confidence limits of the able-bodied population, and it would be hard to predict which chimpanzees suffered significant impairment from their injuries. Two individuals lacked entire hands, yet on this bimanual task they processed leaves as quickly as some of the able-bodied in the population. The same was true of Kewaya, a sub-adult female who has a totally paralysed right hand. Her wrist is hooked at all times, and considerably stretched and twisted round the forearm; the hand is wasted and the fingers contorted so that the middle finger lies overlapping the forefinger. Kewaya's hand is only capable of a certain amount of passive movement—swinging limply about the wrist, with movement confined to a small angle. While Kewaya processed food at relatively normal rates, the adult female Kalema, who shows a similar 'claw hand' deformity, was significantly slowed. Her right hand is rigidly hooked at the wrist and the fingers are flexed and immobile, with the whole hand emaciated and wasted. That two individual chimpanzees with such similar injuries should differ so markedly in processing efficiency is strange, but the pattern among able-bodied chimpanzees is equally varied. When we compared the feeding efficiency of these five injured chimpanzees with the 11 able-bodied chimpanzees studied, although overall the severely injured individuals process food slower than the able-bodied group, there was no simple partition (Stokes 1999). Three of the able-bodied sample processed food significantly *slower* than five able-bodied and three injured chimpanzees. If the sample is divided according to efficiency, there are thus more inefficient individuals—whose processing is significantly impaired compared with the more efficient majority—among the able-bodied than among injured chimpanzees. We have no explanation for this phenomenon, in which apparently normal, able-bodied chimpanzees exhibit efficiencies that would be consistent with severe disablement. The three individuals affected are adult female Zimba, whose dependent infant may have got in her way to some extent; sub-adult male Andy, and adult male Maani, for whom we can think of no possible justification. However, the overlap in competence between severely maimed and intact chimpanzees in feeding efficiency does highlight the extent to which injured individuals can compensate for their disablement.

Such ability to withstand extreme injury by means of low-level flexibility may only be available to those species with extensive capacity to generalize learnt skills to individual circumstances. So far this has only been reported in the great apes and humans, which may well explain why a similar survival rate as a result of comparable injury has not been found in any non-provisioned monkey populations in the wild. (High rates of injury are found in monkey populations that are fed by humans, but it may be that here human compassion acts in favour of injured individuals and artificially elevates their survival chances.)

A primate view of human malingering

To an evolutionist, discovering common features in the cognition of humans and their primate relatives is fascinating, as it allows evolutionary history to be discovered, and to some extent the adaptive causes of the changes can also be understood. Thus, the primate potential to malinger and to comprehend malingering are of interest to evolutionary psychologists—but should they interest those whose primary focus is the phenomenon of malingering in humans? We suggest there are some points that follow from our analyses that may be worth considering.

Firstly, primates have given a vivid demonstration that it is not necessary to understand the causal mechanisms—that is, to intend to create false beliefs—in order to malinger. Malingering is rife among primates, where it pays, but there is no sign that most of the monkey malingerers understand how their tricks work. Most primate malingering is *'unintentional malingering'*, in the sense that the agents typically do not intend to create false beliefs in their audiences, and it would make no sense to treat them as morally guilty. We find that the frequency of primate deception increases with the relative investment in neocortex of the particular primate species, and humans have vastly larger neocortical regions than any of the non-human primates. We therefore suggest that humans should have a great potential for unintentional malingering, regardless of any that they plan deliberately. In some clinical analyses of psychiatric conditions, such as conversion hysteria or factitious disorders, in which there is little to suggest that subjects have intentional comprehension or control of their presentation of themselves as sick, this is already recognized. However, we suggest that unintentional malingering may be commonplace, in much more everyday cases of avoidance of duty or undeserved gain from simulation of illness.

Our analysis of genuinely disabled great apes, who can expect no help or accommodation from their fellow group members, shows that impressive compensation for lost abilities is possible. Despite dramatic maiming of the hands, manual food-processing was slowed only to a quite minor extent or absent altogether, even in complex and demanding tasks. Thus, as with humans, it is possible for an ape to be disabled as a result of injury, yet not be handicapped.

Most relevant for malingering, however, was the remarkable overlap in efficiencies between genuinely disabled and able-bodied apes, and the huge variation in efficiency of the able-bodied population in a task presumably important for survival. Since no help was offered to any of the genuinely disabled apes, none of this variation can be attributed to malingering. Presumably variations in motivation and demeanour are so large that they simply outweigh the (well compensated) effects of serious injuries. However, such great baseline variation in efficiency of performance in our closest relatives bodes ill, for any ideas of objective detection of genuine malingering in humans by comparing a candidate malingerer's efficiency to that of the able-bodied population. In fact, even with primate deception, functionally defined, behavioural scientists have great difficulty in discerning whether *any* cases reflect intention to deceive. Objective, visible markers of intentional deception are few and far between. This task is unlikely to be easier in humans, who are so vastly more intelligent and subtle.

We therefore suggest that if scientific analyses of malingering can be carried out without need to make the difficult discrimination of whether it is done intentionally or not, so much the better. The same applies to measures to combat malingering, as a problem for society. Ideally, perhaps, preventive measures should take no account of intentionality, and simply aim to reduce the overall frequency. Rather than agonizing over the guilt or otherwise of individuals, or trying to devise objective performance tests (in the face of huge baseline variation in efficiency among the unimpaired population), it may be better simply to change the pay-off matrix in such as way that discourages malingering.

References

Barton, R. A. and Harvey, P. H. (2000). Mosaic evolution of brain structure in mammals. *Nature*, **405**, 1055–8.

Boesch, C. (1991). The effects of leopard predation on grouping patterns of forest chimpanzees. *Behaviour*, **117**, 220–42.

Brothers, L. (1990). The social brain: a project for integrating primate behavior and neurophysiology in a new domain. *Concepts in Neuroscience*, **1**, 27–51.

Byrne, R. W. (1993). Do larger brains mean greater intelligence? *Behavioural and Brain Sciences*, **16**, 696–7.

Byrne, R. W. (1996*a*). Machiavellian intelligence. *Evolutionary Anthropology*, **5**, 172–180.

Byrne, R. W. (1996*b*). Relating brain size to intelligence in primates. In *Modelling the early human mind* (eds P. A. Mellars and K. R. Gibson), pp. 49–56. Macdonald Institute for Archaeological Research, Cambridge.

Byrne, R. W. (1997). What's the use of anecdotes? Attempts to distinguish psychological mechanisms in primate tactical deception. In *Anthropomorphism, anecdotes, and animals: the emperor's new clothes?* (eds R. W. Mitchell, N. S. Thompson, and L. Miles), pp. 134–50. SUNY Press, Biology and Philosophy, New York, NY.

Byrne, R. W. (1998). Cognition in great apes. In *Brain and cognition in monkeys, apes and man* (ed. A. D. Milner), pp. 228–44. Oxford University Press, Oxford.

Byrne, R. W. (1999). Cognition in great ape ecology. Skill-learning ability opens up foraging opportunities. *Symposia of the Zoological Society of London*, **72**, 333–50.

Byrne, R. W. (2000). The evolution of primate cognition. *Cognitive Science*, **24**, 543–70.

Byrne, R. W. and Byrne, J. M. E. (1993). Complex leaf-gathering skills of mountain gorillas (*Gorilla g. beringei*): Variability and standardization. *American Journal of Primatology*, **31**, 241–61.

Byrne, R. W., Corp, N., and Byrne, J. M. (2001). Manual dexterity in the gorilla: bimanual and digit role differentiation in a natural task. *Animal Cognition*, **4**, 347–61.

Byrne, R. W. and Russon, A. E. (1998). Learning by imitation: a hierarchical approach. *Behavioral and Brain Sciences*, **21**, 667–721.

Byrne, R. W. and Stokes, E. J. (2002). Effects of manual disability on feeding skills in gorillas and chimpanzees: a cognitive analysis. *International Journal of Primatology*, **23**, 539–54.

Byrne, R. W. and Whiten, A. (1985). Tactical deception of familiar individuals in baboons (*Papio ursinus*). *Animal Behaviour*, **33**, 669–73.

Byrne, R. W. and Whiten, A. (1988*a*). *Machiavellian intelligence: social expertise and the evolution of intellect in monkeys, apes and humans*. Clarendon Press, Oxford.

Byrne, R. W. and Whiten, A. (1988*b*). Towards the next generation in data quality: a new survey of primate tactical deception. *Behavioral and Brain Sciences*, **11**, 267–73.

Byrne, R. W. and Whiten, A. (1990). Tactical deception in primates: the 1990 data-base. *Primate Report*, **27**, 1–101.

Byrne, R. W. and Whiten, A. (1991). Computation and mindreading in primate tactical deception. In *Natural theories of mind* (ed. A. Whiten), pp. 127–41. Basil Blackwell, Oxford.

Byrne, R. W. and Whiten, A. (1992). Cognitive evolution in primates: evidence from tactical deception. *Man*, **27**, 609–27.

de Waal, F. (1982). *Chimpanzee politics*. Jonathan Cape, London.

de Waal, F. B. M. (1989). Food sharing and reciprocal obligations among chimpanzees. *Human Evolution*, **18**, 433–59.

de Waal, F. B. M. (1996). *Good natured: the origins of right and wrong in humans and other animals*. Harvard University Press, Boston, MA.

de Waal, F. and van Roosmalen, A. (1979). Reconciliation and consolation among chimpanzees. *Behavioral Ecology and Sociobiology*, **5**, 55–6.

Fossey, D. (1983). *Gorillas in the mist*. Hodder & Stoughton, London.

Goodall, J. (1971). *In the shadow of man*. Collins, London.

Goodall, J. (1986). *The chimpanzees of Gombe: patterns of behavior*. Harvard University Press, Cambridge, MA.

Hamilton, W. D. (1964). The genetical evolution of social behaviour. I & II. *Journal of Theoretical Biology*, **7**, 1–52.

Humphrey, N. K. (1976). The social function of intellect. In *Growing points in ethology* (eds P. P. G. Bateson and R. A. Hinde), pp. 303–17. Cambridge University Press, Cambridge.

Macphail, E. M. (1985). Vertebrate intelligence: the null hypothesis. In *Animal intelligence* (ed. L. Weiskrantz), pp. 37–50. Clarendon Press, Oxford.

Parker, S. T., Mitchell, R. W., and Boccia, M. L. (1994). *Self-awareness in animals and humans: developmental perspectives*. Cambridge University Press, Cambridge.

Quiatt, D. (1996). Budongo Forest chimpanzees: behavioral accommodations to physical disability. In *XVIth Congress of the International Primatological Society, August 11–16*, Madison, WI.

Quiatt, D. and Reynolds, V. (1994). Budongo Forest chimpanzees: composition of feeding groups during the rainy season, with attention to social integration of disabled individuals. In *XVth Congress of the International Primatological Society, August 3–8*, Kuta-Bali, Indonesia.

Russon, A. E., Bard, K. A., and Parker, S. T. (eds). (1996). *Reaching into thought. The minds of the great apes*. Cambridge University Press, Cambridge.

Skinner, B. F. (1953). *Science and human behaviour*. Macmillan, New York, NY.

Skinner, B. F. (1981). Selection by consequences. *Science*, **213**, 501–4.

Stephan, H., Frahm, H., and Baron, G. (1981). New and revised data on the brain structures in insectivores and primates. *Folia Primatologica*, **35**, 1–29.

Stokes, E. J. (1999). Feeding skills and the effect of injury on wild chimpanzees. PhD Thesis, University of St Andrews, Scotland.

Stokes, E. J. and Byrne, R. W. (2001). Cognitive capacities for behavioural flexibility in wild chimpanzees (*Pan troglodytes*): the effect of snare injury on complex manual food processing. *Animal Cognition*, **4**, 11–28.

Stokes, E. J., Quiatt, D. and Reynolds, V. (1999). Snare injuries to chimpanzees (*Pan troglodytes*) at 10 study sites in East and West Africa. *American Journal of Primatology*, **49**, 104–5.

Trivers, R. L. (1974). Parent–offspring conflict. *American Zoology*, **14**, 249–64.

Whiten, A. and Byrne, R. W. (1988). Tactical deception in primates. *Behavioural and Brain Sciences*, **11**, 233–73.

Yerkes, R. M. (1943). *Chimpanzees*. Yale University Press, New Haven, CT.

Section 3

Conceptual, methodological, and cultural context

5 Conceptual issues and explanatory models of malingering

Richard Rogers and Craig S. Neumann

Abstract

This chapter provides an important overview outlining conceptual issues and explanatory models central to our understanding of malingering and deception. Terminological and classificatory limitations are delineated with cautions against the use of unvalidated or controversial descriptors. Diagnostic distinctions between factitious disorders and malingering are examined critically. From a clinical perspective, the chapter considers how professional assumptions and misassumptions may affect the accurate assessment of response style. An important contribution of the chapter is a re-analysis of extensive data on explanatory models of malingering. This re-analysis reveals a previously observed limitation in the pathogenic model. In addition, it confirms the importance of the adaptational model and a refined criminological model in explaining why persons are likely to malinger mental disorders. Clinical research and practice have devoted extensive efforts to the classification of malingering but have largely avoided its conceptual underpinnings. This chapter selectively addresses conceptual issues relevant to our understanding of malingering and related response styles. In addition, it provides a framework for examining explanatory models that grapple with the primary motivations for feigning. To assist in our understanding of explanatory models, prototypical data from 221 forensic experts (Rogers *et al.* 1998) are re-examined via confirmatory factor analysis (CFA).

Conceptual issues

Malingering and related terms

A major concern in the classification and study of malingering is the widespread use of diagnostic and descriptive terms without meticulous attention to their differences. From the North American perspective, DSM-IV-TR (American Psychiatric Association, 2000) nosology attempts to differentiate the 'V' code classification of malingering from the diagnosis of factitious disorders. Although malingering is not a diagnosis, the medical and psychiatric influences on its classification continue to hold sway. Beyond diagnostic issues, various descriptive terms (e.g. 'over-reporting' and 'suboptimal effort') are employed in clinical assessments to delineate response styles similar to malingering. The relevance of these constructs to malingering deserves close examination. Finally, we have characterized *secondary gain* evaluated as a 'quasi-construct' based on the severe limitations in its conceptualization and validation. Diagnostic issues, descriptive terms, and secondary gain are investigated sequentially in the following three sub-sections.

Malingering versus factitious disorders

Cunnien (1997) cogently questions the complete division of feigning into mutually exclusive categories of malingering and factitious disorders. In particular, Cunnien (1997, p. 24) probed, 'Are the distinctions between putative disorders (e.g. factitious disorder) and deceptive behaviors which are not granted the status of a mental disorder (e.g. malingering) conceptually meaningful and empirically valid?' Conceptually, Rogers *et al.* (1989) question the diagnostic legitimacy of factitious disorders that postulate an intentional production of psychological or physical symptoms in the service of intrapsychic and presumably unconscious motivation to assume a patient's role. This curious admixture of intentional and unintentional motivation is more closely aligned with a psychodynamic formulation than formal diagnosis.

The key difference between malingering and factitious disorders is the requirement that factitial patients are motivated to 'assume the sick role' and 'lack external incentives' for their behaviour (American Psychiatric Association, 2000, p. 517). This attempt to specify a single motivation (i.e. a sick role without external incentives) defies clinical determination. The two basic alternatives (see Rogers *et al.* 1989) for establishing motivation are problematic:

1. Data from individuals with factitial presentations are suspect for two reasons: (a) their established dishonesty; and (b) their assumed incognizance of their intrapsychic motivations.
2. Simplistic inferences by health care professionals about a feigner's motivation based only on its potential consequences (e.g. financial benefits from factitious benefits) do not rise above the level of speculation.

The isolation of a specific motivation may never be knowable and, therefore, not satisfy the basic scientific principle of falsifiability (Popper, 1959). We surmise that clinicians are more likely to classify feigning cases as malingering rather than factitial disorders because the sick role is almost always accompanied by either a reduction of usual responsibilities or material gain. As required by factitious disorders, the isolation of 'sick role' as the sole motivation is difficult to achieve.

The nosological separation of malingering and factitious disorders was first propounded by DSM-III (American Psychiatric Association 1980). After more than two decades, virtually no research has attempted to test the differences between these clinical constructs. A rare exception is research by Rogers *et al.* (1994a) that systematically compared 9 patients with factitious disorders with predominantly psychological symptoms to 25 suspected malingerers and 26 genuine inpatients. This study relied upon a known-groups comparison with forensic experts performing the classifications. Using the well-validated Structured Interview of Reported Symptoms or SIRS (Rogers *et al.* 1992), they found that patients with factitious disorders had: (a) scored higher than genuine patients on six SIRS primary scales; and (b) had no significant differences from suspected malingerers. In contrast, suspected malingerers scored significantly higher than inpatients on all eight SIRS primary scales. With a Bonferroni correction for familywise (FW) error ($\alpha_{FW} = 0.05/122$ or 0.00041), the modest finding was that only two individual SIRS items could distinguish between factitious and malingering cases. These items involved a simple cognitive task (i.e. responding to simple words with opposites) and a rare symptom (i.e. thought broadcasting). Clearly, more research is needed with larger samples on differences in clinical presentation for these two feigning groups.

Employing some of the same participants reported in Rogers *et al.* (1994), Rogers *et al.* (1992) compared 36 suspected malingerers with 11 patients with factitious disorders. They found that most patients with factitious disorders did not have markedly high scores on five SIRS scales. For instance, marked elevations on Blatant Symptoms (i.e. BL > 13) and Inconsistency of Symptoms (INC > 6) occurred infrequently for patients with factitious disorders (12.5 and 10.0 per cent, respectively). In marked contrast, these elevations occurred for nearly one-half (50.0 and 48.5 per cent, respectively) of suspected malingerers. Overall, very high elevations on these scales suggest malingering rather than feigning.

In summary, the clinical distinctions between malingering and factitious disorders are blurred by the lack of clear observable differences in the current inclusion criteria. Invoking only motivation as the crucial dimension is both theoretically suspect[1] and diagnostically ambiguous. On a practical level, clinicians must consider the extremeness of the presentation and the feigner's investment in his or her health care providers. As outlined by Rogers *et al.* (1992), this investment may take several nonexclusive forms, such as excessive admiration, dependency, and feelings of aggrievement.

Descriptive terminology

Practitioners are likely to use distinctive terms, depending on the employed clinical methods, to describe the feigning of psychological symptoms. While malingering is commonly used in diagnostic conclusions, other terms prevail for psychological testing. We explore these differences with two foci: multi-scale inventories and cognitive/neuropsychological measures.

MMPI-2 studies predominate multiscale inventories in their investigations of response styles. From its initial conceptualization, the MMPI-2 incorporated scales to evaluate whether patients were under-reporting or over-reporting their psychological impairment. However, the term 'malingering' is rarely used in accordance with DSM-IV-TR definition. The highly influential work by Greene (2000) routinely uses the term 'over-reporting' to describe the over-endorsement of psychopathology, although he suggests the term may also be applied to socially undesirable responses. Greene's (2000, p. 63) characterization of over-reporting cannot be equated with malingering because he claims that 'a client's motivation for over-reporting or under-reporting may range from being very conscious and intentional to being out of awareness and unconscious.' This description is perplexing because his body of empirical studies on over-reporting (see, e.g. Table 3.26, p. 86) relate to *intentional* feigning. In contrast to Greene, Butcher and Williams (1992) appear to prefer the term 'symptom exaggeration' to describe feigned MMPI-2 profiles. This term seems inapt because the MMPI-2's true–false format lends itself much more to fabrication than exaggeration. Most recently, Friedman *et al.* (2001) appear to equate malingering with the overclaiming of symptoms (p. 34). While partially consistent with DSM-IV-TR, an enduring problem is aligning the discrete categories of DSM-IV classification with the dimensional nature of MMPI-2 indicators.

Beyond the MMPI-2, other multiscale inventories have wrestled with their own descriptive terms. For example, Morey (1991) in his development the Personality Assessment Inventory (PAI) described extreme elevations on the NIM scale as deliberate efforts at 'negative self presentation' (p. 12). For moderate elevations, he is more equivocal about intent ranging presumably from a genuinely negative self-evaluation to deliberate distortions. As a further example, Millon *et al.*'s (1997) work on the MCMI-III ascribes putatively negative judgments to the faking-bad response style. High scores on the Debasement Index are described as 'an inclination to *deprecate and devalue oneself* by presenting more troublesome emotional and personal difficulties than are likely to be uncovered by objective review' (emphasis added, Millon *et al.*

---

[1] We might speculate that the narcissistic needs of clinicians are operative in making this disputable distinction. Deliberate and calculated fabrications to garner health care services are accorded the status of a mental disorder. Identical fabrications for other purposes are pejoratively labelled but not diagnosed.

1997, p. 118). The example from Millon *et al.* adds untested inferences about self-deprecation to the consideration of feigned psychopathology.

The clinical literature on feigned cognitive impairment uses its own descriptive terminology that is at odds with the DSM-IV-TR definition of malingering (Rogers and Bender 2003). Lacking the standardization provided by DSM-IV, these terms also lack any specific parameters for their implementation. The most disparate examples involve effort: 'sub-optimal effort', 'incomplete effort', and 'sub-maximal effort'. These terms are markedly discordant with malingering which provides a functional standard of fabrication or gross exaggeration. In stark contrast, sub-optimal effort implies that anything less than the very best endeavor is suggestive of feigning. As noted by Fishbain *et al.* (1999), the relationship between sub-maximal effort and malingering remains to be investigated. An additional term seen occasionally in disability evaluations is 'symptom magnification'; this designation suggests exaggeration rather than fabrication. However, the level of exaggeration is not specified thereby allowing mild or isolated examples to be equated with feigned cognitive impairment.

In summary, any conceptual framework for malingering must take into account distinct and often dissimilar constructs used in the clinical literature. Professionals must resolve for their own practices the conflicts between Greene's (2000) 'over-reporting' and Friedman *et al.*'s (2001) 'over-claiming' in interpreting MMPI-2's validity indicators. Researchers may wish to test directly: (a) differences between sub-optimal effort and malingering; and (b) potential confounds (e.g. co-morbid depression) contributing to sub-optimal effort.

Secondary gain

The construct of *secondary gain* is sometimes invoked to describe either deliberate or nondeliberate efforts to obtain presumably unwarranted benefits. As delineated by Rogers and Reinhardt (1998), the concept of secondary gain is splintered by professional and theoretical differences (i.e. psychodynamic, behavioural, and forensic). Psychodynamically, secondary gain focuses on the patient's unmet intrapsychic needs. The motivation to satisfy these needs is hypothesized to be mostly unconscious and therefore nonmodifiable by the patient. Behaviourally, secondary gain focuses on the social context of treatment. Health care providers and support systems may unwittingly promote illness behaviour leading to an avoidance of negative stimuli and reinforcement of maladaptive responses. A network of social contingencies often limits the patient's ability to modify secondary gain. Forensically, secondary gain focuses on the patient's inferred motivation to acquire unearned incentives. The forensic model is flawed by faulty logic: potentially should never be equated with actuality. For instance, the inference is untenable that a *potential* incentive (e.g. disability payments) can be equated with the *actual* incentive.[2]

Rogers and Vitacco (2002) argue against the general use of secondary gain in either clinical or forensic evaluations. As noted, implicit conflicts remain unresolved regarding its conceptualization. With particular reference to feigning, the concept of secondary gain is highly speculative and empirically untested.

Problematic issues in the conceptualization and classification of malingering

Current research has largely overlooked the study of how mental health professionals address malingering in their clinical evaluations. Therefore, this section relies primarily on heuristic

---

[2] Offering a different perspective, Shuman (2000) suggests that the legal system with its protracted delays may contribute to secondary gain by perpetuating the sick role via questioning the injured person's credibility and provision of large awards for chronic impairment.

observations of professional practices. We address problematic issues that are likely to result in distorted understandings and unacceptable misclassifications of malingering.

Attributions to the patient or the setting

A cursory examination of DSM-IV-TR indices of potential malingering suggests that malingerers form a deplorably immoral and criminal group. Indices include antisocial personality disorders, ongoing legal involvement, and uncooperativeness. Strong adherents of the DSM-IV-TR model are likely to over-emphasize malingering among 'bad' persons while under-emphasizing it among 'good' persons. Improper generalizations from 'bad' in certain aspects (e.g. criminal background) to 'bad' in other aspects (e.g. malingering) are apt to be examples of the *ad hominem* fallacy (Dauer 1989). Anecdotally, forensic patients that are abrasive and irritating to hospital staff run the risk of being misclassified as malingering based on their general obnoxiousness. Conversely, the *ad hominem* fallacy may lead mental health professionals to overlook malingering among persons of good reputation. For example, Faust *et al.* (1988) found that neuropsychologists missed *every* child case of malingering in research involving a simulation design. A conceivable explanation is that neuropsychologists, implicitly believing in the inherent goodness of youth, simply did not consider adequately issues of malingering, even when forewarned of its possibility.

Professional judgements about malingering and other response styles may also be colored by the setting. For example, some correctional institutions have informal prohibitions against the prescription of certain medications (e.g. anxiolytics and sedatives) because of general fears that some inmates may be feigning. Rather than attempt individual discriminations between genuine and feigned complaints, the tacit assumption is that all inmates are likely to feign for the 'right' medications.

Intuitional perspective

According to Rogers and Bender (2003), intuitional perspective presupposes that malingering cases can be 'intuited' and do not require systematic assessment. Some experienced clinicians adopt an insular view toward malingering, namely 'I know it when I see it.' Such insularity is not open to critical review because no additional data are likely to be sought to confirm or disconfirm such intuitive judgements. Besides not satisfying basic requirements of reliability and validity, intuitional judgements are likely to be inaccurate as evidenced by the classic research by Rosenhan (1973).

Application of base-rates to malingering

Several investigators (Mossman and Hart 1996; Rosenfeld *et al.* 2000; Sweet *et al.* 2000) have argued vigorously for the application of base rates to classificatory models of malingering. Superficially, this advocacy appears to have merit. Unfortunately, the instability of base rates militates against their use. Rogers and Salekin (1998) examined prevalence estimates of malingering furnished by 221 forensic experts. In forensic cases, the M was 17.4 per cent ($SEM = 1.1$ per cent; $SD = 14.4$ per cent). Focusing simply on the distribution (i.e. $M \pm 2SDs$), we can expect that most of the prevalence rates for most forensic settings to fall between 0.0 and 46.2 per cent. Because the distribution for forensic malingering is slightly skewed (i.e. 1.41), we found that 5.6 per cent exceeded this range with 2.8 per cent reporting prevalences ≥ 60 per cent.

Estimations of base-rates for response styles shoulder a greater burden than the typical disease categories. Unlike most disorders, malingering and other intentional distortions often do not appear to be static. Decisions to malinger typically factor in referral issues and situational demands. For referral issues, feigned incompetency-to-stand-trial cannot be accurately captured by a single estimate. For instance, malingering is unlikely to occur for an offense punishable by only a fine. Situational demands may affect dramatically the prevalence of malingering. As an illustration, a male psychiatrist in Toronto was successful in producing 24-hour cures for bogus disorders. He would simply explain to defendants the isolation and hardships they would face at a maximum-security forensic hospital isolated in northern Ontario.

Challenges of classification

Debates regarding the relative merits of categorical versus dimensional classification are well known (Widiger 1992). A categorical model provides a classification of malingering only for compelling cases of feigning. It is silent on marginal and indeterminate cases of malingering. In contrast, the dimensional model provides probabilistic estimates across the continuum. Beyond methodological concerns, practitioners must also consider the *consequences* of their conclusions.

Rogers (1998) expressed apprehension about the dimensional classification of malingering. On most psychological measures, malingering can only be excluded completely (i.e. 0.0 per cent probability) for a very small percentage of clinical referrals. For example, Shea *et al.* (1996) found only 7.8 per cent of male pre-trial defendants had low scores on the MMPI-2 F scale. Therefore, practitioners must consider what would be the real-world consequences of providing probability estimates of malingering, even when these estimates are low. Rogers (1998) suggested that low estimates might have devastating consequences in legal proceedings; for example, a 20 per cent estimate of malingering might derail an otherwise successful insanity defense.

Explanatory models of malingering

The bulk of the malingering literature (see Rogers 1997) addresses issues of clinical classification. Beyond classification, explanatory models have been proposed to elucidate the primary motivations for why certain persons malinger. Rogers (1990*a, b*) put forth three non-mutually exclusive explanatory models (i.e. pathogenic, criminological, and adaptational) described in next section. Following their description, results and commentary on two prototypical analyses are presented. Finally, we re-examine Rogers *et al.* (1998) data using confirmatory factor analysis (CFA).

Original conceptualization

Rogers (1990*b*) synthesized the existing literature and proposed three explanatory models for explaining the primary motivations of malingering. The motivations include: (a) an underlying psychopathology coupled with a deteriorating course (pathogenic model); (b) a manifestation of antisocial behaviour and attitudes (criminological model); and (c) an attempt to respond to adversarial circumstances that takes into account other alternatives (adaptational model). While described separately for the purposes of clarity, these models are not conceptualized as mutually exclusive.

The pathogenic model, influenced by psychodynamic thought, posits that ostensible motivations are insufficient to explain acts of malingering. Rather, malingering results from intrapsychic and possibly unconscious needs. From the pathogenic perspective, the crumbling of ineffective defenses leads to further deterioration. With increasing impairment, overtly intentional acts of malingering are gradually transformed to involuntary behaviour.

The criminological model was first articulated in DSM-III (American Psychiatric Association 1980) and subsequently reaffirmed in successive editions (DSM-III-R, American Psychiatric Association 1987; DSM-IV, American Psychiatric Association 1994; DSM-IV-TR, American Psychiatric Association 2000). The criminological model is represented by four indices that includes one *diagnostic* variable [antisocial personality disorder (APD)], one *contextual* variable (medicolegal evaluation), and two *presentational* variables (uncooperativeness and discrepancies with objective findings). What accounts for this peculiar amalgamation of indices? According to Rogers (1990*a, b*), the unifying theme for three indices is badness. It is composed of a *bad* individual (diagnosis of APD) in a *bad* situation (medicolegal evaluation) participating *badly* (uncooperative). As observed by Rogers and Bender (2003), the basic notion of the criminological model is that antisocial persons are generally deceptive. These deceptions are especially salient when the stakes are high (e.g. avoidance of criminal sanctions or acquisition of undeserved rewards). Malingering is thus viewed by the criminological model as a variation of deception capitalizing on situational opportunities.

The adaptational model was proposed by Rogers (1990*a*) to avoid the monistic explanations of the malingering, namely mad (pathogenic) and bad (criminological). It assumes that most malingerers attempt to resolve difficult circumstances via some form of cost–benefit analysis. In some instances, this analysis is very straightforward. A criminal defendant, facing an avalanche of incriminating evidence, might simply conclude that he or she has 'nothing to lose'. As observed by Rogers (1997), many simulators feigning mental disorders have an inaccurate appraisal of their ability to malinger. Nevertheless, malingerers likely weigh their options and potential success, whether accurately or inaccurately, before adopting this response set.

Prototypical analysis

Rosch (1978) promoted the use of prototypical analysis for the explication of fuzzy constructs that cannot be defined by a conclusive set of necessary and sufficient features. Because explanatory models of malingering lack clear parameters, Rogers *et al.* (1994*b*, 1998) performed two prototypical analyses. These studies shared two common features. First, very experienced forensic experts were recruited in both studies from postdoctoral workshops sponsored by the American Academy of Forensic Psychologists. Second, both studies utilized the same list of prototypical characteristics: (a) pathogenic items addressed underlying psychopathology, continued deterioration, and development of genuine symptoms; (b) criminological items included DSM indices supplemented by psychopathic characteristics as delineated by Psychopathy Checklist: Screening Version (PCL:SV; Hare *et al.* 1994); and (c) adaptational items focused on the adversarial context and cost–benefit analysis.

Rogers *et al.* (1994*b*) conducted a principal components analysis (PCA) of prototypical ratings from 320 forensic experts who averaged more than 1000 evaluations (i.e. 312 forensic and 746 non-forensic) in their professional careers. The PCA yielded a three-factor solution with nearly all the prototypical items (96.9 per cent) evidencing high (>0.50) and unique loadings consistent with the proposed explanatory models. The adaptational model was the most prototypical followed by the criminological and pathogenic models.

Rogers *et al.* (1998) performed a second prototypical analysis with 221 forensic experts. Applying the clearest and most representative examples, experts were asked to identify their most prototypical cases including one each from their forensic and nonforensic practices. These cases were grouped by the *type* of feigning into three categories: mental disorders, cognitive impairment, and medical syndromes. With a principal axis factoring (PAF), the optimum solution yielded a four-factor solution. The principal difference with the earlier prototypical analysis was the division of the adaptational model into two meaningful dimensions: cost–benefit analysis and adversarial setting. With this modification, separate exploratory analysis yielded consistent results across forensic and non-forensic solutions (*M* congruence coefficients = 0.91). In addition to the PAF, differences in the type of feigning were explored. Focusing on non-forensic cases, the pathogenic model was the least applicable to feigned cognitive impairment. In addition, adversarial context appeared more applicable to simulated mental disorders than either feigned cognitive impairment or bogus medical syndromes. Gender differences were also observed with the criminological model applying more to males than females in both forensic and non-forensic cases.

Re-analysis of Rogers et al. (1998)

For the purposes of this chapter, the Rogers et al. (1998) data were re-analysed. The foremost issue to address was whether CFA could provide additional empirical support for either the three or four factor solutions. In addition, we investigated predictor variables for experts based on the level of malingering found in their forensic practices. For use with clinical data, we focused on two fit indices: the comparative fit index (CFI) and the robust comparative fit index (RCFI) (Bentler 1995). We also examined the root mean square error of approximation (RMSEA) to assess how well the model fits the data in the population.

We tested the original three-factor model by Rogers et al. (1994b). This model resulted in a poor fit for the data in both forensic and nonforensic samples (see Table 5.1). We also failed to confirm the four-factor solution for the original PAF analysis by Rogers et al. (1998). While approaching an adequate fit (see Table 5.1), the fit indices fell clearly short for both forensic (CFI = 0.83; RCFI = 0.85) and non-forensic (CFI = 0.84; RCFI = 0.86) solutions. We observed several problems in confirming the four-factor model: (a) the pathogenic items tended to have modest factor loadings; and (b) most of the criminological items reflected dimensions of psychopathy (i.e. Arrogant and Deceitful Interpersonal (ADI) Style, Deficient Affective Experiences (DAE), and Impulsive and Irresponsible Behavioural (IIB) Style; see Cooke and Michie 2001). While the elimination of pathogenic items improved the fit, this option was conceptually unappealing. A more attractive alternative involved a refinement of criminological model treating the three dimensions (i.e. ADI, DAE, and IIB) as parcels (i.e. the summing of items within each category). With conceptually related items, parcels have been shown to be more reliable and valid indicators of their CFA factors when compared with individual items (Bagozzi and Heatherton 1994; Greenbaum and Dedrick 1998). The modified four-factor models (see Table 5.1) resulted in generally good fit for both forensic (RCFI = 0.90; RMSEA = 0.07) and non-forensic (RCFI = 0.94; RMSEA = 0.06) prototypic ratings. Table 5.2 provides standardized factor loadings and error terms separately for the forensic and non-forensic models.

The cost–benefit factor appears to be related to other dimensions of malingering. A positive relationship was found with the criminological factor (forensic, $r = 0.43$, $p < 0.001$; non-forensic,

Table 5.1 CFA for explanatory models of malingering: a re-analysis of Rogers et al. (1998)

Model	Setting	x^2	d.f.	CFI	RCFI	RMSEA
1994 three-factor*	Forensic	727	347	0.76	0.77	0.09
1994 three-factor*	Non-forensic	791	347	0.77	0.80	0.10
1998 four-factor[†]	Forensic	514	269	0.83	0.85	0.08
1998 four-factor[†]	Non-forensic	572	269	0.84	0.86	0.09
Modified four-factor[‡]	Forensic	225	113	0.86	0.90	0.07
Modified four-factor[‡]	Non-forensic	181	113	0.93	0.94	0.06

* The three factors are criminological, pathogenic, and adaptational.
[†] The four factors are criminological, pathogenic, cost–benefit, and adversarial context.
[‡] The four factors are criminological (modified into three parcels), pathogenic, cost–benefit, and adversarial context.

Table 5.2 CFA of Rogers et al. (1998) explanatory models of malingering with forensic and non-forensic prototypes: standardized parameter loadings

	Forensic					Non-forensic				
	F1	F2	F3	F4	Error	F1	F2	F3	F4	Error
Criminological factor (F1)										
Arrogant and Deceitful Interpersonal Style	0.86				0.51	0.85				0.52
Deficient Affective Experiences	0.87				0.49	0.89				0.45
Impulsive and Irresponsible Interpersonal Style	0.70				0.71	0.76				0.65
Pathogenic factor (F2)										
Malingered as attempt to control pathology		0.69			0.73		0.76			0.65
Malingered, feigned symptoms became real		0.63			0.78		0.61			0.79
Control of psychosis by producing symptoms		0.52			0.86		0.65			0.76
Feigned symptoms to avoid real pathology		0.79			0.62		0.80			0.60
Malingering is early or prodromal phase		0.61			0.80		0.61			0.79
Feigned symptoms to ward off emotional crisis		0.47			0.89		0.75			0.67
Compelled to feign by unconscious forces		0.52			0.86		0.59			0.81
Cost–benefit factor (F3)										
Appeared to make rational decision to malinger			0.85		0.53			0.90		0.44
Weighed alternatives before feigning			0.78		0.62			0.74		0.68
Assessed circumstances and likelihood of success			0.57		0.82			0.49		0.87
Adversarial-context factor (F4)										
Malingered as a way to cope a difficult situation				0.95	0.32				0.92	0.39
Tried to meet needs in unsympathetic system				0.47	0.87				0.56	0.83
Tried to make best of bad situation				0.60	0.80				0.52	0.85
Could not find better way of getting what needed				0.34	0.94				0.46	0.89

Note: All factor and error loadings are significant ($p < 0.5$ to < 0.001).

$r = 0.48$, $p < 0.001$), suggesting that individuals with psychopathic characteristics may use cost-benefit analysis in deciding to malinger. Conversely, cost–benefit analysis is less likely to be seen in non-forensic cases ($r = -0.58$, $p < 0.001$) among malingerers with prominent pathogenic characteristics.

Based on the current CFA, the criminological model is best understood as dimensions of psychopathy (ADI, DAE, IIB). In the original conceptualization, this dimension also included the four DSM indices of malingering. Given that only one item (APD) loaded consistently in earlier analyses, it is not surprising that DSM indices were not included in the current CFA analyses.

In conclusion, the current CFA's provide general support for three refined explanatory models of malingering with the adaptational model being composed of two dimensions. However, an important question remains whether experts' understanding of explanatory models influences their findings in either forensic or non-forensic cases.

To test for potential influences, we explored differences for forensic experts between those less likely and more likely to classify evaluatees as malingerers. If explanatory models substantially influence malingering classifications, we expected that they could be used to predict prevalence rates. With nearly one-half (45.6 per cent) of the experts having estimated prevalence rates of malingering between 10 and 20 per cent,[3] we selected 50 experts with low prevalence rates (i.e. < 10 per cent; $M = 3.9$ per cent) and 48 experts with moderate prevalence rates (i.e. ≥25 per cent; $M = 36.6$ per cent). We tested via stepwise discriminant analyses whether explanatory models could significantly predict low versus moderate prevalence rates. We were surprised at the consistently nonsignificant results.[4] None of the variables associated with the explanatory models reached even the minimal significance to be entered into a discriminant function. DAE approached significance but only accounted for a minuscule 2.4 per cent of the variance (i.e. $\lambda = 0.9760$). Adding background variables (e.g. years of post-doctoral experience and percentage of forensic practice) did not improve the discriminant function.

Explanatory models are likely to be useful in understanding the underlying motivations of various malingerers. However, the total lack of any explanatory-based predictors for classifying low- and moderate-prevalence experts suggests that explanatory models do not exert any systematic bias on malingering classifications. Pending confirmation, this finding is heartening in suggesting that experts' perceptions of explanatory models are unlikely to influence their clinical decisions.

Concluding remarks

The assessment of malingering is a multi-faceted process that challenges experts with both its complex conceptualization and demanding clinical tasks. This chapter underscores these intricacies in its examination of diagnostic classification and terminological confusion. Of special concern is the widespread use of controversial terms, such as secondary gain, that are found lacking on both theoretical and empirical grounds.

An important contribution of this chapter is its explication of explanatory models. Based on prototypical analysis, we re-examine pathogenic, criminological, and adaptational models of malingering. As before, we find the pathogenic model to be generally lacking in salience and prototypicality. We add further refinements to criminological model and confirm the adaptational model. Finally, we do not find any systematic evidence of these explanatory models biasing forensic evaluations.

References

American Psychiatric Association. (1980). *Diagnostic and statistical manual of mental disorders*, 3rd edn. American Psychiatric Press, Washington, DC.

American Psychiatric Association. (1987). *Diagnostic and statistical manual of mental disorders*, 3rd edn, revised. American Psychiatric Press, Washington, DC.

American Psychiatric Association. (1994). *Diagnostic and statistical manual of mental disorders*, 4th edn. American Psychiatric Press, Washington, DC.

---

[3] Because 41 participants did not provide estimates, these prevalence rates are based on 180 forensic experts.

[4] Discriminant analyses based on a single sample often capitalize on chance variation and may produce spuriously significant results.

American Psychiatric Association. (2000). *Diagnostic and statistical manual of mental disorders: text revision*, 4th edn. American Psychiatric Press, Washington, DC.

Bagozzi, R. P. and Heatherton, T. F. (1994). A general approach to representing multifaceted personality constructs: application to state self-esteem. *Structural Equation Modeling*, **1**, 35–67.

Bentler, P. M. (1995). *EQS structural equations program manual*. Multivariate Software, Inc., Encino, CA.

Butcher, J. N. and Williams, C. L. (1992). *Essentials of MMPI-2 and MMPI-A interpretation*. University of Minnesota Press, Minneapolis, MN.

Cooke, D. J. and Michie, C. (2001). Refining the construct of psychopathy: towards a hierarchical model. *Psychological Assessment*, **13**, 171–88.

Cunnien, A. J. (1997). Psychiatric and medical syndromes associated with deception. In *Clinical assessment of malingering and deception* (ed. R. Rogers), 2nd edn, pp. 23–46. Guilford, New York, NY.

Dauer, F. W. (1989). *Critical thinking: an introduction to reasoning*. Barnes and Noble, New York, NY.

Faust, D., Hart, K., and Guilmette, T. J. (1988). Pediatric malingering: the capacity of children to fake believable deficits of neuropsychological testing. *Journal of Consulting and Clinical Psychology*, **56**, 578–82.

Fishbain, D. A., Cutler, R. B., Rosomoff, H. L., and Rosomoff, R. S. (1999). Chronic pain disability exaggeration/malingering and submaximal effort. *The Clinical Journal of Pain*, **15**, 244–74.

Friedman, A. F., Lewak, R., Nichols, D. S., and Webb, J. T. (2001). *Psychological assessment with the MMPI-2*. Lawrence Erlbaum, Mahwah, NJ.

Greenbaum, P. E. and Dedrick, R. F. (1998). Hierarchical confirmatory factor analysis of the Child Behavior Checklist. *Psychological Assessment*, **10**, 149–55.

Greene, R. L. (2000). *The MMPI-2/MMPI: an interpretive manual*. Allyn and Bacon, Boston, MA.

Hare, R. D., Cox, D. N., and Hart, S. D. (1994). *Manual for the Screening Version of Psychopathy Checklist Revised (PCL-SV)*. Multi-Health Systems, Toronto.

Millon, T., Davis, R., and Millon, C. (1997). *The Millon Clinical Multiaxial Inventory-III manual*, 2nd edn. National Computer Systems, Minneapolis, MN.

Morey, L. C. (1991). *Personality Assessment Inventory: professional manual*. Psychological Assessment Resources, Inc, Tampa, FL.

Mossman, D. and Hart, K. J. (1996). Presenting evidence of malingering to courts: Insights from decision theory. *Behavioral Sciences and the Law*, **14**, 271–91.

Popper, K. (1959). *The logic of scientific discovery*. Basic Books, New York, NY.

Rogers, R. (1990*a*). Development of a new classificatory model of malingering. *Bulletin of the American Academy of Psychiatry and Law*, **18**, 323–33.

Rogers, R. (1990*b*). Models of feigned mental illness. *Professional Psychology: Research and Practice*, **21**, 182–8.

Rogers, R. (ed.) (1997). *Clinical assessment of malingering and deception*, 2nd edn. Guilford, New York, NY.

Rogers, R. (1998). The uncritical acceptance of risk assessment: a dangerous enterprise in forensic evaluations. Paper presented at the *American Psychology-Law Society Biennial Conference*, Redondo Beach, CA.

Rogers, R., Bagby, R. M., and Dickens, S. E. (1992). *Structured Interview of Reported Symptoms (SIRS) and professional manual*. Psychological Assessment Resources, Inc., Odessa, FL.

Rogers, R., Bagby, R. M., and Rector, N. (1989). Diagnostic legitimacy of factitious disorder with psychological symptoms. *American Journal of Psychiatry*, **146**, 1312–14.

Rogers, R., Bagby, R. M., and Vincent, A. (1994*a*). Factitious disorders with predominantly psychological signs and symptoms: a conundrum for forensic experts. *Journal of Psychiatry and Law*, **22**, 99–106.

Rogers, R. and Bender, S. D. (2003). Evaluation of malingering and deception. In *Comprehensive handbook of psychology: forensic psychology* (ed. A. M. Goldstein), Vol. 11, pp. 109–29. Wiley, New York, NY.

Rogers, R. and Reinhardt, V. (1998). Conceptualization and assessment of secondary gain. In *Psychologist's desk reference* (eds G. P. Koocher, J. C., Norcross, and S. S. Hill, III), pp. 57–62. Oxford University Press, New York, NY.

Rogers, R. and Salekin, R. T. (1998). Beguiled by Bayes: a re-analysis of Mossman and Hart's estimates of malingering. *Behavioral Sciences and the Law*, **16**, 147–53.

Rogers, R., Salekin, R. T., Sewell, K. W., Goldstein, A., and Leonard, K. (1998). A comparison of forensic and nonforensic malingerers: A prototypical analysis of explanatory models. *Law and Human Behavior*, **22**, 353–67.

Rogers, R., Sewell, K. W., and Goldstein, A. (1994*b*). Explanatory models of malingering: A prototypical analysis. *Law and Human Behavior*, **18**, 543–52.

Rogers, R. and Vitacco, M. J. (2002). Forensic assessment of malingering and related response styles. In *Forensic psychology: From classroom to courtroom* (ed. B. Van Dorsten). Kluwer Academic/Plenum Publishers, Boston, MA.

Rosch, E. (1978). Principles of categorization. In *Cognition and categorization* (eds E. Rosch and B. B. Lloyd), pp. 27–48. Erlbaum, Hillsdale, NJ.

Rosenfeld, B., Sands, S. A., and Van Gorp, V. G. (2000). Have we forgotten the base rate problem? Methodological issues in the detection of distortion. *Archives of Clinical Neuropsychology*, **15**, 349–59.

Rosenhan, D. (1973). On being sane in insane places. *Science*, **172**, 250–8.

Shea, S. J., McKee, G. R., Craig-Shea, M. E., and Culley, D. C. (1996). MMPI-2 profiles of male pretrial defendants. *Behavioral Sciences and the Law*, **14**, 331–8.

Shuman, D. W. (2000). When time does not heal: understanding the importance of avoiding unnecessary delay in the resolution of tort cases. *Psychology, Public Policy, and Law*, **6**, 880–97.

Sweet, J. J., Wolfe, P., Sattlberger, E., Numan, B., Rosenfeld, J. P., Clingerman, S., and Nies, K. J. (2000). Further investigation of traumatic brain injury versus insufficient effort with the California Verbal Learning Test. *Archives of Clinical Neuropsychology*, **15**, 105–13.

Widiger, T. A. (1992). Categorical versus dimensional classification: implications from and for research. *Journal of Personality Disorders*, **6**, 287–300.

6 The social cognition of intentional action

Bertram F. Malle

Abstract

Malingering is defined as an intentional social act of simulating or exaggerating illness. However, determinations of intentionality are often met with suspicion, and among experts in malingering nobody quite likes to make intentionality judgements. A serious medical, legal, and political management of malingering, however, must confront the problem of intentionality. Both malingerers (in planning their deception) and examiners (in trying to detect it) rely on a folk concept of intentionality that has evolved over a million years and has been refined in everyday social practice. Though folk judgements of intentionality are not perfect, they are well grounded in a systematic conceptual framework and thus provide the starting point for a comprehensive analysis of malingering as a social act. This chapter discusses the folk-conceptual and cognitive underpinnings of intentionality judgements and offers implications for a better understanding and handling of malingering. Important distinctions are introduced, such as between intentions (the mental state of being committed to act) and intentionality (the skilful and conscious performance of an intended action), and factors are identified that increase or decrease the validity of intentionality judgements. The picture of malingering painted here is one of a complex but tractable type of intentional action that is, in principle, no more elusive than other intentional actions people perceive and manage every day.

Introduction

Malingering is typically defined as the intentional attempt to simulate or exaggerate illness symptoms in order to reach a consciously desired goal (e.g. health benefits or release from military duty). Because of its intentional and conscious quality, malingering is more blameworthy in our social and legal system than hypochondria, hysteria, or related disorders, which count as unintentional because their illness symptoms are caused by nonconscious factors (e.g. anxiety). However, the distinction between intentional and unintentional behaviour is often treated with suspicion. In particular, within the complex web of individuals and institutions who deal with the problem of malingering, nobody wants to make intentionality judgements. Investigators for the insurance industry or the government are only interested in 'facts', not judgements (even though, naturally, brute facts do not have the causal power to deny benefits or demand repayment; they have causal power only insofar as individuals judge them as relevant and decisive for the question at issue). Physicians focus on describing illness symptoms and organic deficits (or their absence) and claim that judgements about intentional deception lie beyond their professional expertise—they are the lawyers' province. Lawyers, on their part, argue that they are no experts at distinguishing malingering from hysteria and would rather have the physicians make that call.

This avoidance of intentionality is misguided, and for two reasons. First, if malingering is distinct from hypochondria and if one of the distinguishing features is intentionality, then no party involved can ignore the issue of intentionality. Second, intentionality judgements are made every day, by all social agents, and that has been the case for probably about a million years (Malle 2002; MacWhinney 2002). Judging the intentions and goals of other people is a common social practice, and as such it is neither metaphysically impossible (as some philosophers have it) nor completely reliable. But if it were not the case that most people are correct in their intentionality judgements a good part of the time, social interaction would be impossible, and the evolution of humankind would have been halted long ago.

An adequate foundation for social and professional dealings with malingering must involve a clear concept of intentionality. However, scholars of various disciplines have long argued about the meaning of intentionality without reaching a consensual understanding of this phenomenon. Rather than add to the numerous expert definitions, I suggest a different approach, namely to focus on the social cognition of intentionality. Social cognition comprises the tasks and tools involved in the human interpretation of behaviour, and judgements of intentionality play a central role therein. These judgements have been rendered reliable and socially shareable (see Freyd 1983) by the evolution of a folk concept of intentionality. A folk concept operates like a filter that classifies certain perceptual input into significant categories and thus frames or interprets the perceptual input in ways that facilitate subsequent processing, including prediction, explanation, evaluation, and action (Malle in press). At least some folk concepts are historically and cross-culturally stable, and there is good reason to believe that intentionality is one of them (Malle and Knobe 1997; Ames 2001; Malle and Nelson in-press).

Three reasons make this approach compelling. First, malingering agents act in accordance with their folk concept of intentionality—that is, they generate action that is intentional in their minds. Second, malingering agents conceal the true motives of their actions in light of what they consider to be other people's perceptions of intentionality—that is, they try to behave in ways that do *not* appear intentional to others. And third, social perceivers of malingering behaviour, such as physicians, insurance agents, jury members, or judges, cannot help but use their folk concept of intentionality to distinguish malingering from genuine illness.

In this chapter, I thus introduce a definition of intentionality that is grounded in people's social practice of judging intentionality, and I examine some of the features on which people base such judgements. This contribution does not solve the problem of judging intentionality in any particular case, but it lays the groundwork for an adequate approach to malingering in general by providing a systematic conceptual language that can be used in social as well as legal contexts.

The concept of intentionality

In court and in daily interactions, people regularly make judgements of intentionality. However, surprisingly little research has been devoted to the concept that underlies these judgements. A number of researchers have offered theoretical discussions (Heider 1958; Jones and Davis 1965; Shaver 1985; Fiske 1989), but their respective models disagree on the specific components that make up intentionality. Malle and Knobe (1997) therefore relied on an empirical approach to reconstruct the folk concept of intentionality, using qualitative and experimental methods.

In a first study, participants read descriptions of 20 behaviours and rated them for their intentionality, using an 8-point scale ranging from 'not at all' (0) to 'completely' (7) intentional. About one-half of the participants received a working definition of intentionality before they rated the 20 behaviours. The definition read: 'What do we mean by *intentional*? This means that the person had a *reason* to do what she did and that she *chose* to do so.' The assumption was that if people used their own folk concept to rate the behaviours, then there should be high agreement among participants with or without an experimenter-provided definition. Agreement was high in the whole sample. Any two people's intentionality ratings showed an average inter-correlation of $r(20) = 0.64$, and any one person showed an average correlation of $r(20) = 0.80$ with the remaining group, resulting in an inter-rater reliability of $\alpha = 0.99$. More important, the experimenter-provided definition had absolutely no effect on average agreement, so it appears that people share a folk concept of intentionality and spontaneously use it to judge behaviours.

The question now becomes what specific components, or 'necessary conditions', this folk concept has. Malle and Knobe (1997) answered this question in two steps. The first was to examine people's direct and explicit definitions of intentionality; the second was to experimentally manipulate components of intentionality and thus demonstrate their reliable effect on judgements of intentionality.

A sample of 159 undergraduate students provided explicit definitions in response to the question 'When you say that somebody performed an action *intentionally*, what does this mean?' Twenty participants (13 per cent) provided only synonyms of the term *intentionally* (e.g. 'on purpose', 'purposefully', 'deliberately'). Of the remaining 139 participants, 54 per cent mentioned exactly one component, 31 per cent mentioned two or more. After initial inspection of the definitions, two coders classified them into various categories, of which four reached substantial frequencies accounting for 96 per cent of the meaningful definitions. These four categories were *desire, belief, intention*, and *awareness*. To qualify for the desire category, a definition had to mention the desire for an outcome or the outcome itself as a goal, purpose, or aim (e.g. 'He did it in hopes of getting some result'). To qualify for the belief category, a definition had to mention thoughts about the consequences of the act or about the act itself (e.g. 'She thought about the act and its effect'). To qualify for the intention category, a definition had to mention the intention to perform the act, or states of intending, meaning, deciding, choosing, or planning to perform the act ('She made a decision to perform the action'). Finally, to qualify for the awareness category, a definition had to mention awareness of the act while the person is performing it (e.g. 'He knows what he is doing').

Each of these four categories was mentioned by a quarter to a half of participants, but none of the participants mentioned all four components, presumably because the instructions to this study ('What does it mean that . . .') did not encourage exhaustive definitions. Significantly, however, those who mentioned two or more components drew careful distinctions between them. They distinguished, for example, between intention and desire: 'The person meant to act that way and was motivated to do so'; between belief and intention: 'Someone gave thought to the action beforehand and chose to do it'; between belief and awareness: 'This person thought about the action before he did it and was fully aware of performing the action while he was doing it'; and between intention and awareness: 'They decided to do something and then did it with full awareness of what they were doing'.

The folk concept of intentionality, as reconstructed from explicit definitions, thus encompasses four components. For an agent to perform an action intentionally, the agent must have: (a) a desire for an outcome; (b) beliefs about an action that leads to that outcome; (c) an intention to perform the action; and (d) awareness of fulfilling the intention while performing the action. To illustrate these components with a malingering behaviour, suppose person P wants to receive disability benefits (desire). He learns that those benefits are given, for example, to workers who have done hard labour of at least 5 years (which is true for P) and display severe immobility in their joints or spine (beliefs). He therefore plans to display exactly those symptoms to the company's physician (intention). During the exam, P executes his plan with specific attention to displaying immobility (awareness).

Some theoretical models of intentionality postulate a fifth component of skill or ability (e.g. Mele and Moser 1994), but people did not mention this component in their own definitions. Malle and Knobe (1997) therefore conducted an initial study to explore whether skill may be implicitly used in people's intentionality judgements, even if it was not explicitly mentioned.

In a vignette presented to 141 undergraduate students, a novice at darts surprisingly hits triple 20 (a very difficult throw) on his first try. His partner dismisses the throw as a fluke, so the novice tries again, this time missing badly. Surely, he *wanted* and *tried* to hit the triple 20 each time? Most participants (77 per cent) agreed. But would people infer that he hit the triple 20 *intentionally* the first time? This was not the case, as only 16 per cent said that he hit it intentionally. So most people felt that the novice *tried* or *intended* to hit the target, but, without any evidence of skill, they did not feel that he hit it *intentionally*. Instead, he got lucky. When the scenario was altered to suggest that the novice did have skill—he hit the triple 20 twice in a row—a significantly greater number of participants (55 per cent) were willing to grant that he hit it intentionally even on his first try ($p < 0.001$).

These initial results suggested that people were sensitive to skill information when making judgements of intentionality. The skill component may have been omitted from explicit definitions because people focused on social behaviours, for which skill can be assumed, in contrast to, say, artistic or athletic behaviours, for which skill cannot be assumed. A more systematic study explored this possible fifth component of intentionality (Malle and Knobe 1997, Study 3).

If skill indeed plays a role, it could only be a necessary condition of intentionally performing an action, not a necessary condition of forming an intention. Forming an intention requires only a desire for an outcome and beliefs about an action leading to that outcome (and of course a process of reasoning to combine desires and beliefs; see Malle and Knobe 2001). Once the agent tries to execute that intention, however, skill will be necessary for successfully acting as intended—to perform the action intentionally (not just out of luck or by accident). Thus, the prediction was that a skill component should be necessary for judgements of *intentionality* (whether the agent truly performed the action intentionally) but not for judgements of *intention* (whether the agent merely tried or planned to act a certain way).

A sample of 132 undergraduate students read a vignette that described a person named David flipping a coin to land on tails, which settled a debate among David and his friends over whether they should go to a movie or not. Additional information was experimentally manipulated to provide information about the presence or absence of David's skill of making the coin land on the side he wants ('he has not been able to do better than chance' versus 'by now, he almost always succeeds'); desire ('he wants to see the movie' versus 'he does not want to see the movie'); and belief (David hears the suggestion that 'tails' stands for going to the movie versus he does not hear it). The awareness component was always implied to be present. Participants then answered two questions: 'Do you think that David *tried* to make the coin land on tails?' and 'Do you think that David made the coin land on tails *intentionally*?' (Some people were asked only one questions, others both, but the results were identical.)

As predicted, the presence of both belief and desire was necessary for an ascription of intention (81 per cent for belief and desire versus 21 per cent for desire only, and 31 per cent for belief only), and the presence of skill was necessary for an ascription of intentionality (76 per cent for belief and desire and skill versus 3 per cent for belief and desire only). This finding not only shows skill as a genuine component of intentionality but also highlights that people distinguish between judgements of *intention* (a mental state of planning or trying) and judgements of *intentionality* (the quality of an action performed intentionally). To return to the earlier malingering example of a person P trying to gain disability benefits, P must be capable of faking an immobile spine or joint restrictions. If he happens to actually have an immobile spine (without knowing it and even

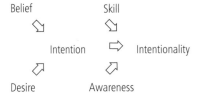

Figure 6.1 A model of the folk concept of intentionality (adapted from Malle and Knobe 1997).

without trying to pretend immobility), then he was not malingering intentionally, even though he had the *intention* to malinger in the first place.

Malle and Knobe (1997) thus proposed a five-component model of the folk concept of intentionality, displayed in Figure 6.1. According to this folk conception, the direct cause of an intentional action is the mental state of intention. For it to be ascribed, at a minimum a desire (for an outcome) and a belief (about the action–outcome link) must be present. For an action to be seen as performed intentionally, however, skill and awareness have to be present as well. The awareness component specifies the agent's state of mind at the time of acting (knowing what he or she is doing), and the skill component refers to the agent's ability to actually perform the action as he or she intended.

Occasionally, I meet experts in the law or sciences who are incredulous toward the finding that judgements of *intention* are distinct from judgements of *intentionality*. There cannot possibly be a meaningful difference, they argue, between intention and intentionality. But this incredulity appears to be a consequence of sloppy habits of speaking and thinking about the phenomena surrounding intentional action. In their role as ordinary social perceivers, I am confident, these experts will distinguish between someone who merely intended (planned, tried) to do something and another who also performed the planned action intentionally. To be convinced that the first agent had an intention they need only establish certain motives and beliefs and signs of a committed plan; they need not see her perform the action. To be convinced that the second person actually performed the action intentionally, more information is needed. Just learning that the agent had an intention to so act is not enough, for the action itself could have been an accident or a lucky fluke. A skilful (i.e. controlled) and conscious performance is what makes the action intentional.

Cases in which agents had an intention but did not intentionally perform the planned action are not too hard to find. Consider the therapist who intends to cure her patient from severe depression. Now suppose the patient undergoes spontaneous remission. Did the therapist *intend* to cure the patient? Most definitely. Is the patient now cured? Indeed. Did the doctor intentionally cure the patient? Not so. She was merely lucky in getting the outcome she had hoped for. Less lucky is a prospective malingerer who intends to feign an illness but, surprisingly, contracts the very illness he tried to feign. Just because the person had an intention to malinger, we would not be justified in denying him an insurance benefit, because the person did not intentionally display his illness symptoms. Similarly, a person who has what she considers slight back pains might plan to present more severe pain during a medical exam. To that end, she walks in a hunched-over manner, but in so doing, falls when entering the physician's office, acquiring through natural cause the severe back pains she had planned to feign. This person clearly does not malinger, even though she intended to. The folk distinction between intention and intentionality entails that an intention to malinger without conscious, skilful performance does not constitute intentional malingering.

A precise model of the folk concept of intentionality also highlights factors that help with the detection of malingering attempts. For example, the specific role of beliefs can be exploited. An agent who forms an intention to act must have certain beliefs about the link between her action and the desired outcome. If these action–outcome beliefs are altered, then the agent's behaviour, insofar as it is intentional, will likely be altered as well. For example, if an agent presents with an illness from class A but is made to believe (falsely) that illnesses of class B yield greater insurance benefits or are less stringently probed by the pertinent institutions, then the agent may be induced to 'switch' to illness B, thereby revealing intentionality. Similarly, if an agent is made to believe that the illness with which he is presenting characteristically includes symptom S (but in reality S never co-occurs with that illness), then the agent might begin to present with S and thereby expose his intentional control over the presentation.

In addition, because intentionality presupposes skill, a convincing illness deception will require a certain amount of sophistication, intelligence, and self-control. If the agent in question clearly lacks these attributes—for example, because of age, education, resources, mental capacity, or the like—an act of malingering becomes rather unlikely.

Judgements of intentionality

By recognizing intentionality as a central concept of social cognition and analysing its defining components, we have made some progress in offering a clear and systematic vocabulary to discuss the phenomenon of malingering in medical and legal contexts. But a clear concept of intentionality is only one condition for the adequate study of illness deception. The second condition is to facilitate reliable detection of intentionality, which involves inferences of those mental states that define intentional action, particularly belief, desire, and intention.

Mental state inferences are made every day by human agents, and it is curious that experts often emphasise that one cannot really *know* what is in another person's mind—with the tacit implication that one should not bother trying. But what notion of *knowing* is assumed here—certainty, without any room for doubt? If such certainty were required, there could be no guilty verdicts, no weather forecasts, and no medical diagnoses. For millions of years, humans have learned to infer what others think, feel, or intend to do. Of course, these inferences are fallible, but had early hominids given up trying to infer mental states merely because they could not reach certainty, *Homo sapiens* would be without language, civilization, and complex social relationships (Malle 2002).

There is consensus in cognitive science that the perception of intentional action is a key component of human social cognition, that it has evolved for its adaptive value in social interaction, and that it develops rather rapidly in the early years of childhood (Baron-Cohen 1999; Zelazo *et al.* 1999; Malle *et al.* 2001). We also know that adults judge intentionality automatically and with ease (Heider and Simmel 1944; Smith and Miller 1983) and that these judgements both regulate attention in social interaction and guide explanations and evaluations of behaviour (Malle 1999; Malle and Pearce 2001; Malle and Nelson in press). So how do people make these judgements?

Development and practice of intentionality judgements

During the first year of life, infants begin to identify intentional behaviour by attending to self-propelled movement (Premack 1990), eye-gaze (Farroni *et al.* 2000), and basic hand movements such as grasping or putting (Woodward *et al.* 2001). During the second year of life, they parse streams of behaviour into units that correspond to initiated or completed intentional actions (Baldwin *et al.* 2001), and they seem able to infer intentions or goals from incomplete action attempts (Meltzoff 1995). But early intentionality judgements also suffer from limitations. Children consider all outcomes that match a person's desire as brought about intentionally (Shultz and Wells 1985), which shows their insensitivity to both the desire–intention distinction (Astington 2001; Moses 2001) and the skill component of intentionality.

In adulthood, we see an enriched concept of intention. Whereas desires are understood as mental states that can be directed at any conceivable object (even non-existent ones), intentions are regarded as mental states directed only at one's own actions. Intentions, but not desires, are furthermore understood to result from a process of reasoning and to yield a characteristic commitment to action (Malle and Knobe 2001). In trying to detect intentions (and thereby often intentionality), social perceivers therefore look for indicators of reasoning and commitment, which are features that can be observed even before an action is performed.

Another later-developing indicator of intentionality is what Heider (1958) called equifinality—the characteristic pattern of intentional action to be repeated until its desired goal is reached. A homeowner who forgot her keys and therefore cannot enter her house through the door will look for an open window—seeking a different path toward the unchanging goal. A persistent malingerer will 'adopt' a new illness if the initial professed illness did not lead to the desired benefits.

Adults also increasingly base their inferences of intentionality on heuristic principles, general knowledge, or social scripts. For example, certain contexts, classes of behaviour, or types of agents may so strongly suggest intentionality that the perceiver does not even process the relevant component information (presence of beliefs, desires, etc.) but simply presumes intentionality. This tendency makes the judgement process faster and more efficient but also exposes it to serious distortions (cf. Crick 1995; Dodge and Schwartz 1997). For instance, angry affect in conflict situations, partisanship, and prejudice often lead to biased intentionality judgements. It should be noted, however, that novel, ambiguous, and high-stakes situations are likely to encourage a more systematic strategy of observing behavioural details and gathering information about the agent's mental states.

In search of objective markers of intentionality

So far, I have focused on the perceiver's conceptual assumptions and cognitive strategies in inferring intentionality. But are there objective features of intentional action that can be used to make one's intentionality judgements more accurate? The evolutionary significance of intentionality perceptions would suggest that at least some of the perceiver's assumptions and strategies will validly correspond to a reality of intentional action, just as colour perception shows a correspondence with the physical reality of light (Shepard 1994). But we must keep in mind that intentionality may be, in part at least, a social construction that *characterizes* certain behaviour patterns as intentional, whether or not they truly are intentional (and whether or not intentionality is a genuine attribute of human behaviour). This is, however, exactly where the strength of the folk-conceptual approach lies: It examines the conditions under which people (workers, lawyers, physicians, and all the rest) ascribe intentionality, and these conditions are located both in the head of the perceiver and in the head (or body) of the agent. Research on the latter is rather slim, but we can identify at least some candidates of intentionality indicators (Dittrich and Lea 1994; Carpenter *et al.* 1998; Baird and Baldwin 2001).

Coordination of body parts moving relative to each other

Here, the classic case is hand–eye coordination, which is a developmental achievement during infants' first year. Coordination indicates integration of motor plans with sensory information, making the resulting behaviour more responsive to the environment, better controlled through a corrective feedback loop, and thus more skilled and intentional. Another case of coordinated patterns is the gaze shift in preparation for action. Before humans perform an action that involves movement (e.g. getting up from a chair to close the window), they tend to first turn their head and gaze in the direction of the planned move, indicating the early phase of executing an intention. Talented athletes in basketball, soccer, football, and the like take advantage of the ordinary perceiver's strong response to these intention indicators when they use head fakes and body fakes to make the other move in one direction while they swiftly move in the other direction.

Systematic object interactions

Many intentional actions involve the interaction with and manipulation of objects. These objects are often represented in the contents of the agent's mental states (desire, belief, intention) and thus reveal something about the means and ends of the action in question. Object manipulations can also reveal the level of skill and control involved in a behaviour, and patterns of disengaging and re-engaging with objects signify equifinality.

Spatial information of the moving body

Whereas many unintentional behaviours are non-directed and display sudden and unpredictable speed shifts, intentional actions show clearer direction, more even speed, and smoothness of execution. These features can sometimes convey the agent's goals and specific action plans, but more reliably they highlight the level of skill involved in the behaviour. Close replication of movement patterns also indicates skill and is reliably used by people to assess intentionality (Malle 1994; Malle and Knobe 1997).

Emotional reactions to action completions

A successful intentional action is executed as intended and brings about the outcome that was desired. This match between mind and world typically leads to expressions of pleasure, such as smiles, nods, and approving exclamations ('there!'; 'all right'). By contrast, mismatches are typically followed by expressions of displeasure, such as frowns, turning away in disgust, head shakes, and distancing exclamations ('oops'; 'oh no!'). The problem with this indicator set, however, is that it cannot by itself distinguish between an outcome that happens to match one's desire and an outcome that was intentionally brought about. The soccer player's high-arching free kick that suddenly drops under the crossbar will be celebrated with fist pumps whether it was intentional or a wind-swept fluke. Additional indicators of movement, execution, and environmental interference will always have to complement the interpretation of emotional reactions.

Conclusions

Social, political, and legal dealings with malingering require clarity about the phenomenon of intentionality. The approach taken here does not rely on specialized definitions of intentionality often found in legal or other expert contexts. Instead, it focuses on the folk concept of intentionality that underlies ordinary people's perceptions of human behaviour. Consequently, the picture of malingering painted here is one of a complex but nevertheless tractable kind of intentional action that is, in principle, no more elusive than other intentional actions that people perceive and manage every day.

I have argued that the ordinary social cognition of intentional action—by jury members, physicians, or lawyers—is a good starting point for assessments of intentionality. Lay judgements of intentionality are based on a reliable and sophisticated folk concept that offers a systematic vocabulary with which to examine the phenomenon of malingering. In addition, over a period of millions of years, humans have evolved to detect intentionality and to infer mental states; and though far from being perfect, they are overall quite successful at this task.

Empirical research is also emerging that specifies which factors increase or decrease the success of people's intentionality judgements. On the side of increasing success are such factors as explicit deliberations about each component of intentionality, attendance to equifinality, and careful observation of behaviour preparation, movement execution, and subsequent emotional reactions. On the side of decreasing success are such factors as the perceiver's self-interest in the outcome of the judgement, negative affect toward the agent, and reliance on heuristics, scripts, and categorical assumptions. Physicians, investigators, and lawyers involved in the problem of malingering are therefore well advised to have a basic trust in their lay judgements of intentionality but also to become sensitive to the factors that moderate the quality of these judgements.

Acknowledgements

Preparation of this chapter was supported by NSF CAREER award SBR-9703315.

References

Ames, D. R. (2001). *Cultural concepts of intentionality: American and Chinese folk concepts.* Unpublished manuscript, Berkeley, CA.

Astington, J. W. (2001). The paradox of intention: assessing children's metarepresentational understanding. In *Intentions and intentionality: foundations of social cognition* (eds B. F. Malle, L. J. Moses, and D. A. Baldwin), pp. 85–104. MIT Press, Cambridge, MA.

Baird, J. A. and Baldwin, D. A. (2001). Making sense of human behaviour: action parsing and intentional inference. In *Intentions and intentionality: foundations of social cognition* (eds B. F. Malle, L. J. Moses, and D. A. Baldwin), pp. 193–206. MIT Press, Cambridge, MA.

Baldwin, D. A., Baird, J. A., Saylor, M. M., and Clark, M. A. (2001). Infants parse dynamic action. *Child Development,* **72**, 708–17.

Baron-Cohen, S. (1999). The evolution of a theory of mind. In *The descent of mind: psychological perspectives on hominid evolution* (eds M. C. Corballis and S. E. G. Lea), pp. 261–77. Oxford University Press, New York, NY.

Carpenter, M., Akhtar, N., and Tomasello, M. (1998). Fourteen- through 18-month-old infants differentially imitate intentional and accidental actions. *Infant Behaviour and Development,* **21**, 315–30.

Crick, N. R. (1995). Relational aggression: the role of intent attributions, feelings of distress, and provocation type. *Development and Psychopathology,* **7**, 313–22.

Dittrich, W. J. and Lea, S. E. G. (1994). Visual perception of intentional motion. *Perception,* **23**, 253–68.

Dodge, K. A. and Schwartz, D. (1997). Social information processing mechanisms in aggressive behaviour. In *Handbook of antisocial behaviour* (eds D. M. Stoff and J. Breiling), pp. 171–80. Wiley, New York, NY.

Farroni, T., Johnson, M. H., Brockbank, M., and Simion, F. (2000). Infants' use of gaze direction to cue attention: the importance of perceived motion. *Visual Cognition,* **7**, 705–18.

Fiske, S. T. (1989). Examining the role of intent: toward understanding its role in stereotyping and prejudice. In *Unintended thought: limits of awareness, intention, and control* (eds J. S. Uleman and J. A. Bargh), pp. 253–83. Guilford, New York, NY.

Freyd, J. J. (1983). Shareability: the social psychology of epistemology. *Cognitive Science,* **7**, 191–210.

Heider, F. (1958). *The psychology of interpersonal relations.* Wiley, New York, NY.

Heider, F. and Simmel, M. (1944). An experimental study of apparent behaviour. *American Journal of Psychology,* **57**, 243–59.

Jones, E. E. and Davis, K. E. (1965). From acts to dispositions: the attribution process in person perception. In *Advances in experimental social psychology* (ed. L. Berkowitz), Vol. 2, pp. 371–88. Erlbaum, Hillsdale, NJ.

Malle, B. F. (1994). *Intentionality and explanation: a study in the folk theory of behaviour*. Doctoral dissertation, Stanford University, Stanford, CA.

Malle, B. F. (1999). How people explain behavior: A new theoretical framework. *Personality and Social Psychology Review*, **3**, 23–48.

Malle, B. F. (2002) The relation between language and theory of mind in development and evolution. In *The evolution of language from pre-language* (eds T. Givón and B. F. Malle). pp. 265–84. John Benjamins, Amsterdam.

Malle, B. F. (in press) The folk theory of mind: conceptual foundations for social cognition. In *The new unconscious* (eds R. Hassin, J. S. Uleman, and J. A. Bargh). Oxford University Press, New York, NY.

Malle, B. F. and Knobe, J. (1997). The folk concept of intentionality. *Journal of Experimental Social Psychology*, **33**, 101–21.

Malle, B. F. and Knobe, J. (2001). The distinction between desire and intention: A folk-conceptual analysis. In *Intentions and intentionality: foundations of social cognition* (eds B. F. Malle, L. J. Moses, and D. A. Baldwin), pp. 45–67. MIT Press, Cambridge, MA.

Malle, B. F., Moses, L. J., and Baldwin, D. A. (eds). (2001). *Intentions and intentionality: foundations of social cognition*. MIT Press, Cambridge, MA.

Malle, B. F. and Nelson, S. E. (in press). Judging mens rea: the tension between folk concepts and legal concepts of intentionality. *Behavioural Sciences and the Law*.

Malle, B. F. and Pearce, G. E. (2001). Attention to behavioural events during social interaction: Two actor–observer gaps and three attempts to close them. *Journal of Personality and Social Psychology*, **81**, 278–94.

MacWhinney, B. (2002). The gradual emergence of language. In *The evolution of language from pre-language* (eds T. Givón and B. F. Malle). pp. 233–63. John Benjamins, Amsterdam.

Mele, A. R. and Moser, P. K. (1994). Intentional action. *Nous*, **28**, 39–68.

Meltzoff, A. N. (1995). Understanding the intentions of others: re-enactment of intended acts by 18-month-old children. *Developmental Psychology*, **31**, 838–50.

Moses, L. J. (2001). Some thoughts on ascribing complex intentional concepts to young children. In *Intentions and intentionality: Foundations of social cognition* (eds B. F. Malle, L. J. Moses, and D. A. Baldwin), pp. 69–83. MIT Press, Cambridge, MA.

Premack, D. (1990). The infant's theory of self-propelled objects. *Cognition*, **36**, 1–16.

Shaver, K. G. (1985). *The attribution of blame*. Springer, New York, NY.

Shepard, R. N. (1994). Perceptual–cognitive universals as reflections of the world. *Psychonomic Bulletin and Review*, **1**, 2–28.

Shultz, T. R. and Wells, D. (1985). Judging the intentionality of action-outcomes. *Developmental Psychology*, **21**, 83–9.

Smith, E. R. and Miller, F. D. (1983). Mediation among attributional inferences and comprehension processes: Initial findings and a general method. *Journal of Personality and Social Psychology*, **44**, 492–505.

Woodward, A. L., Sommervile, J. A., and Guajardo, J. J. (2001). How infants make sense of intentional action. In *Intentions and intentionality: foundations of social cognition* (eds B. F. Malle, L. J. Moses, and D. A. Baldwin), pp. 149–70. MIT Press, Cambridge, MA.

Zelazo, P. D., Astington, J. W., and Olson, D. R. (eds). (1999). *Developing theories of intention: social understanding and self-control*. Erlbaum, Mahwah, NJ.

7 Malingering and criminal behaviour as psychopathology

Adrian Raine

Abstract

Malingering is not a clinical disorder as listed in the *Diagnostic and Statistical Manual-IV* (DSM-IV), but is instead listed in the appendix as a condition requiring further attention. The main goal of this paper is to assess whether malingering is a clinical disorder. A model for this approach is provided from the argument that repeated, recidivistic behaviour is a clinical disorder. Nine criteria previously used to define psychopathology are outlined, which make up an overall gestalt of psychopathology against which criminality and malingering can be compared. A comparative analysis between criminality and malingering against disorders currently listed in DSM-IV is made to help assess the relative extent to which malingering and criminality meets these combined criteria. The construct validity approach which represents a second important approach to assessing psychopathology is also outlined. It is argued that while criminality does indeed meet many criteria for assessing disorder, there is currently insufficient empirical data on malingering to establish whether it too fulfils these criteria. Future research on malingering needs to focus more on the question of *why* people malinger in order to better understand the biopsychosocial aetiology on what may in the future prove to be a meaningful clinical syndrome.

Introduction

Malingering is not included in the *Diagnostic and Statistical Manual-IV* (DSM-IV; American Psychological Association 1994) as a clinical disorder, but in the appendix it is listed and assigned a 'V' code to mark it as a condition that requires further attention and elucidation. In this context, malingering is defined as 'The intentional production of false or grossly exaggerated physical or psychological symptoms, motivated by external incentives such as avoiding military duty, avoiding work, obtaining financial compensation, evading criminal prosecution, or obtaining drugs' (p. 683). Guidelines are given to suggest malingering would be suspected if it is present in a medicolegal context, if there is a marked discrepancy between claimed stress and disability and objective findings, if the individual lacks cooperation in either evaluation or treatment protocols, or if there is concomitant presence of Antisocial Personality Disorder. DSM guidelines on malingering have, however, been criticized by Rogers (1990) on the grounds that studies have shown that they correctly identify malingerers in only 20 per cent of cases.

Importantly, malingering is discriminated from factitious disorders. Those with factitious disorders also feign physical or psychological signs of thinking, but in these cases there is a lack of external incentives for such behaviour and instead the primary driving goal appears to be to take on the sick role. In contrast, malingering appears at one level to be more 'understandable' in that there are clear, concrete, motivational goals that drive the behaviour. At one level, malingering can be conceptualized as one manifestation of the wider syndrome of antisocial, criminal behaviour. As with malingering, antisocial criminal behaviour is also a V code in DSM-IV, whereas its associated condition, Antisocial Personality Disorder is defined as a disorder.

The main goal of this paper is to explore the possibility that malingering is a clinical disorder (similar to other personality disorders), albeit not necessarily the same type of disorder that malingerers are claiming to have. A model for this approach is provided from the argument that has been made that repeated, recidivistic behaviour is a clinical disorder (Raine 1993). Nine criteria which have been used by Raine (1993) to define psychopathology will be outlined, which, when taken together, make up an overall gestalt of psychopathology against which criminality and malingering can be compared. This argument that recidivistic crime is a disorder will in part be based on assessment of the extent to which criminal behaviour fits definitions of psychopathology, but also, and perhaps more importantly, on empirical data which indicate differences between criminals and non-criminals on biological, psychological, and social variables.

A comparative analysis between criminality and malingering against disorders currently listed in DSM-IV will then be made to help assess the relative extent to which malingering and criminality meets these combined criteria. The construct validity approach which represents a second important approach to assessing psychopathology will then be outlined. It will be argued that while criminality does indeed meet many criteria for assessing disorder, there are not enough empirical data on malingering to establish whether it too fulfils these criteria. The critical question to be answered is essentially, are malingers 'bad'—or are they 'mad' and have an underlying condition or disorder which predisposes them to cheat in a medicolegal context for material gain. This approach places more emphasis on an empirical approach to defining disorder in contrast to merely relying on sociological and societal judgements of what is 'mad' or merely 'bad' and which can be more arbitrary and subjective.

Those who repeatedly engage in life-long non-trivial criminal behaviour constitute the key population to which the psychopathology argument is being applied to, whether they be caught offenders who reside in prisons or whether they are undetected, repeated offenders residing in the community. Similarly, it is those who knowingly and deliberately feign physical or mental illness for gain who constitute the target population of malingerers. It is important to recognize, however, that mental disorders are more likely to be dimensional in nature and less likely to form water-tight, discrete categories. Just as there are differing degrees to which an individual may be characterized as depressed or anxious, so in turn there are individual degrees to which individuals express non-trivial criminal behaviour. At this stage, drawing very discrete boundaries to whom the psychopathology argument can be applied would be both misleading and inconsistent with the nature of disorder.

Defining disorder

Not only is it almost impossible to conclusively demonstrate that crime or malingering constitute psychopathologies, but also it is equally difficult to demonstrate that they are *not* disorder. The reason for this paradox is simple; experts in psychiatry and psychology have found it exceedingly difficult to outline an acceptable definition of psychopathology. As indicated by Frances *et al.* (1991): 'There have never been any very convincing definitions of illness, disease, or mental disorder' (p. 408). DSM-III-R (American Psychiatric Association 1987) states that 'no definition adequately specifies precise boundaries for the concept of "mental disorder" ' (p. xxii). If psychopathology cannot be defined, one cannot definitively say whether or not criminal behaviour, or any other behaviour for that matter, falls into this category. The difficulties in defining psychopathology will soon become apparent, but these difficulties have not prevented professionals and the public alike from easily accepting the view that conditions such as depression and schizophrenia are clearly disorders or psychopathologies. Psychiatry continues to make these judgments, and society to accept them, because pragmatic decisions inevitably need to be made about who to treat and who not to treat—who is guilty by reason of insanity and who is not.

Although no single definition clearly delineates psychopathology, the many definitions, when taken together, create a general 'gestalt' or picture of what constitutes a psychopathology. Seen within the context of this gestalt, depression and schizophrenia appear to be disorders, even though neither can adequately meet all definitions. The key question is whether these definitions provide any degree of 'fit' to malingering and criminal behaviour. To the extent that they provide some fit, the notion that malingering and crime may be psychopathologies becomes a possibility. This notion of a gestalt for defining psychopathology constitutes a central idea in this chapter, and although individual definitions of psychopathology will be presented and a critique provided, the argument that must be borne in mind is that, ultimately, it is the *overall* fit of a condition to the totality of these criteria which may provide the best assessment for what constitutes a psychopathology.

Definitions of clinical disorder

Deviation from a statistical norm

This first definition is a simple and relatively clear-cut attempt to define abnormal behaviour as behaviour which is statistically infrequent. Schizophrenia, for example, affects approximately only 1 per cent of the population and as such would be viewed as a disorder on the grounds that it is relatively rare. Amongst the personality disorders, lifetime risk for schizotypal personality disorder is approximately 6 per cent (Baron and Risch 1987), although other sources estimate it to be higher at approximately 10 per cent (Meehl 1989). Prevalence rates for major depression range from 9 to 26 per cent for females and from 5 to 12 per cent for males, while lifetime risk for alcohol abuse or dependence is approximately 13 per cent (American Psychiatric Association 1987).

Recidivistic criminal behaviour meet the criterion of deviation for a statistical norm reasonably well. A significant number people have committed some criminal offence at some time in their lives. For example, 16.8 per cent of the English population have been convicted of a criminal offence (London Home Office, 1985), while Visher and Roth (1986) in an extensive review of participation rates in criminal careers concluded that the best available estimates indicate that 25–35 per cent of urban males will be arrested for at least one index offence during their lives. On the other hand, a small minority tend to repeatedly commit offences and account for the bulk of serious offending. Mednick (1977) reported that about 1 per cent of the male population accounted for more than half the criminal offences committed by a Copenhagen birth cohort of over 30 000 men. Wolfgang *et al.* (1972) report the same type of finding for the city of Philadelphia. The notion that crime is a psychopathology is best applied to this relatively small group of recidivistic, serious offenders because they are more likely to have some intrinsic predisposition to crime relative to one-time offenders whose antisociality may be more transient and situation specific. One of the difficulties with this criterion for disorder lies in the vagaries of the operational systems that define crime and malingering. In the case of recidivistic crime, for example, the base-rate will be a function of characteristics of the criminal justice system such as police clearance rates.

It is even more difficult to obtain accurate assessments of the base-rates in society for malingering. One survey of forensic experts estimates that a mean of 17.4 per cent of forensic patients (SD = 14.4 per cent) are thought to be malingerers (Rogers and Neumann, Chapter 5). Given that this is a very select sample, it is likely that the base rate of malingering in the general population is relatively modest, and would fit the definition of deviation from statistical norm as well as many other disorders listed in DSM-IV. Similarly, Boden (1996) estimates malingering at 3 per cent in injured workers. On the other hand, Halligan *et al.* (Chapter 1), argue that if one construes malingering as one form of deception, then given the fact that deception is relatively widespread, malingering in turn would be more prevalent than first imagined. Establishing a base-rate of malingering is difficult because definitions of malingering vary from study to study, detection of malingering is imperfect, and base rates are underestimated because they do not include 'successful' malingerers who escape detection.

Deviation from ideal mental health

A parallel criterion to that of statistical infrequency is the notion of deviation from ideal mental health. The World Health Organization has defined health as 'a state of complete physical, mental, and social well-being, and not merely the absence of disease or infirmity'. This definition has been evaluated as both comprehensive and meaningless (Lewis 1953). More specific than this all-encompassing statement are six criteria of positive mental health drawn up by Jahoda (1958), which include self-actualization, resistance to stress, autonomy, competence, accurate perception of reality, and an appropriate balance of psychic forces.

Criminal behaviour meets this criterion for disorder fairly easily. Very few criminals could be characterized as being in a state of robust physical, mental, and social well-being, and certainly do not as a group present as self-actualizers who have achieved full realization of their own unique psychological, scientific, and artistic potential (Allman and Jaffe 1978). Criminals are characterized by major social, cognitive, and biological deficits which clearly preclude them from achieving this ideal state of well-being (Raine 1993), although this may not be true of 'successful' criminals who are not caught and punished.

Malingerers presumably do not meet this state of perfect well-being, although there appears to be little or no empirical data on social, cognitive, and biological well-being of malingerers. As it stands, only a minority of the general population could be described as being in this optimal state of well-being. This criterion of disorder is probably viewed best as a fine goal for society and at worst as a relatively weak criterion for psychopathology due to its lack of specificity.

Deviation from the social norm

This criterion is again a parallel to the statistical infrequency criterion, but instead of defining abnormality as deviation from a statistical, objective norm, it is defined in terms of the norms laid down by society. Using this definition, behaviour that lies outside the bounds of social acceptability and which violates the prevailing social norm is judged to be abnormal or disordered (Gorenstein 1984). In some senses this is a powerful criterion. Social deviance has the feeling of being central to the definition of disorder because deviation from the social order is a fundamental concept in society which is understood and shared by almost everyone, except perhaps by criminals themselves (Scheff 1970). A social definition appears to capture some essential ingredient in the way the concept of illness is applied in real terms in society. The limitation of this definition is that these social norms which evolve over time within the group and which are reinforced by the criminal justice system vary both across and within countries and are culture specific.

Criminal behaviour very clearly fits within this definition of disorder. Criminal activities are clearly viewed as lying outside the norm of social acceptability. Those who both break the norm and are caught face being ostracized and isolated from society by being sent to prison. Indeed, criminal behaviour probably fits this definition as well as any other mental disorder; while there is an increasing degree of social acceptability to suffering from a disorder such as anxiety, depression, and alcoholism which make these illnesses fit less well to this criterion, criminal behaviour has become no more acceptable, and as such is a good fit. Similarly, many forms of malingering are viewed as socially deviant and would fit this criterion for disorder. On the other hand, other forms of malingering are viewed as socially deviant but are nevertheless practiced by a large proportion of the normal population

Distress/suffering to self or others

Using this criterion, individuals who experience suffering, psychological distress, discomfort, or unhappiness are deemed to be 'suffering' from a mental disorder. This again is a relatively more powerful criterion because it has a high degree of face validity, stemming directly from the medical model of illness; individuals usually go to doctors because they experience physical discomfort which is interpreted as a direct symptom of some underlying pathology. As such, patients complaining of psychological discomfort (e.g. depression, anxiety) are viewed as suffering from a disorder that produces these symptoms.

This simple definition has been extended to include behaviours that causes distress to others as well as to the self (Altrocchi 1980; Adams and Sutker 1984). The reason for this extension is that there are many syndromes that are commonly viewed as disorders yet which do not meet the simple criterion of distress to self. For example, patients suffering from bipolar disorder often feel ecstatic, full of energy, feel an increase in goal-directed activity during the manic phase, have high self-esteem, and would not report being unhappy. Indeed, such states frequently tempt patients to stop taking medication so that they can experience these temporary 'highs'. Schizophrenics with predominantly negative residual symptomatology (social isolation, blunted emotions, lack of interests, poor personal hygiene) may also not express any particular psychological discomfort or unhappiness.

Criminal behaviour fits the extended aspect of this definition in that it clearly creates distress; people do not enjoy being robbed or assaulted. Again, it probably fits the second half of this criterion better than any other established disorder. On the other hand, it is not obvious that criminal behaviour fits the first part of this definition. Criminals are not obviously distressed or personally unhappy. Although criminals do not verbalize distress in their lives, there is behavioural evidence that they are in reality suffering from distress. Criminals have higher than normal rates of suicide, and are exposed to a high degree of life stress include trauma, abuse, downward social mobility, homelessness, disturbed marital relationships, and social isolation (Raine 1993). For malingering, the issue is more complex. They do not appear to create significant distress in others, and there is simply no empirical data on whether malingerers are in a state of psychological suffering.

Seeking out treatment

This definition is an extension of the distress/discomfort criterion in that it defines disorder in terms of whether an individual seeks out treatment. This is a deceptively appealing definition which again stems from the medical model; just as medical doctors treat individuals with diseases and other physical ailments, psychiatrists and psychologists treat people with psychological disorders. Those seeking out clinical treatment are therefore viewed as disordered.

Criminal behaviour does not meet this criterion because a criminal will only very rarely turn himself in because he recognizes that he is psychologically disturbed and in need of some form of treatment. In contrast, malingerers very clearly meet this criterion. They may not actually want medical treatment for the disorder that they are feigning (they instead want financial or other rewards), but they do nevertheless seek out treatment for their feigned disorder and consequently meet the criterion.

Impairment in functioning/efficiency

This criterion defines psychopathology in terms of functioning and efficiency: impairments in social, occupational, behavioural, educational, and cognitive functioning or efficiency are thought to be indicative of disorder. The functioning definition is a close relative of the distress and seeking treatment definitions in that those who seek out treatment and are distressed frequently suffer impairments in their ability to function in the world. The impairment in functioning definition also shares common ground with the distress definition in that it too originates from the classical medical model of physical illness. Impairments in the functioning of the heart, liver, kidneys, and other body organs play a central role in the definition of medical disorders, and by the same token, psychological disorders can be seen as involving impairments in psychological functioning. Its limitation, like many other definitions, is that it is non-specific insofar as individuals can have impaired functioning without suffering from a mental disorder.

This criterion has been cited by many researchers in discussing the nature of disorder, and is seen as a key element in any definition. Klein (1978) defines mental illness as 'a sub-set of all illnesses that present evidence of cognitive, behavioural, affective, or motivational aspects of organismal functioning' (p. 52). Frances et al. (1990) also cite disability as one of the many terms used to help define disorder, while Spitzer and Endicott (1978) also include disability ('impairment in functioning in a wide range of activities', p. 23) and disadvantage ('in interacting with aspects of the physical or social environment', p. 23) in their definition of disorder.

Criminality meets this criterion of mental illness. With respect to cognitive functioning, there is strong evidence for cognitive dysfunction in criminals as indicated by cognitive and neuro-psychological tests (Raine 1993). A standard finding in the literature, for example, has been that criminals and delinquents have IQ scores that are consistently lower than controls (Wilson and Herrnstein 1985; Quay 1987). These IQ deficits may in turn underlie a number of other functional deficits such as communication skills which may predispose to crime. In terms of functional deficits in learning, there is substantial evidence that antisocials, criminals, and psychopaths possess deficits in both classical and instrumental learning (Raine 1993). With respect to educational functioning, criminals are characterized by a history of learning disability, while school failure has been found to be an important predictor of later criminal offending (Raine 1993). In terms of social functioning, criminals are more likely to have either no wife or co-habitee, or to be divorced/separated. Deficits in social skills documented in delinquents, sex offenders, and violent offenders may well underlie some of these social deficits (Henderson and Hollin 1983; Huff 1987; McGurk and Newell 1987). In terms of occupational functioning, delinquents and criminals have poorer work records and have frequent periods of unemployment (Wilson and Herrnstein 1985; Ashmore and Jarvie 1987; Farrington and West 1990).

The case for malingering is currently much weaker. Unlike recidivistic crime, there appears to be no evidence for or against the notion that malingerers have impairments in functioning and efficiency. At one level, by definition of the term 'malingering' they do not have the impairments in functioning that they claim to have. Nevertheless, it could be hypothesized that malingerers suffer from social and occupational impairments of the type outlined above that increases their motivation to obtain financial benefits, and that consequently they do suffer impairments in psychosocial functioning. No study to date appears to have been conducted to assess this issue.

Listing in DSM-IV

Defining mental disorder as any behavioural syndrome that is outlined in DSM-IV is a very unequivocal criterion as it essentially avoids the main problems with many of the above criteria. DSM-IV is published by the American Psychiatric Association (1994) and provides a listing of all disorders recognized by the psychiatric profession with explicit diagnostic criteria. The manual is used extensively by clinicians and researchers alike to diagnose and classify mental disorders. It claims to be both neutral with regard to aetiology, and usable across varied theoretical orientations to psychopathology (Spitzer 1991), although such claims have been disputed.

Superficially, it would seem that criminal behaviour does not meet this criterion because it does not list a disorder called 'crime'. Surprisingly, it actually meets this criterion very well on the basis that there are many disorders listed in DSM-III-R which, taken together, encapsulate most people who commit criminal behaviour. These disorders include antisocial personality disorder, conduct disorder, psychoactive substance abuse/dependence, paedophilia, exhibitionism, frotterurism, sexual sadism, voyeurism, pyromania, kleptomania, and intermittent explosive disorder. The very large majority of institutionalized criminals will fall into one of the above categories.

In contrast, malingering is only contained in DSM-IV as a 'V' code and as such does not meet this specific definition of disorder. On the other hand, malingering is a *symptom* of antisocial personality disorder. Specifically, the second diagnostic feature of antisocial personality disorder listed in DSM-IV consists of 'deceitfulness, as indicated by repeated lying, use of aliases, or conning others or failure to plan ahead' (p. 650). The question that remains unanswered so far concerns whether there is truly a clustering of signs and symptoms in malingerers which form a coherent and unique clinical *syndrome*, rather than merely representing a single behavioural trait.

Biological dysfunction

This simple and pragmatic view suggests that a disorder may arise when there has been a disturbance to normal biological regulatory functions (Goodstein and Calhoun 1982; Roth and Kroll 1986) and again stems directly from the medical model of illness. In the seventeenth and eighteenth centuries, the classification of diseases was modelled on the classification of plants, but during the nineteenth century developments in morbid anatomy and pathology indicated evidence that illness was often correlated with biological disturbances or 'lesions' (Kendell 1986). As knowledge increased over the next century, this notion expanded to include biological and physiological abnormalities.

Criminality meets this definition of psychopathology. Criminals do appear to differ from non-criminals on a number of biological functions that may be aetiologically related to crime. Studies have demonstrated differences between criminal and non-criminal groups on genetic, psychophysiological, biochemical, neuropsychological, neurological, and brain imaging measures. Although there is fairly clear evidence to support such associations, the question of whether these biological differences cause crime are just as much open to debate as whether many social correlates of crime are causal factors. Consequently, such evidence does not unequivocally confirm that crime meets this biological criterion of disorder.

This last issue outlines the main difficulty with this definition of mental illness. Most mental illnesses simply cannot be defined in terms of some underlying biological difference because the etiology of most illnesses are currently unknown. Furthermore, it is highly unlikely that mental illness is commonly caused by some discrete biological process acting independently of psychological, social, and cultural forces. Many commentators have further argued that this notion of 'mental' illness tends to foster an outdated mind–body dualism. As Frances *et al.* (1991) point out, there is much that is physical about 'mental' disorders, and much that is mental about 'physical' disorders; minds do not exist independent of bodies, and vice versa. These issues are highly pertinent to criminal behaviour and malingering. It is highly likely that neither biological nor social forces alone will provide a complete explanation for criminal behaviour because such behaviour is driven by a complex, interactive system involving diverse biological and social factors (Raine *et al.* 1997). This is probably also true for many mental disorders, and possibly malingering.

Again, the problem with trying to apply this criterion to malingering is that there seems to be no data. Studies simply have not been conducted to assess whether malingerers show the type of biological deficits that have now been well documented in criminal populations. If malingering is part of a wider construct of antisocial, cheating behaviour, one would expect that it would share at least some of the biological correlates of crime. Whether this is actually true remains to be seen.

DSM-III-R definition of 'mental disorder'

The above eight criterion each represent single conceptual units individually attempting to delineate psychopathology. This last definition is more comprehensive in that it aggregates across some of these individual criteria. DSM-III-R (American Psychiatric Association 1987) acknowledged the many difficulties involved in providing a working definition of mental disorder, but nevertheless offered a definition that influenced decision-making regarding what should and should not be included in the manual, a definition that has been repeated in DSM-IV. This definition conceptualizes mental disorder as a 'clinically significant behavioural or psychological syndrome' that is associated with distress or disability or an increased risk of suffering death, pain, disability, or an important loss of freedom. This syndrome must not be a response that is expected to a specific event such as death of a relative. It must also be considered a 'manifestation of a behavioural, psychological, or biological dysfunction in the person'. Finally, conflicts that are primarily between the individual and society are not seen as disorders unless they are a symptom of 'a dysfunction in the person, as described above' (p. xxii).

Recidivistic crime meets this definition. Recidivistic criminal behaviour is certainly clinically significant. It is clearly behavioural in nature and there is extensive research showing that it encapsulates a constellation of features which form a meaningful syndrome. It clearly increases the risk of an important loss of freedom (i.e. imprisonment). Criminals have also been found to be more prone to physical injury than non-criminals. As outlined earlier, they have disabilities and impairments in multiple social, cognitive, educational, and occupational functioning. Crime is not an expected response to a particular event, such as a death in the family, and is can be viewed as a manifestation of a behavioural, psychological, or biological dysfunction in the person (Raine 1993). Finally, although criminality can be construed as a conflict between the individual and society, it meets the definition because it is an outgrowth of biological, psychological, and behavioural dysfunction within the individual.

With respect to malingering, a case can be made for malingering being clinically significant, although as mentioned earlier it is unclear whether it constitutes a syndrome. It is also unclear if it is associated with true distress/disability, or at least there are no empirical data to support this position so far. There is no significant loss of freedom as malingerers are rarely prosecuted in the United Kingdom (Sprince, chapter 18) and while they may be more likely to be prosecuted in the United States, they are rarely institutionalized. Similarly, there are no studies to date on whether malingering is a manifestation of a behavioural, psychological, or biological dysfunction within the person. As such, malingering at best only partly meets this criterion for disorder.

Overview of definitions and their fit to criminal behaviour and malingering

The above nine attempts to define mental disorder vary in their completeness, face validity, and practical utility. The first eight represent more or less single faces of a multi-faceted concept, while the ninth draws on several of these single features to obtain a more complete definition. To provide a general overview of the conclusions drawn from the preceding analysis, Table 7.1 lists these nine criteria and the extent to which recidivistic criminal behaviour and malingering meets them. Because there are no precise definitions of these criteria (e.g. how infrequent is statistically infrequent) no precise assignments can be given to fit, and as such it must be emphasized that this table is best viewed as illustrative rather than definitive. Fit of each criteria to criminal behaviour is assessed as 'good', 'bad', or 'moderate'.

Criminal behaviour does not fit the seeking treatment criterion. It partly meets three other criteria (statistical infrequency, distress/suffering, and biological functioning), but it is a good fit for five others (ideal health, deviation from social norm, impaired functioning, listing in DSM-III-R and definition in DSM-III-R).

To provide some comparisons, Table 7.1 also provides fit assessments for schizotypal personality disorder, schizophrenia, caffeine intoxication, and malingering. Schizotypal personality disorder is chosen as one comparison because it represents a non-trivial personality disorder but which is undoubtedly viewed as a significant disorder within psychiatry. Schizophrenia is chosen because it is an Axis I disorder, which is a classic illustration of an established, debilitating mental disorder. Caffeine intoxication is chosen because it is a relatively non-serious, ubiquitous condition that may help establish a base level for what may be viewed as a disorder.

Schizotypal personality disorder only partly meets the statistical infrequency criterion because its base rate in the population is approximately 6–10 per cent (Baron and Risch 1987; Meehl 1989). Schizotypals are not, however, in a state of ideal mental health given their unusual perceptual experiences, ideas of reference, and magical thinking. Schizotypals are odd and eccentric, but do not break social norms in a major way and are largely accepted in society because they tend to keep to themselves and avoid social contact; they only partly meet the criterion of deviation from social norm. Schizotypals rarely if ever seek help for their condition largely because they have only

Table 7.1 Extent to which criminal behaviour, malingering, and three other DSM conditions meet criteria for disorder

	Crime	Schizotypal personality	Schizophrenia	Caffeine intoxication	Malingering
1. Statistical	Moderate	Moderate	Good	Poor	Moderate
2. Ideal health	Good	Good	Good	Poor	Unknown
3. Deviation from social Norm	Good	Moderate	Good	Poor	Good
4. Distress/suffering	Moderate	Poor	Good	Moderate	Unknown
5. Seek treatment	Poor	Poor	Moderate	Poor	Good
6. Impaired functioning	Good	Moderate	Good	Poor	Unknown
7. Listing in DSM-IV	Good	Good	Good	Good	Poor
8. Biological functioning	Moderate	Moderate	Good	Poor	Unknown
9. Definition: DSM-IV	Good	Good	Good	Poor	Moderate

partial insight into their peculiarities, partly because of their discomfort in social interactions, and also because they are not unduly troubled by their disorder. Schizotypals are relatively functioning and only moderately impaired (American Psychiatric Association 1987), and currently evidence for impaired biological functioning is much less than for either schizophrenia or crime (although see Siever *et al.* 1984).

In contrast, schizophrenia meets all of the criteria well, with the one exception that many paranoid schizophrenics are unlikely to receive treatment. As with any disorder, it must be remembered that there will always be some schizophrenics who as individuals meet these criteria less well, who are much less impaired, who are able to function acceptably well in the community, and indeed who do not come to medical attention.

Those with caffeine intoxication may suffer some degree of distress/suffering, and it is a disorder listed in DSM-III-R, but otherwise they tend not to meet these criteria. Hughes *et al.* (1991) found caffeine withdrawal symptoms in about 50 per cent of those who drank more than two cups of coffee per day; since 89 per cent of the American population regularly drink coffee or tea daily (Gilbert 1976), one would expect lifetime risk for this disorder not to be statistically infrequent. The disorder is not severe enough to warrant clinical attention, and the degree of distress associated with it is minimal (American Psychiatric Association 1987). It is not viewed as a deviant act, and it does not meet the definition given in DSM-III-R because there is currently little evidence that it stems from a behavioural, biological, or psychological dysfunction within the individual.

For malingering, the lack of systematic studies assessing characteristics of these individuals makes it impossible to draw any definitive conclusion. Clearly, they seek treatment and deviate from the social norm, but even in seeking treatment they are not seeking treatment because they are truly suffering. For many of the definitions of disorder, there is to date no empirical data that can shed light on the question. In contrast, if one compares recidivistic criminal behaviour to these three disorders, it does not meet criteria as well as schizophrenia. On the other hand, it meets criteria slightly better than schizotypal personality disorder, and considerably better than caffeine intoxication.

The way forward: the construct validity approach to defining psychopathology

Assessing the extent to which malingering and criminal behaviour fit proposed definitions of mental disorder is one way of evaluating whether they can be viewed as a psychopathology. A second approach which can help address this issue and which is gaining increasing importance is that of empirical validation (Carson 1991; Frances *et al.* 1990, 1991; Morey 1991; Widiger *et al.* 1991).

Many critics of DSM have reiterated the issue that there has been an overemphasis on expert opinion and issues of reliability at the expense of construct validity (Blashfield and Livesley 1991; Carson 1991; Millon 1991). For example, Carson (1991) states 'there has been and seemingly remains an unaccountable neglect of specifically directed efforts to establish networks or correlated variables that in the aggregate affirm and support the concept to which any proposed diagnosis must be presumed to refer' (p. 306). The argument in favour of a construct validity approach to psychiatric classification lies in the fact that named disorders are constructs in much the same way as IQ or personality dimensions, and as such are essentially hypothetical constructions. This argument applies much less to those medical disorders where the aetiology is known.

In the absence of a known etiology, one way to establish the validity of a mental disorder is to establish a 'nomological network' of relationships between it and other constructs and observable behaviour (Chronbach and Meehl 1955). To the extent that this can be achieved, the measure of behaviour in question could be said to have construct validity. This approach is certainly not new. An influential paper by Robins and Guze (1970) suggested essentially the same approach, but used the term 'diagnostic validity' as opposed to construct validity. This approach is, however, being increasingly used in classification in mental disorders and seems likely to play an even greater role in the future, with revisions to DSM increasingly emphasizing systematic reviews of the research literature in addition to data analyses and field trials in order to provide rationale and support for current and proposed disorders.

Traditionally, the diagnostic validity approach in psychiatry and psychology has emphasized data from family and genetic studies, biological studies, response to drug treatment and course of illness, and psychological test data (Robins and Guze 1970; Frances *et al.* 1991). While genetic and biological data are clearly important elements of such validation, it is equally clear that social, environmental and cultural data are just as integral in any modern-day analysis of the construct validity of a mental disorder.

The critically pressing issue that malingering research needs to address is the surprising absence of even simple empirical data on the characteristics of groups of malingerers compared to well-matched control groups. Apparently, even the simplest facts on the backgrounds of malingerers is unknown. As a group, have malingerers grown up in impoverished home backgrounds where their parents out of necessity have modelled such 'cheating' behaviour? Are they more likely to come from families who have suffered significant family adversity where malingering for financial gain has been a necessity for economic survival and which the child models in the future adult life? Are they economically impoverished? Have they poor occupational and educational functioning? It appears that there are no, or very few studies which have systematically assessed groups of malingers, perhaps because clinicians and practitioners usually deal with individual malingerers rather than groups.

Is most malingering normative within the sub-culture in which it takes place? If this were so, the case for a psychopathological model of malingering is misplaced and erroneous and a sociological perspective may be more appropriate. Alternatively, is malingering simply the tip of an 'antisocial iceberg', with such individuals have a deep-seated disturbance in psychological functioning with concomitant neurobiological underpinnings which warrants classification as a disorder? Even this simple question cannot be answered because there appears to be no systematic research on the backgrounds of malingerers. Practitioners have traditionally focused on the question on whether individuals are malingering or not, not on *why* they malinger, what has caused them to malinger, and whether such behaviour is more symptomatic of a core insidious pattern of cheating, conning, manipulative, and parasitic lifestyle. The description of malingering in DSM-IV would have us believe that these individuals have antisocial personality disorder, but clearly there are forms of malingering (e.g. taking sick days off work when one is not sick or over-exaggerating of actual symptoms) that are relatively common and not symptomatic of antisocial personality disorder. Would these forms of malingering *not* be associated with neurocognitive, psychophysiological, and brain impairments that have been associated with criminal behaviour and antisocial personality?

Confounding this lack of knowledge is a clear definition of what malingering really is. The definition in DSM-IV is a reasonable starting point, but 'The intentional production of false or grossly exaggerated physical or psychological symptoms, motivated by external incentives such as avoiding military duty, avoiding work, obtaining financial compensation, evading criminal prosecution, or obtaining drugs' (American Psychiatric Association 1994, p. 683) does not help much in defining the boundaries of malingering. Feigning a whiplash injury to obtain financial compensation in a law-case is clearly malingering. But what about exaggerating an innocuous cold to justify a day off work? Is malingering categorical in nature (i.e. the population can be unequivocally divided into malingerers and non-malingerers), or is it dimensional (i.e. there are individual differences in the *degree* to which we all malinger at some point in our lives). What frequency and severity criteria should be used for establishing status as a malingerer?

Without clear answers to these assessment issues, it is going to be difficult to conduct the type of systematic research studies that can provide us with the much-need basic information on the biopsychosocial characteristics of malingers. In turn, without this information, the question of whether malingering is a clinical disorder will remain elusive. Currently, malingering is little more than a description of one specific form of antisocial criminal behaviour, and not a clinical disorder. To emphasize the point made by Halligan *et al.* (Chapter 1), this field needs less opinion and more rigorous empirical research. Malingering may simply be the free, wilful choice to cheat and manipulate for personal gain, but the possibility also remains that future development, clarification, and elaboration of malingering will give rise to a syndrome that will ultimately become viewed as a meaningful clinical disorder.

Establishing the biological and social correlates of a construct, in and of itself, cannot establish that construct as a disorder. Constructs such as extraversion and intelligence have relatively well-established nomological networks, but they could not be regarded as disorders because neither even begin to fulfil some of the criteria of mental disorder discussed earlier. If malingering is viewed as meeting some of these criteria *and* if a specific network of biological and social factors can be identified which may be of aetiological significance to malingering, then this would constitute grounds to consider the possibility that malingering either constitutes a psychopathology or constitutes a sub-diagnosis of a broader antisocial construct.

Acknowledgements

This review was written with support from an Independent Scientist Award from NIMH (K02 MH01114-01).

References

Adams, H. E. and Sutker, P. B. (1984). *Comprehensive handbook of psychopathology*. Plenum, New York, NY.

Allman, L. R. and Jaffe, D. T. (1978). *Abnormal psychology in the life-cycle*. Harper and Row, New York, NY.

Altrocchi, J. (1980). *Abnormal behavior*. Harcourt, Brace, Jovanovich, New York, NY.

American Psychiatric Association (1987). *Diagnostic and statistical manual of mental disorders*, 3rd edn revised. American Psychiatric Association, Washington, DC.

American Psychiatric Association (1994). *Diagnostic and statistical manual of mental disorders*, 4th edn. American Psychiatric Association, Washington, DC.

Ashmore, Z. and Jarvie, J. (1987). Job skills for young offenders. In *Applying psychology to imprisonment: theory and practice* (eds B. J. McGurk, D. M. Thornton, and M. Williams), pp. 329–40. HMSO, London.

Baron, M. and Risch, N. (1987). The spectrum concept of schizophrenia: evidence for a genetic–environmental continuum. *Journal of Psychiatric Research*, **21**, 257–67.

Blashfield, R. K. and Livesley, W. J. (1991). Metaphorical analysis of psychiatric classification as a psychological test. *Journal of Abnormal Psychology*, **100**, 262–70.

Boden, L. I. (1996). Work disability in an economic context. In *Psychological aspects of musculo-skeletal disorders in office work* (eds S. Moon and S. L. Sauter), pp. 287–94. Taylor and Francis, London.

Carson, R. C. (1991). Dilemmas in the pathway of the DSM-IV. *Journal of Abnormal Psychology*, **100**, 302–7.

Chronbach, L. J. and Meehl, P. E. (1955). Construct validity in psychological tests. *Psychological Bulletin* **52**, 281–302.

Farrington, D. P. and West, D. J. (1990). The Cambridge study in delinquent development: a long-term follow-up study of 411 London males. In *Criminality: personality, behavior, and life history* (eds H. J. Kerner and G. Kaiser), pp. 115–38. Springer-Verlag, Berlin.

Frances, A. J., First, M. B., Widiger, T. A., Miele, G. M., Tiley, S. M., Davis, W. W., and Pincus, H. A. (1991). An A to Z guide to DSM-IV conundrums. *Journal of Abnormal Psychology*, **100**, 407–12.

Frances, A. J., Pincus, H. A., Widiger, T. A., Davis, W. W., and First, M. B. (1990). DSM-IV: Work in progress. *American Journal of Psychiatry*, **147**, 1439–48.

Gilbert, R. M. (1976). Caffeine as a drug of abuse. In *Research advances in alcohol and drug problems* (eds R. J. Gibbons, Y. Israel, H. Kalant, R. E. Popham, W. Schmidt, and R. G. Smart), Vol. 3, pp. 49–176. Wiley, New York, NY.

Goodstein, L. D. and Calhoun, J. F. (1982). *Understanding abnormal behavior*. Addison-Wesley, Reading, MA.

Gorenstein, E. E. (1984). Debating mental illness: implications for science, medicine and social policy. *American Psychologist*, **39**, 50–6.

Henderson, M. and Hollin, C. R. (1983). A critical review of social skills training with young offenders. *Criminal Justice and Behavior*, **10**, 316–41.

Huff, G. (1987). Social skills training. In *Applying psychology to imprisonment: theory and practice* (eds B. J. McGurk, D. M. Thornton, and M. Williams), pp. 227–58. HMSO, London.

Hughes, J. R., Higgins, S. T., Bickel, W. K., Hunt, W. K., Fenwick, J. W., Gulliver, S. B., and Mireault, G. C. (1991). Caffeine self-administration, withdrawal, and adverse effects among coffee drinkers. *Archives of General Psychiatry*, **48**, 611–17.

Jahoda, M. (1958). *Current concepts of positive mental health*. Basic Books, New York, NY.

Kendell, R. E. (1986). What are mental disorders? In *Issues in psychiatric classification* (eds A. M. Freedman, R. Brotman, I. Silverman, and D. Hutson), pp. 23–45. Human Sciences Press, New York, NY.

Klein, D. F. (1978). A proposed definition of mental illness. In *Critical issues in psychiatric diagnosis* (eds R. L. Spitzer and D. F. Klein), pp. 41–72. Raven Press, New York, NY.

Lewis, A. J. (1953). Health as a social concept. *British Journal of Sociology*, **4**, 109–24.

London Home Office (1985). Criminal careers of those born in 1953, 1958 and 1963. *Home Office Statistical Bulletin*. Home Office Statistical Department, London.

McGurk, B. J. and Newell, T. C. (1987). Social skills training: case study with a sex offender. In *Applying psychology to imprisonment: theory and practice* (eds B. J. McGurk, D. M. Thornton, and M. Williams), pp. 219–26. Her Majesty's Stationery Office, London.

Mednick, S. A. (1977). A bio-social theory of the learning of law-abiding behavior. In *Biosocial bases of criminal behavior* (eds S. A. Mednick and K. O. Christiansen). Gardner Press, New York, NY.

Meehl, P. E. (1989). Schizotaxia revisited. *Archives of General Psychiatry*, **46**, 935–44.

Millon, T. (1991). Classification in psychopathology: rationale, alternatives, and standards. *Journal of Abnormal Psychology*, **100**, 245–61.

Morey, L. C. (1991). Classification of mental disorder as a collection of hypothetical constructs. *Journal of Abnormal Psychology*, **100**, 289–93.

Quay, H. C. (1987). Intelligence. In *Handbook of juvenile delinquency* (ed. H. C. Quay), pp. 106–17. Wiley, New York, NY.

Raine, A. (1993). *The psychopathology of crime: criminal behavior as a clinical disorder*. Academic Press, San Diego, CA.

Raine, A., Brennan, P., Farrington, D. P. and Mednick, S. A. (eds) (1997). *Biosocial bases of violence*. Plenum, New York, NY.

Robins, E. and Guze, S. B. (1970). Establishment of diagnostic validity in psychiatric illness: Its application to schizophrenia. *American Journal of Psychiatry*, **126**, 983–7.

Rogers, R. (1990). Models of feigned mental illness. *Professional Psychology: Research and Practice*, **21**, 182–8.

Roth, M. and Kroll, J. (1986). *The reality of mental illness*. Cambridge University Press, Cambridge.

Scheff, T. J. (1970). Schizophrenia as ideology. *Schizophrenia Bulletin*, **2**, 15–19.

Siever, L. J., Coursey, R. D., Alterman, I. S., Buchsbaum, S., and Murphy, D. L. (1984). Impaired smooth-pursuit eye movements: vulnerability marker for schizotypal personality disorder in a normal volunteer population. *American Journal of Psychiatry*, **141**, 1560–6.

Spitzer, R. L. (1991). An outsider–insider's views about revising the DSMs. *Journal of Abnormal Psychology*, **100**, 294–6.

Spitzer, R. L. and Endicott, J. (1978). Medical and mental disorder: proposed definition and criteria. In *Critical issues in psychiatric diagnosis* (eds R. L. Spitzer and D. F. Klein), pp. 15–40. Raven Press, New York, NY.

Visher, C. A. and Roth, J. A. (1986). Participation in criminal careers. In *Criminal careers and career criminals* (eds A. Blumstein, J. Cohen, J. A. Roth, and C. A. Visher), pp. 211–91. National Academy Press, Washington, DC.

Widiger, T. A., Frances, A. J., Pincus, H. A., Davis, W. W., and First, M. B. (1991). Toward an empirical classification for the DSM-IV. *Journal of Abnormal Psychology*, **100**, 280–8.

Wilson, J. Q. and Herrnstein, R. (1985). *Crime and human nature*. Simon & Schuster, New York, NY.

Wolfgang, M. E., Figlio, R. F. and Sellin, T. (1972). *Delinquency in a birth cohort*. University of Chicago Press, Chicago, IL.

8 Alternatives to four clinical and research traditions in malingering detection

David Faust

Abstract

Some commonly accepted prescriptions for research and clinical practice in malingering detection disregard complementary and, at times, potentially more productive approaches that can be derived from the study of decision making and clinical judgement, and from work in epistemology and philosophy of science. I discuss four such popular views or clinical dictates, which are central to work in malingering detection, and then present possible alternative or adjunct views. These include the following: (a) when reaching clinical conclusions, combine all of the data, with particular attention to patterns or configurations; versus, only utilize data that produce incremental validity; (b) nothing can substitute for experience in learning how to detect malingering; versus, nothing like experience in the context of discovery; nothing like research in the context of verification; (c) determining whether malingering is a category or taxon is mostly a matter of convenience and is of little practical use; versus, determination of taxonicity is not arbitrary, really does matter, and can provide practical help to researchers and clinicians; and (d) research requires a 'gold standard' (unambiguous criteria) to make real progress; versus, it is scientifically commonplace to make progress without a gold standard.

Introduction

The best scientific methodology does not ensure success, nor the worst failure, as the soundness of methodology and the productiveness of scientific efforts are linked probabilistically (Faust and Meehl 2002). However, the odds of a positive yield may be enhanced, or greatly enhanced, depending on the methodology employed. The detection of malingering presents some intellectually fascinating and deep methodological challenges, and our capacity to meet them may determine, more than anything else, the productivity and success of our research and, ultimately, of our clinical efforts in this domain.

My ruminations about applied clinical and scientific problems in malingering detection, and more particularly about methodological issues, start from what might seem an odd combination of involvement in research and writing in clinical decision making, and in epistemology and philosophy of science (e.g. see Faust 1984; Faust and Meehl 1992, 2002). In both areas, my focus has been on judgemental processes—whether it be the judgement of clinicians deciding upon a diagnosis, or of a scientist appraising a body of research or a theory—and in the design of methods to increase the accuracy of decisions and the synthesis of information. Study of these areas some-times suggests normative advice that differs from certain popular philosophical or methodological positions in psychology and psychiatry, or from common adages in clinical decision-making. It is my concern and contention that some received views disregard complementary and, at times, more productive alternatives for research and clinical decision-making in malingering detection. In the text that follows, I will discuss four such popular methodological views or clinical dictates, which I consider central to work in malingering detection, and then present possible alternatives or adjunct views.

(1.) When reaching clinical conclusions, combine all of the data, with particular attention to patterns or configurations <u>versus</u> only utilize the data that yield incremental validity

When attempting to identify malingering (or perform most any other diagnostic task), clinicians are commonly advised to combine or integrate all of the available data. They are also often urged to be particularly attentive to patterns or configurations in the data, such as whether the obtained results fit with a known pattern of disorder.

This notion of combining all of the data is so frequently articulated that it has become almost like breathing, a component of our clinical consciousness that is so ensconced it draws minimal thought or evaluation; rather, it is a taken-for-granted and seemingly self-evident truth. However, if one takes a step back, armchair analysis, particularly when viewed in conjunction with a considerable body of pertinent research, raises serious questions about this methodological dictate.

Imagine that one is conducting a study on some topic, such as memory proficiency following at least 20 hours of sleep deprivation. Research participant Jones performs poorly on the memory measure. Upon interview, however, he admits that he was out at a bar the entire night before, that his last recollection is finishing his sixth pint of beer before the blackout period started, and that the five aspirin pills he took before the testing did nothing for his pounding headache. Would we still maintain at this point that we need to consider or integrate all of the data, and thus should not exclude Jones's results in the analysis? Likewise, what about the control group subject who forgot her glasses, misaligned her answers on the recording sheet, and consequently obtained a memory test score of zero?

The reader might object that these examples are extreme, and that in a parallel clinical situation a practitioner with any judgement would not include obviously contaminated or worthless information. But this is exactly my point: we should not necessarily combine all of the data, but only the data that have some merit or potential utility.

If we accept this simple proposition for limiting ourselves to the useful information (e.g. that which contributes to an accurate diagnosis), the question that naturally arises is: How can we determine which information this might be? Here research (see Faust 1984) suggests that our clinical beliefs or intuitions are not necessarily the best guide, and that discernment and utilization of informational value can be enhanced by applying certain analytic and conceptual tools, and by exercising greater selectivity.

For purposes of the present discussion, I wish to focus on dichotomous decisions, such as whether a person is or is not feigning psychosis, and bypass other conceptual issues that will occupy us later, such as whether the thing we seek to identify is truly a category. It is understood that nature does not necessarily break down into neat dichotomies, and that other judgements, such as those involving breadth and magnitude of a condition, may be critical. However, we are often faced with dichotomous decision (e.g. brain damaged or not; hospitalize or do not hospitalize, medicate or do not medicate), and limiting the present analysis to these judgements should aid conceptual clarity.

When contemplating whether to consider or disregard some type of information or variable in reaching a decision, a basic question is whether it shows a true association with the condition of interest. For example, we might ask whether certain odd voice qualities are associated with malingering. If the answer to this question is negative, the variable should be dropped from further consideration. However, despite what may be contrary intellectual instincts, a positive answer is *not* dispositive. Indeed, the assumption that valid information will necessarily contribute to accuracy, and, therefore, that the more information one considers or combines the better, is simply wrong and can exert a destructive influence on diagnostic accuracy.

Accuracy is not, strictly speaking, cumulative, and more is not necessarily better. Additional valid information may not increase, and can even decrease, accuracy (e.g. see Faust and Nurcombe 1989). Rather than just asking whether a sign or indicator has a true association with a condition, we also need to ask what happens when we add this variable to other available, valid indicators. It may increase accuracy, it may be neutral, and it also may *decrease* accuracy, with the latter two results occurring far more often than might be anticipated. It is the frequency of negative outcomes that makes asking this question about adding information, and properly evaluating impact, so critical.

The possibility that valid information can *decrease* accuracy seems paradoxical or counter-intuitive, which partly explains why the suggestion to combine all of the information is so common and so often taken for granted. However, whether or not a valid variable increases accuracy depends in part on how well we can do, or are doing, without it. Assume, for example, a diagnostic indicator that achieves 70 per cent accuracy. If the best we can achieve with other available information is 60 per cent accuracy, then the addition of this new indicator (or even its substitution over other information) will increase accuracy. However, if we are already achieving 80 per cent accuracy without it, it may not be helpful at all or may even decrease accuracy. A valid indicator, hence, may not increase accuracy when it is added to valid predictors that are already available. Whether a new variable increases accuracy above that achieved by other available predictors is often described as the property of 'incremental validity'.

To further explain this seeming paradox, imagine you consult a cardiologist who achieves 90 per cent accuracy in identifying congestive heart failure. To be on the safe side, you consult a second cardiologist, who is also outstanding, although not quite as good as the first one and rather achieves 80 per cent accuracy. Both are accurate, but this does not mean that adding the opinion of the second cardiologist to the first cardiologist will help matters. More likely, the opposite will result.

If the two cardiologists agree, or the second agrees with the first, the initial conclusion remains unaltered. Hence, the situation of greatest interest will usually be the one in which there is disagreement. It is exactly in these situations, however, that the first cardiologist is twice as likely to be right as the second cardiologist (because the error rate of the second is twice that of the first, or 20 versus 10 per cent). Thus, each time one countervails the first cardiologist's diagnosis based on disagreement with the second cardiologist, the likelihood of error has been doubled.[1] Note that we are dealing here with a circumstance in which, when they disagree, both cannot be right. The patient either does or does not have the condition, and the judgements of the two physicians are inconsistent or opposed.

Although there are conceivable schemes for combining the judgement of the two consultants in the hopes of increasing accuracy (e.g. there might be a way to identify a subset of cases in which the judgement of the first cardiologist is inferior), such schemes often require a level or type of

[1] Even this statement about increasing the likelihood of error two-fold is not precisely correct or complete. It would be more exact to say that the chances of error are *at least* doubled, and could be greater than this rate. For example, the two cardiologists may only disagree on 10 cases. In the 90 instances of agreement, both might be right in 80 of the 90 cases and both wrong in 10 of the 90 cases. In the 10 instances of disagreement, the first cardiologist might be right each time and the second wrong each time, resulting in total accuracy rates of 90% and 80%, respectively.

knowledge that is superior to that of either of the two decision makers. This is usually the very knowledge that we lack and that leads us to seek the opinions of the physicians in the first place. The ability to identify when error occurs usually requires knowledge or accuracy superior to that of the better diagnostician. And, if such superior knowledge existed, one would probably just tap into it and not seek out the consultants.

Assume now a situation in which, rather than two consultants or diagnosticians, there are multiple diagnostic indicators, and we are trying to determine whether an individual is malingering. When various available indicators all point in the same direction, the decision is easy and it will not matter if our judgement rests on only one, as opposed to all, of the variables. However, as commonly happens, all indicators do not coincide, and some may be in direct conflict with one another, precluding a true synthesis of information. Rather, we must decide which variables to bet upon and which to disregard. If we rely on valid but weaker variables, or if we allow weaker variables to override stronger variables, our overall accuracy will not increase and quite possibly will decline.

In many such situations like this, when diagnostic indicators point in opposing directions, one must select one or some over others, no legitimate synthesis can be achieved, and a composite that includes the total pool of variables will do no better, and may well do worse, than use of the stronger indicators alone. The point remains that additional valid information does not necessarily produce an increment in accuracy and rather may have the opposite affect.

How can we determine what information, or combination of information, produces and maximizes incremental validity? Research yields helpful insights into this matter. First, for many decision tasks, one often approaches, or reaches, a ceiling in accuracy once a surprising limited amount of information is taken into account (Faust 1984; Dawes *et al.* 1989). For example, when making a diagnosis in psychology or psychiatry, distinguishing one condition from another, or judging the severity of disorder, about three to five of the most valid and non-redundant variables, if combined properly, often approaches or equals the level of accuracy achieved by considering greater amounts of information.

Part of the explanation for restriction in gain as additional information is added is the redundancy of many predictors. For example, as seems to be the case in malingering detection now that so much productive research has been conducted, there is often a wide range of valid indicators (e.g. see Rogers 1997). Many of these indicators, however, are likely to be highly redundant with one another and consequently to add little unique predictive information.[2] Highly correlated or redundant variables usually produce little gain in accuracy over the use of the variables in isolation. Rather, improvement is achieved to the extent variables are valid *and* do not overlap or are not correlated (Goldberg 1991). By analogy, albeit an extreme one that serves to illustrate the point, suppose we are trying to determine something about a person's health, and we know that weight is a valid indicator of health status. If one has an accurate scale that measures weight in pounds, a second accurate scale that measures weight in kilograms adds no unique information and will not enhance our diagnostic or predictive accuracy.

If there are multiple predictors, many of which are highly redundant, and if a ceiling in predictive accuracy is often approached or reached by utilizing about three to five variables, it follows that failure to incorporate one of these multiple predictors when reaching a conclusion will typically have little or no adverse affect on accuracy. Thus, errors of exclusion often are not serious. In contrast, inclusion of a relatively weaker, and especially an invalid predictor, is potentially much more serious. A weaker or invalid predictor may well disagree with the better predictors, and to

---

[2] Redundancy, in a context like this, is not an all-or-nothing thing, but rather refers to the extent of overlap or, more precisely, the level of shared variance. For example, two variables that are highly correlated with one another, say, at a coefficient of 0.85, may be said to be largely or highly redundant. Mathematical procedures can be used to formally determine the extent of redundancy. If there are multiple potential variables and accuracy or validity were strictly cumulative, we often should be able to predict with over 100% accuracy, an obvious absurdity. For example, to simplify a bit, if four variables each achieved 60% accuracy and validity were strictly cumulative, we should be able to predict with 240% accuracy!

the extent judgement is swayed by these weaker predictors, overall accuracy is likely to decrease. For example, suppose three strong indicators suggest that an individual is malingering but that two other, weaker predictors, suggest otherwise. On average, across cases, to the extent the weaker predictors influence judgement, accuracy will decline. Again, the widely accepted dictate to 'consider and integrate all of the information' is probably non-optimal, if not potentially poisonous.

None of this would be much of a problem if it were simple to determine the validity and redundancy of variables and then to direct oneself to decide accordingly. However, considerable research shows that subjective identification of such matters as the extent of redundancy among variables is very difficult, and that it is even more difficult still to determine whether, or the extent to which variables produce incremental validity (Faust 1984; Dawes *et al.* 1989). In fact, it is often problematic to determine whether a variable is valid at all: many studies show how prone even highly trained clinicians are to developing false beliefs about the association between variables and diagnoses or outcomes (e.g. see Chapman and Chapman 1967, 1969). Research also strongly suggests that certain variables may have more, and others less, influence then we believe or intend in our decision making. Therefore, even if we have an optimal scheme for including and combining information, we still may fail to execute the plan that we intend (Fischhoff 1982; Faust 1984).

It is asking much of the human mind to discern just how valid a variable is, to perform precise comparative judgements (e.g. to analyse whether the Jones Sign is about the same, a little better, or modestly better than the Smith Sign within the clinical population of interest), to judge level of redundancy, and then to determine how to best combine the indicators that remain. Such judgements can be greatly assisted by formal studies on such matters as redundancy among variables, incremental validity, and optimal means of data combination. Indeed, voluminous research shows that the accuracy of such difficult judgements can be bolstered by various decision aids that analyse and incorporate the needed information (see Dawes *et al.* 1989; Grove and Meehl 1996; Meehl 1996; Faust and Ackley 1998; Grove *et al.* 2000).

It is commonly assumed that success in clinical judgement rests on the analysis of patterns or configurations in the data. However, from a methodologic (versus an ontologic) standpoint, this matter is not at all clear. In psychology and psychiatry at least, and perhaps in more areas of physical medicine than might be realized, schemes for data combination that disregard patterns or configurations can often reproduce decisions that are reached, or purportedly reached, through pattern analysis (see Dawes and Corrigan 1974; Faust 1984). (I will not enter into the reasons that may underlie this common research result, except to note that high level pattern analysis is often extremely difficult and that the resultant cognitive inefficiencies and inaccuracies frequently allow simpler data combination schemes to equal or exceed the success of such approaches.) From a practical standpoint, for many diagnostic and predictive undertakings in the clinic, it is probably as, if not more important to identify the best and non-redundant predictors, and to recognize and exclude the weaker or invalid predictors, then it is to focus on patterns. Even the relative weights attached to different variables may not matter a great deal. Mathematical and conceptual analyses (e.g. Wilks 1938; Dawes and Corrigan 1974) show that the same final decision or judgement is often reached whether variables are differentially weighted, equally weighted, or even assigned random weights!

It is helpful to separate out the completely reasonable ontological belief that nature often forms patterns from the practical question of how to reach the most accurate conclusions. Whether or not nature is patterned does not necessarily tell us whether, at present, the best diagnostic or predictive results are achieved by focusing on patterns or configurations. For example, nature may tolerate over-simplification to a certain, or even considerable, extent (e.g. the simplifying assumption that planetary motion is elliptical worked rather well). An over-simplification (e.g. such as that involved in merely adding together variables that in truth form a pattern) may still achieve decent results, whereas an attempt to discern patterns, if faulty, may lead to more frequent error.

There are surely many circumstances in which patterns may exist but the identification of an entity does not necessarily depend on pattern recognition. For example, one could still identify and distinguish zebras with some accuracy by calculating a white-to-black ratio. We would almost surely do better by looking for a pattern of alternating black and white stripes. However, suppose we had not reached a state of knowledge in which we knew about this pattern, or if identification of pattern was very difficult and frequently lead to misjudgements. In such circumstances, a simple additive approach might well produce greater success than attempts at pattern recognition.

Pattern recognition in science, and especially in applied clinical sciences that focus on human behaviour, is often far more difficult and hazardous than assumed (Faust 1990). Much research in the mental health field suggests that 'patterns' clinicians believe they observe are often artefacts, and that attempts at pattern analysis, despite subjective impressions to the contrary, often do not contribute much to diagnostic or predictive accuracy (see Faust 1984). Thus, in malingering detection, the common advice to look for patterns and to consider all of the data may not maximize success.

The agenda for researchers seems very clear here. First, studies on incremental validity are urgently required. We probably have limited need for additional studies which show that yet another sign or indicator has some utility in malingering detection. There is probably something approaching an unlimited universe of potential variables that show some association with malingering. We are almost certainly reaching a point at which most new variables are highly redundant with already existing ones, and it is of much greater practical importance to determine which variables to use in which combination. Second, as follows, related studies are needed on optimal methods for data combination. Do we need to differentially weight variables? Do we need to consider patterns? Are there disjunctive or conjunctive strategies that may prove useful? For example, if someone scores well below chance on a measure, do we override other measures that show good cooperation? Should a subject who is cooperating be expected to score above a certain level on all malingering measures? Again, if the adage to integrate all of the information is probably not sound and a strategy in which one focuses on incremental validity is much better, how are we to proceed if the needed research and knowledge base is lacking?

(2.) Nothing can substitute for experience in learning how to detect malingering <u>versus</u> nothing like experience in the context of discovery; nothing like research in the context of verification

Benjamin Franklin is often (mis)quoted (in the United States at least) as saying through Poor Richard that 'experience is the best teacher'. Franklin actually said that experience is a 'dear' teacher (meaning a costly one) and that 'fools learn from no other'. For reasons to be described, it seems exceedingly unlikely that experience, such as repeated opportunities to assess for the presence of deception, is the best teacher in learning to detect malingering. Over-reliance on experience is likely to lead to the under-weighting or disregard of research on malingering detection, which, in turn, is likely to increase the rate of false-positive and false-negative errors. Unlike Franklin's homily, however, the one bearing the dear cost is not the originator but the subject of the error, such as a person incapacitated by a brain injury who has been mislabelled a fraud.

Experience is of course of indisputable value for many undertakings. Experience may lead to the identification of possible signs and indicators of malingering that would not have been discovered otherwise. The problem and difficulty, however, is in determining the true utility, if any, of the potential indicators that have been identified. Some of them may turn out to be quite valuable, and others of less value or worthless. Also, in lines with the prior section, it is insufficient, by itself, to determine if a sign has a true association with malingering. One also wishes to investigate all of the other matters that go into a determination of incremental validity.

The history of medicine and psychology shows that experience may be a wonderful basis for *discovering* things of potential value, but that it is far from the best means for testing or verifying these same possibilities. Medicine, for example, is littered with treatments that were thought to be useful or superior on the basis of clinical experience, but that turned out to be something less than this: just inefficacious perhaps, but sometimes harmful or lethal.

When attempting to identify or verify means for malingering detection on the basis of experience, the problem is especially acute. In medicine at least, what befalls the patient is often relatively clear (even if causal mechanisms are not). For example, if the patient survives, there is unlikely to be much debate about whether the patient is or is not dead. In malingering detection, we often do not know whether our judgements are correct. It is not logically sound to test the accuracy of one's judgement by determining whether one agrees with one's own judgement. It is like saying I have verified that Ms. Jones is an alien because I concluded that she is an alien, and in turn suggesting that this and other like instances of verification permit one to appraise the accuracy and utility of the signs and indicators upon which one relies.

There may be select or unusual cases in which one receives relatively clear feedback about judgemental accuracy. For example, an examinee might confess that he is feigning insanity, or a person the clinician believes is faking lower extremity weakness may be caught on video in the building stairway handing his cane to his spouse and taking the steps three at a time. However, the chances are poor that isolated cases in which we receive clear feedback provide a basis for verifying or appraising the accuracy of our judgements *across* cases, or of the diagnostic indicators upon which we rely. The cases on which we receive such relatively unambiguous feedback are unlikely to be representative of our cases as a whole, or to provide sufficient numbers to formulate reliable estimates.

Suppose, for example, that we receive clear feedback about 5 per cent of the time. Even if a sign achieved a 95 per cent rate of accuracy across all of our cases, the feedback in each of these specific instances could be that the sign was wrong. Alternatively, the accuracy of the sign could be 5 per cent, and yet the feedback each time could indicate that the sign was right. It should be clear that although estimates are unlikely to be off by these extreme levels, the potential for a large degree of error is great and, even worse, we have almost no trustworthy means for determining what the level of error might be.

The problem with obtaining useful or representative feedback is not limited to restrictions in sample size. An equal or greater problem is that the sample of individuals on whom we receive feedback will probably be skewed. Obtaining a representative sample typically depends substantially on random selection. However, the group of individuals on whom we receive feedback is unlikely to be a random composition but rather to be atypical in some way, one that is systematically related to the probability of receiving feedback. For example, they may be the least skilful malingerers and thus the most likely to be caught. This is the type of person who runs to his car in the parking lot, despite having just been in the clinician's examining room with the big picture window overlooking this exact spot. As a consequence, the feedback may seem to verify an indicator that only tends to work in the situations in which we least need help, that is, with poor malingerers who are likely to be detected in any of a variety of ways. Further, this very same indicator will be unlikely to help where assistance is most needed, that is, when malingering is more difficult to detect. As also follows, estimates of accuracy based on these selective cases is likely to misrepresent, perhaps by a wide margin, success over cases as a whole.

Additionally, we are not merely trying to determine if a sign is valid, but also how it compares to other signs and whether it produces incremental validity. What are the chances that occasional or rare feedback on what are likely to be atypical cases will help us determine in a trustworthy manner that Variable A produces, say, 9 per cent greater accuracy than Variable B, but that Variable B, by virtue of lesser redundancy with the combination of variables C, D, and E, produces greater incremental validity when weighted 0.5 than Variable A? And yet these are exactly the types of key determinations that are necessary to provide practical help in the clinic.

Again, none of this should be mistaken as a general argument against the value of experience. There is no substitute for experience for a number of purposes, and discoveries or hypotheses that emerge may later gain strong support and prove to be of tremendous utility. These successes could not occur unless judgements based on experience had the potential to decipher phenomena correctly. My point is that clinical experience is not the best means for testing or verifying hypotheses, and all too often can be misleading, especially in the area like malingering detection. When we need to test or verify beliefs and hypotheses, formal and properly conducted scientific study is clearly the superior option.

Given difficulties learning from experience in this domain, it perhaps is not surprising that research raises doubts about clinicians' capacity to detect malingering, especially when such judgements are made without the benefit of specialized methods designed for this purpose. In contrast, the best available techniques demonstrate greater consistency and success. For example, Rogers *et al.*'s (1994) meta-analysis of studies with the Minnesota Multiphasic Personality Inventory (MMPI) lists indicates fairly large or robust effect sizes. This differential level of success mirrors a very large volume of literature which shows: (a) that clinical experience often produces less, or much less gain in judgemental accuracy than may be assumed (Garb 1997); and (b) that judgements based primarily on empirically established relations (e.g. actuarial or statistical judgements) almost always equal, and often surpass experientially based judgements (Dawes *et al.* 1989; Grove and Meehl 1996; Grove *et al.* 2000).

In a domain like malingering detection, in which the clinician usually operates under such severe disadvantages as gross deficiencies in feedback, formal decision methods that are based on well-corroborated research are almost sure to equal or exceed the success of experientially based learning or decisions. This is not a negative commentary on human capability. On the contrary, it recognizes the considerable obstacles to experiential learning that exist and the human capacity to nonetheless progress through the genius of the scientific method.

There are, at the same time, reasons to be concerned about how well some of the more positive research findings hold up when methods are applied in real clinical life (something I will have more to say about below). There is a clear trend towards decreased accuracy as studies move closer to the discriminations or conditions of interest in the clinic. Although the advantage of research-based methods over clinical experience *may* not be as great as is suggested by some of the more positive studies, this should not be twisted into an argument from a vacuum (see Dawes 1994). That is, some would claim that because studies have limits, this argues *for* the advantages of clinical judgement, as if such problems as ambiguity of study criterion do not at least equally plague the practitioner. Studies that have examined the capacity of clinicians to detect malingering absent specialized or research-based methods are not encouraging, and there is an enormous body of research favouring actuarial judgement or research-based methods over experientially based or clinical judgement. Thus, although it is possible that studies, taken as a whole, *may* overestimate the advantage of research-based and statistical methods over clinical judgement in malingering detection, even conservative interpretation of the findings still clearly favours the former. Further, before one makes too much of the point that studies can produce inflated hit rates to argue for alternative approaches, one might ask whether subjective, and largely untested clinical impressions about accuracy might not be *at least* equally subject to error.

(3.) Determining whether malingering is a category or taxon is mostly a matter of convention and is of little practical use <u>versus</u> determination of taxonicity is not arbitrary, really does matter, and can provide practical help to researchers and clinicians

If malingering is a category or categories, it obviously differs from a category like 'frog', or one with direct physical indicia or referents.[3] However, contemplation of categories that lack direct material referents often leads individuals to draw questionable conclusions. For example, it is frequently assumed that determining whether malingering is a category is arbitrary or based merely on some convention, and that even if taxometric status could be decided through other than artificial means, it would be of little practical scientific impact or meaning.

I think most would agree that malingering is unlikely to be reduced to a direct set of physical referents, at least not in the near future, and may never be fully reduced to physiology or chemistry before the sun burns out. This does not mean that whatever else one might say or learn about classification is merely convention and of limited intrinsic scientific meaning (based on the presumption that any seemingly reasonable and clear approach is about as good as any other). Categories or taxons need not have direct physical referents or manifestations to be identifiable, or to be scientifically meaningful or useful. For example, categories may reflect social conditions or orders, examples being Orthodox Jew, democrat, and neurologist. Suppose that almost all persons we identify as falling within the category of neurologist perform neurological examinations, know the 12 cranial nerves, and can recite features that distinguish migraine from tumour headaches, and that few individuals who fall outside this class exhibit these features. Would we say the category 'neurologist' is arbitrary and a mere convention? Or would we say the category was meaningful and of potential use, as in a situation in which we needed to know whether our head pain required aspirin or a CT scan?

What advantages are gained by determining whether something is a true taxon and knowing how to identify when instances of that taxon occur? One is efficiency. Knowing taxonicity may facilitate the prediction of multiple characteristics or features, and thus making a single determination— whether someone or something falls within that category—permits a range of judgements. For example, assume there is such a category as 'hard-core sociopath'. If one can identify a person as belonging to the class, this single determination will likely permit reasonably trustworthy judgements about a number of things (e.g. you would not allow your 15-year old son or daughter to date this person, would not confide potentially damaging personal information in conversation, would not loan him or her one of your favourite books, much less your car, and probably would not be able to effect a cure through psychotherapy). Consider, in contrast, the effort that would be required if each of these types of judgements required separate inquiry or predictive formulae.

Knowing taxonicity also can greatly facilitate efforts to identify distinguishing features, estimate population base-rates, and conduct various types of research, such as that aimed at determining course, prognosis, intervention, or features that distinguish one taxon from another. I will not enter into discussion here about such matters as whether multi-dimensional ratings can substitute for categories, as the issues are too complex (see Meehl 1992, 1995; Waller and Meehl 1998, for detailed discussion). I will limit myself to the assertion that if something is a true category or taxon, it is usually best to identify it as such and to assume that multi-dimensional ratings do not provide comparable benefits or information.

---

[3] See Faust and Ackley (1998) for further discussion of conceptual issues involved in categorization of malingering, such as whether the intention is deceive should be one of the defining characteristics.

Most conventional methods in social sciences for examining taxonicity (e.g. expert judgement, cluster analysis, factor analysis) have serious shortcomings. However, Meehl (1992, 1995, 1999, 2001) and Waller and Meehl (1998) have developed a method that provides a viable means for determining taxonicity and which was been successfully employed or corroborated by multiple independent researchers. Strong *et al.* (2000) applied the method to analysis of malingering on the MMPI, and obtained impressive results that go a long way towards clarifying certain classification issues that other approaches have done little to resolve after years of effort. Meehl's methods do require fairly large samples and have certain other practical restrictions but, if used properly, could be of great benefit in malingering research. These methods can help clarify whether malingering is one or multiple taxons, aid in identifying distinguishing features, and assist in estimating base rates.

(4.) Research requires a gold standard (unambiguous criteria) to make real progress (Corollary: without cleanly separated experimental and control groups, research is not going to get too far) <u>versus</u> it is scientifically commonplace to make progress without a gold standard (Corollary: demanding cleanly separated groups may limit study to largely irrelevant subjects; impure groups are not fatal if dealt with appropriately and may be unavoidable if one is to study various important problems)

In many circumstances, if investigators had a 'gold standard' (GS) for identifying malingering, that is, an infallible or practically infallible method for separating populations of interest into malingering and non-malingering groups, the planned research on detection methods would not need to go forward. This is because we would already have a solution to our problem, this being the very method used to form study groups. There might be conditions under which our for-sure, or almost for-sure method had drawbacks, thereby motivating efforts to develop alternative procedures. For example, the existent method might be impractical in typical clinical circumstances. It might be very expensive or require access to information that is usually unavailable until after a case has been resolved. As such, use of the method might be restricted mainly to (well-funded) research studies, and it would serve as a standard for evaluating the success of more practical procedures. However, none of these qualifications might apply and, as is presently the case in most work on malingering, to demand a GS is to require a solution to the very problems we most want to resolve and that drove the research in the first place.

The presumption that we need a GS to make much progress is essentially self-invalidating, for were this the case, how could the original GS have been developed? Developing a GS itself requires some type of (and sometimes considerable) progress or advance, but such advance would be precluded if one needed a GS in order to achieve it. Thus, a strict argument about the necessity of a GS sets forth a requirement that cannot literally be true for, if it were, it would preclude having a GS. If GSs were required to make progress, we could not progress because we could not create GSs.

Indeed, it is not unusual in science, especially in developing areas or lines of research, to proceed for a period of time, which may can stretch into years, decades, or even indefinitely, with valid but fallible criteria. These indicators need to be sufficiently valid or accurate to tell us whether we are getting somewhere. For example, when the thermometer was first being developed, results could be checked against touch. Although touch is obviously an imperfect or fallible way to tell temperature and can be distorted by various influences (e.g. order effects), it was good enough to tell us whether we might be on the right track with this measurement tool. Along similar lines, IQ tests were initially compared to teacher judgements.

Ironically, or paradoxically, what initially serve as criteria for validating new measuring tools may be replaced by those tools, which in turn become the standard against which subsequent methods are compared. Although it simplifies matters somewhat, proper study may help us to determine which of the measures is best (and might best serve as the standard) by the orderliness of the data revealed. For example, our background knowledge may help us create experiments that appraise the instruments. We might know something about the pliability of materials and hence can determine whether feel or the thermometer shows better correspondence with material properties as something is cooled. Or we might be able to gather long-term outcome information, such as autopsy results, which tells us whether Method A or B was more accurate in identifying general paresis. In important ways, assessing and verifying measurement tools is like appraising a theory. For example, over time, it may become clear that one or the other method shows greater predictive accuracy in novel domains or stronger correspondence with other known things and, therefore, provides superior measurement. None of these developments or advances necessarily require a GS. Attempts to create one, especially in initial stages when one is exploring less well-known or understood phenomenon, often requires artificiality or considerable distortion, limits study to areas of minimal interest, and *impedes* progress.

In malingering research, it is possible to have a GS, or something close to it, but this usually forces one to study domains of little practical importance. For example, one can have normal individuals respond to a questionnaire twice, on one occasion answering honestly and the other time faking psychosis. Even such groups may not be all that pure because, for example, some individuals might not comply with instructions. However, simple steps, such as a manipulation check, may keep such problems from becoming too acute, and only a fanatic would take the position in a soft science that *no* errors can occur in separating individuals into groups in order to conduct meaningful research. That supposed GSs in malingering research may be more realistic-ally viewed as 'silver standards' (SSs) would not seem to materially alter any of the issues I am describing here.

The core problem that is created by a demand for GSs (or a close approximation) is that, given the current state of the art, it usually precludes study of the problems of greatest or ultimate clinical relevance. Ironically, it is these very problems, such as the development of effective detection methods, that this same research is intended to address. Let us return, for example, to the type of study just described in which normals are asked to respond honestly on one occasion and to fake insanity on another. In a courtroom or real-life case that involves the insanity plea, how often does the clinician encounter a normal person who feigns no problems? In the improbable event that such a person were seen, would we expect the clinician to struggle to distinguish that individual from one feigning insanity and require the assistance of research on the topic?

Perhaps the main function of GSs in this context is to provide a weak, but usually convenient, initial test of a method. If the method cannot pass such an easy test, it will likely need to be modified or abandoned. However, such a study will not reveal much about the efficacy of the method in the situations in which we need it or might employ it, such as in distinguishing between a person with psychosis and one feigning psychosis, or between a psychotic individual who reports that he was delusional during the crime and is, or is not, telling the truth. Similarly, how difficult is it to tell the difference between a normal person feigning no symptoms of brain damage versus one faking symptoms, and how often is this the task before the forensic evaluator?

Most clinically relevant, and challenging, decisions require one to distinguish between someone who appears to have some type of problem (e.g. brain damage) and does versus someone who appears to have this problem and does not or has some other type of problem or explanation for his/her presentation (e.g. malingering, somatoform disorder, depression). As will be further discussed, it is usually problematic to determine whether these studies with GSs provide diagnostic guides that generalize to clinical settings and tasks (thereby rendering such work of little practical value), and accuracy rates are very likely to be artificially inflated.

It might be thought that studies involving malingerers who are caught provide a GS, or something approaching it anyway. Typically, however, these are individuals who 'fail' multiple malingering measures and/or are caught doing things that they should not possibly be able to do if they had the condition they are claiming. For example, I had a case in which an individual supposedly was experiencing marked confusion and various other symptoms that would indicate a severe psychosis. Yet, during a supposedly florid period, he had secretly attended advanced lectures on his (purported) disorder and took copious, lucid, and highly organized notes.

As already described, there are strong grounds to believe that these types of malingerers who are caught are not representative of malingerers as a whole and may well be rather atypical. They are especially likely to differ from those we are not detecting and are the main target of our research. Stated differently, if, in order to create a GS or supposed GS, we only study those demonstrating nearly unequivocal signs of malingering, we are restricting ourselves to those we already know how to catch and probably need not study. These individuals most likely will differ systematically from those we have not caught because assignment as a member into the respective groups is largely determined by the same features that lead to either being caught or not caught. This is contamination between group assignment and standing on the *dependent* variables at its worst, a methodological problem that alone can easily doom a study or line of research. The problem is typically made even worse by limiting the investigation to those who are caught, and by not including some type of contrasting or control group. A deeper problem is the nearly complete inability to measure or determine representativeness. Thus, even if, due to luck or other factors, the group was actually representative in some way, there would be no way to know it.

There is a clear trends towards decreased accuracy, with the rates sometimes plummeting, as one moves from more artificial to more realistic situations (e.g. see Vickery *et al.* 2001 review). These trends obviously suggest that variables or indicators uncovered in artificial situations often do not generalize strongly to more realistic situations. Problems achieving satisfactory generalization are likely to occur when one attempts to create GSs by studying artificial experimental groups or, given present methodologies, naturalistic groups of individuals caught malingering. It should be recognized, at the same time, that it is often hard to separate out the extent to which diminished accuracy stems from lack of generalization versus the increased impurity of groups as one moves from more artificial to more realistic groups. (There are some potential strategies for achieving this separation that will be described momentarily.) For example, with a perfect method of identification, one would achieve 100 per cent accuracy with true GS groups, that is, groups in which, for example, *every* individual in the malingering group is a malingerer and *every* individual in the non-malingering group is a non-malingerer. Accuracy would drop to 80 per cent, however, if 20 per cent of the subjects in each group had been accidentally misassigned (i.e. 20 per cent in the malingering group were non-malingerers and 20 per cent in the non-malingering group were malingerers). As studies move closer to realistic discriminations, situations, and settings, methods for separating individuals into malingering and non-malingering groups often are likely to be less precise or accurate.

If attempts to create GSs often preclude meaningful advance, and if fallible indicators and impure groups, although creating certain methodological stomach aches, are usually not fatal and allow study of critical problems, the choice between the two is typically pretty clear. Who cares about gaining a lot of precise information that is of very limited use? It is better to have imprecise or impure, but potentially quite informative data. This is not to underestimate the seriousness of group impurity, the need to deal with it properly and intelligently, and the realization that it will sometimes exceed manageable levels.

There are various approaches for dealing with a lack of GSs and resultant group impurity. For example, Dawes and Meehl's (1966) mixed group validation method allows the investigator to compensate for group impurity in order to appraise the accuracy and utility of diagnostic signs. This method has been put to good use in malingering detection research by Frederick (2002, personal communication).

Researchers have also used contrasting group methods with some success. In augmenting such methods, certain approaches might help sharpen estimates of malingering, or differential rates of malingering, across groups. For example, one could use methods with limited sensitivity but low, or very low false-positive rates. Lack of sensitivity can then adjusted for in calculating frequencies. For example, suppose one uses a forced-choice method to identify performances that are well below chance. Although two in three malingerers might be missed, positive identifications will usually be accurate. There is also a reasonable chance that rates of false-negative error will be relatively consistent across the contrasting groups and, therefore, will allow one to estimate in a straightforward manner the differential frequency of malingering across the groups. (I understand that a group with a higher rate of malingering may have a greater percentage of individuals who know how to beat methods, but there are other factors that are likely to offset this difference and, in any case, should it be necessary, there are ways to compensate for this potential problem.)

Suppose, for example, that 20 per cent of the subjects in the group with a presumed high rate of malingering (e.g. disability applicants with seemingly minor injuries that are re-applying for benefits) obtain positive results on forced-choice testing. In comparison, in a group of individuals with comparable injuries who are undergoing examination by their general practitioners and are not applying for disability benefits, 2 per cent obtain a positive result. Comparing these two rates leads one to estimate a 10-fold greater frequency of malingering in the first group. Also, considering the false-negative rate of the forced-choice method, one might go a little further and estimate a rate of malingering in each group that is about two to three times higher than the obtained figures, or about 40–60 per cent versus about 4–6 per cent.

As Dawes and Meehl (1966) pointed out, if one can form reasonable estimates of the differential frequency of the condition of interest in groups, then group impurity can be adjusted for in various respects. In the present situation, for example, one can estimate that the rate of malingering differs by about 10-fold across the groups. One can also estimate that about 50 per cent of subjects in the first group are not malingerers (do not really belong in the group), and that about 5 per cent of the subjects do not belong in the second group. Such estimates can also help distinguish between reduction in accuracy that is due to alteration in the effectiveness of methods as we approach more realistic conditions versus simple artefact, that is, increasingly impure or mixed groups.

As another example, I have previously proposed a method that may allow us, through sufficient effort, to recruit representative groups of malingerers. The method may help counter problems that plague studies involving malingerers who are caught, in particular the likelihood of obtaining atypical samples and the inability to measure representativeness. In principle, representativeness requires random sampling, which can be conceptualized as a situation in which all members of a group or class have an equal chance of being selected. In the usual study of malingerers who are caught, these individuals have not been 'selected' by chance, but more likely because they are atypical, that is, atypically bad malingerers. However, although it does not commonly happen, some malingerers are detected mainly by chance, for example, they happen to be caught on camera by a particularly persistent detective.

In many circumstances in which malingerers are caught, there is sufficient information to estimate the level of chance involved. Take, for example, the individual who fakes so foolishly that he almost cannot be missed versus the aforementioned individual who has the misfortune of being trailed by an incredibly persistent detective. If estimates of the level of chance involved in detection possess even a modest degree of validity, something that does not seem all that difficult to achieve if one avoids more ambiguous cases, there are various ways to calibrate the likely representativeness of groups. Ideally, one would try to focus efforts on individuals whose detection seems to have been almost entirely a product of chance (which, given the low frequency of occurrence, would likely require some pooling of data). Recruiting representative samples, or at least having a method for estimating level of representativeness, would allow for many fruitful studies, for example, How often do certain findings appear on measures? What features best distinguish between malingering and non-malingering groups? Do most malingerers use a single strategy or multiple strategies? Further discussion of the 'Group Membership by Chance' method can be found in Faust (1997) and Faust and Ackley (1998).

Conclusions

The soundness of our methodology will largely determine the success of our research efforts and, ultimately, our clinical evaluations of malingering. Very considerable strides have been made in research on malingering detection. Much of this progress can be traced to a willingness to acknowledge and confront the problems that we face: first, that malingering occurs with sufficient frequency and costs that it had better not be ignored and, second, that clinical impression and routine procedures do not seem to achieve satisfactory detection rates (and may be hard to defend in the courtroom). Thus, self-scrutiny and critique, and a sober realization of problems and limitations, can be seen as a core contributor to progress. In my view, while difficult challenges remain, much additional progress can and will be made. Again, one of the launching points may be a recognition that certain received views and proposed solutions are not necessarily the best or most productive ones. Different thinking about means for combining information in reaching judgements about malingering in the clinic, learning from experience in this domain, the nature of classification issues and their solution, and the relative merits of chasing 'gold standards' at this time versus finding means of compensating for group impurity could turn out to be healthy and productive medicine.

References

Chapman, L. J. and Chapman, J. P. (1967). Genesis of popular but erroneous psychodiagnostic observations. *Journal of Abnormal Psychology*, **72**, 193–204.

Chapman, L. J. and Chapman, J. P. (1969). Illusory correlation as an obstacle to the use of valid psychodiagnostic signs. *Journal of Abnormal Psychology*, **74**, 271–80.

Dawes, R. M. (1994). *House of Cards*. The Free Press, New York, NY.

Dawes, R. M. and Corrigan, B. (1974). Linear models in decision making. *Psychological Bulletin*, **81**, 95–106.

Dawes, R. M. and Faust, D., and Meehl, P. E. (1989). Clinical versus actuarial judgement. *Science*, **243**, 1668–74.

Dawes, R. M. and Meehl, P. E. (1966). Mixed group validation: a method for determining the validity of diagnostic signs without using criterion groups. *Psychological Bulletin*, **66**, 63–67.

Faust, D. (1984). *The limits of scientific reasoning*. University of Minnesota Press, Minneapolis, MN.

Faust, D. (1990). Data integration in legal evaluations: can clinicians deliver on their premises? *Behavioral Sciences and the Law*, **7**, 469–83.

Faust, D. (1997). Of science, meta-science, and clinical practice: the generalization of a generalization to a particular. *Journal of Personality Assessment*, **68**, 331–54.

Faust, D. and Ackley, M. A. (1998). Did you think it was going to be easy? Some methodological suggestions for the development of malingering detection techniques. In *Detection of malingering during head injury litigation* (ed. C. R. Reynolds), pp. 1–54. Plenum, New York, NY.

Faust, D. and Meehl, P. E. (1992). Using scientific methods to resolve questions in the history and philosophy of science: some illustrations. *Behavior Therapy*, **23**, 195–211.

Faust, D. and Meehl, P. E. (2002). Using meta-scientific studies to clarify or resolve questions in the history and philosophy of science. *Philosophy of Science*, **29**, S185–S196.

Faust, D. and Nurcombe, B. (1989). Improving the accuracy of clinical judgement. *Psychiatry*, **52**, 197–208.

Fischhoff, B. (1982). Debiasing. In *Judgement under uncertainty: heuristics and biases* (eds D. Kahneman, P. Slovic, and A. Tversky), pp. 422–44. Cambridge University Press, Cambridge.

Garb, H. N. (1997). Race bias, social class bias, and gender bias in clinical judgement. *Clinical Psychology: Science & Practice*, **4**, 99–120.

Goldberg, L. R. (1991). Human mind versus regression equation: five contrasts. In *Thinking clearly about psychology: Essays in honor of Paul E. Meehl: Vol. 1. Matters of public interest* (eds D. Cicchetti and W. M. Grove), pp. 173–84. University of Minnesota Press, Minneapolis, MN.

Grove, W. M. and Meehl, P. E. (1996). Comparative efficiency of informal (subjective, impressionistic) and formal (mechanical, algorithmic) prediction procedures: the clinical/statistical controversy. *Psychology, Public Policy, and Law*, **2**, 1–31.

Grove, W. M., Zald, D. H., Lebow, B. S., Snitz, B. E., and Nelson, C. (2000). Clinical vs. mechanical prediction: a meta-analysis. *Psychological Assessment*, **12**, 19–30.

Meehl, P. E. (1992). Factors and taxa, traits and types. Differences of degree and differences in kind. *Journal of Personality*, **60**, 117–74.

Meehl, P. E. (1995). Bootstrap taxometrics: solving the classification problem in psychopathology. *American Psychologist*, **50**, 266–75.

Meehl, P. E. (1996). *Clinical versus statistical prediction*. Aronson, Northvale, NJ. (Original work published 1954 by University of Minnesota Press, Minneapolis, MN.)

Meehl, P. E. (1999). Clarifications about taxometric method. *Journal of Applied and Preventive Psychology*, **8**, 165–74.

Meehl, P. E. (2001). Comorbidity and taxometrics. *Clinical Psychology: Science and Practice*, **8**, 507–19.

Rogers, R. (ed.) (1997). *Clinical assessment of malingering and deception*, 2nd edn. Guilford, New York, NY.

Rogers, R., Sewell, K. W., and Salekin, R. T. (1994). A meta-analysis of malingering on the MMPI-2. *Assessment*, **1**, 227–37.

Strong, D. R., Greene, R. L., and Schinka, J. A. (2000). A taxometric analysis of MMPI-2 infrequency scales [F and F(p)] in clinical settings. *Psychological Assessment*, **12**, 166–73.

Vickery, C. D., Berry, D. T. R., Inman, T. H., Harris, M. J., and Orey, S. A. (2001). Detection of inadequate effort on neuropsychological testing: A meta-analytic review of selected procedures. *Archives of Clinical Neuropsychology*, **16**, 45–73.

Waller, N. G. and Meehl, P. E. (1998). *Multivariate taxometric procedures: distinguishing types from continua*. Sage, Newbury Park, CA.

Wilks, S. S. (1938). Weighting systems for linear functions of correlated variables when there is no dependent variable. *Psychometrika*, **3**, 23–40.

9   Characteristics of the sick role

Lindsay Prior and Fiona Wood

Abstract

Parsons' (1951) conceptualization of the 'sick role' identified sickness as a social as much as a physiological event. Yet despite its uses, the model neglects the ways in which sickness is mediated through lay culture. As Freidson (1970) points out, it is usually only after lay consultation (in particular, with family members) that sickness gets presented to medical professionals. Indeed, sickness as a social performance is tied up with lay notions of what does and does not constitute proper illness.

   This chapter examines what lay people consider appropriate to 'take to the doctor'. It draws on data derived from an all-Wales (United Kingdom) study that attempted to understand why people might be reluctant to disclose the symptoms of minor psychiatric disorder to a primary care practitioner. Malingering was not a topic that was covered explicitly in the research. However, in discussing why people should or should not consult with a doctor, our respondents also talked about what was and what was not a 'proper' illness. Insofar as the declared symptoms of a malingerer are subject to public scrutiny and sanction, our research should throw light on the kinds of symptoms that are most likely to be enrolled (or rejected) into a performance of sickness.

Disease, illness, and sickness

> Cléante (a visitor): Monsieur I am delighted to find you up and to see that you are better.
> Toinette (a servant): What do you mean by better? It is false. Monsieur is always ill.
> Cléante: I was told that Monsieur was better, I think he looks well.
> Toinette: What are you thinking about with your 'looking better'?... He has never been so
>   bad... Monsieur is very bad... he walks, sleeps, eats and drinks just like others; but that does
>   not prevent him from being very ill.
> Argan (The Monsieur in question): It's true.
>
> Molière *Le Malade Imaginaire*. Act 2. Scene. 2.

The extract, above, serves to highlight an essential feature of sickness. Namely, that it is embedded in social relationships. In the words of Bellaby (1999), 'Sickness is inherently to do with conduct in social relations'. This is partly because, as Moliere's play illustrates, sickness requires collusion. In *Le Malade Imaginaire* such collusion involved relatives, servants, friends, and doctors. The latter all too ready to recommend duff remedies for imaginary illness at inflated prices. (Other chapters in this volume have identified more modern agents of collusion, see, for example, Chapter 15 by Wynia). Sickness is also about social relations in so far as it involves a socially mediated performance (Frankenberg 1986). And, as one might expect, such performances vary—often markedly—from one human group to another.

Using the lexicon of medical anthropology it is possible to distinguish between three related, but distinct phenomena; disease, illness, and sickness. In terms of this distinction, 'disease' refers to (primarily biological) forms of pathology. 'Illness' concerns the subjective experience of being diseased. Whilst sickness involves the process of being ill. It refers, as it were, to the *performance* of illness (on the distinction between disease and illness see, Kleinman 1973; Eisenberg 1977; Hahn 1983; Mayou and Sharpe 1995).

How people perform when they are ill is as much a product of culture as it is of individuals, and different cultures provide different scripts for being sick. Thus, Lewis (1975) indicates how, among the Gnau, a sick person begrimes himself or herself with dust and ashes and lies alone in a dark hut, eats alone, and rejects normal foods. To be sick, then, is to look the part. It is also to play the part.

In the Western world, probably the most famous description of being sick was that provided by Parsons (1951) in his description of the sick role. The Parsonian image of sickness highlighted four features: (a) the socially sanctioned withdrawal of the sick person from routine duties and the expectations of others; (b) the exemption of the sick person from responsibility for their illness; (c) the requirement on the sick person to do all in their power to get better—in particular by (d) seeking of competent care from medical professionals.

Despite its uses, Parsons' image is somewhat weak at the core—especially insofar as it says little about the role of the body and bodily symptoms in illness. What is more, it is clear that in positing a direct link between sick people and medical professionals, Parsons left little room for a study of the ways in which sickness is mediated through lay culture. For, as Freidson (1970) was to emphasize some decades later, it is usually only after lay consultation (in particular, with family members) that sickness gets presented to medical professionals. Indeed, sickness as a performance is very much tied up with lay notions of what does and does not constitute a proper illness. Yet, despite such criticisms (and for other criticisms see Alexander 1982; Turner 1987), the Parsonian analysis has a particular strength. That strength relates to the emphasis that is placed on sickness as a contractual relationship. The contract presumed is one that binds patient to doctor and, more importantly, the sick person to the community of which he or she is a member. By emphasizing such contractual features, the Parsonian notion of the sick role is much more useful for an understanding of sickness than is, say, the concept of 'illness behaviour' (Pilowsky 1993). This is especially the case in so far as the latter, by implication, emphasizes individual and bodily rather than social aspects of illness. In terms of malingering, it implies that fakers have to recruit people as well as symptoms to underpin their cause.

The notion, then, that sickness is part of a moral order—a social contract—is one that needs to be kept in mind throughout the ensuing analysis. As far as deception is concerned, however, a key practical question for any intending deceiver is how best to play the game. It is a key question because in order to feign sickness we have to know what a proper performance of sickness looks like—and so also do significant others who might support fake presentations of illness. Yet, as with role performances in general, the sick role is multi-faceted. In order to examine those facets, we intend to borrow some ideas developed during the very earliest part of the twentieth century by the French anthropologist Arnold van Gennep.

Van Gennep (1960) was primarily interested in transition rites, so called *rites de passage*—say, from childhood to adulthood. Transition implies movement, and van Gennep saw such movement as involving three stages. Separation from the old world, a relatively short period or phase of transition, and a phase of re-integration into a new world. A tri-partite route such as this is clearly discernible in most cases of chronic and of acute illness. The middle phase (what Turner

1982 would later call the 'liminal' phase) often coinciding with a period of hospitalization, or a somewhat long-drawn out period of uncertainty prior to a diagnosis. Whilst exit into the new social world often coincides with the adoption of a new sickness identity—as, say, with someone who is considered 'diabetic', 'schizophrenic', HIV positive, or just chronically ill.

This dynamic image of the sick role—an image of the role in transition—means that we can profitably examine any one of the attendant phases in detail. Thus, we might choose to examine: (a) the entry points into sickness; (b) the liminal phase of uncertainty; or (c) the exit points. In what follows, we have elected to examine how people might gain entry into the sick role. That is to examine what lay people might recruit, by way of symptoms, on to their passport to sickness. Our data are drawn from a study of lay understandings of illness that was undertaken in Wales during 1999–2000. As we shall see, members of the lay community have quite distinct ideas about what are and what are not symptoms of a 'real' and proper illness. In particular, we shall note how physical and psychiatric symptoms are treated in markedly different ways. The differences affect both aspects of sickness performance and of the social contract between individuals and community that we alluded to above.

Disclosing symptoms

Entry to the 'sick role' requires symptoms of sickness. And as we have suggested above, such symptoms have to pass a community test. The community in question is the lay community. Commonly, members of the lay community hold views on what is and what is not real illness and what is and what is not appropriate to take to the doctor. Before people ever get to a doctor (and receive that all-important imprimatur of illness, the sickness certificate) they are most likely to have their symptoms filtered and vetted through a lay referral system (Freidson 1970). The latter comprises relatives, friends, and possibly work-mates.

In the work that we report upon here, illness deception was not the focal point of the research (see, Pill *et al.* 2001). Instead, the research question was geared to determine some of the reasons why people who show symptoms of mild to moderate depression and related illnesses fail to disclose them in consultations with the primary care physician. (In the United Kingdom, such physicians are called General Practitioners or GPs.) For example, it is estimated that around half of those who have such symptoms go undetected in the primary care practitioner's clinic (Goldberg and Huxley 1992). Naturally, part of the detective work depends on the skills of the physician, and there has been a lot of work undertaken on how rates of detection might be improved. Equally, it is clear that the patient has a central role in matters of illness detection, and that if patients were more ready to openly declare their emotional symptoms, then detection would be easier.

So why do patients hide their symptoms? One common answer is that they fear that they will be stigmatized—by the doctor, by employers, and by members of their community. The implications of real or imagined stigma are not to be underestimated, but their existence should not be used to rule out the investigation of other possibilities to explain the problem of disclosure. One such possibility is that the lay community (in the United Kingdom at least) does not commonly regard symptoms of psychological distress as symptoms of illness. As a consequence they feel that such symptoms cannot be used for entry into the sick role, nor as a component of that unwritten social contract to which Parsons drew our attention.

How the research was done

Focus group methodology was used to determine why members of the lay public might/might not disclose emotional problems to their general practitioner. The crucial distinction between focus groups, (i.e. group discussions organised to explore a specific set of issues), and the broader category of group interviews is the explicit use of group interaction as research data. The technique enables the researcher to 'examine people's different perspectives as they operate within a social network and explore how accounts are constructed, censured, opposed and changed through social interaction' (Morgan 1992).

Compared to the two more well-known methods of data collection, such as questionnaires and one-to-one interviews, focus groups are better for exploring how points of view are constructed and expressed in public settings. Group norms and priorities can be highlighted and differences in assumptions thrown into relief by the questions people ask of each other, the sources they cite and what explanations appear to sway opinions of the group (Bloor *et al.* 2000). Focus groups are especially appropriate for the study of attitudes and experiences around specific topics and exploring the participants' priorities, their language, and concepts. Kitzinger (1995) argues that this method can 'reach the parts that other methods cannot reach, revealing dimensions of understanding that often remain untapped by more conventional data collection techniques'.

Using age–sex registers of primary care practitioners, 18 groups of people were recruited. (There was some difficulty in recruiting young men for the study and they were subsequently recruited through community contacts.) Participants were selected equally from three types of community (rural/agricultural; old industrial and working class; modern middle class suburban) reflecting major aspects of Welsh society. Within each area groups were selected on the key variables of age (18–25, 45–55, and 65–75 years) and gender, reflecting the known importance of these factors on health attitudes and behaviour. Some indication of membership of such groups is provided in Table 9.1.

The focus group discussions (average length over 90 min) were tape-recorded, with permission, and later transcribed. The same general format was followed for all the meetings. While waiting for late arrivals a simple questionnaire was given about presenting symptoms to the doctor (some results are contained in Table 9.1). The moderator then introduced herself, restated the purpose of the meeting and the way it would be run, and dealt with any question put to her. A series of tasks then followed which were designed to elicit the importance attached to a range of symptoms and the interpretations put on them, the perceived appropriateness of different kinds of professional intervention and the acceptability of case-finding questionnaires.

The first stimulus for discussion was contained on (three) cards, each with a short description of the basic demographic characteristics, current situation, and symptoms experienced of a named individual (an example is provided in Fig. 9.1). Vignettes were deliberately varied to include a wide range of social, physical, and emotional problems and cues, some of which psychiatrists would regard as indicative of common mental disorder. The aim was to explore the participants' stories and interpretations of what was going on, the options perceived open to the individuals, and the assumptions and judgements underpinning the debate. For the second exercise, participants

Miss Jones is a 29 year-old single parent with two small children. They live on a fairly run down estate and rely on social security benefits. She feels low in energy, has lost weight, is not sleeping properly and feels terrible in the mornings. She also feels that she has no self-confidence and that the future holds nothing for her. At times, if it were not for the children she wonders if it would be worth going on. Her relatives visit her from time to time but they are not prepared to contribute to childcare.

Figure 9.1 An example of a vignette.
Source: Lloyd *et al.* (1998) and used in the research project with permission.

Table 9.1 Percentage of respondents stating that they would go to the doctor with the following symptoms

	% All N = 111	Males N = 57	Female N = 54	18–25 N = 32	35–45 N = 23	55–70 N = 56	Urban N = 33	Rural N = 43	Industrial N = 35
Chest pains	87	88	85	72	78	98	85	88	86
Breathlessness	71	68	74	66	70	75	70	72	71
Backache	55	58	52	63	52	52	55	47	66
Suicidal thoughts	47	32	63	56	39	45	49	47	46
Weight loss	38	35	41	19	39	48	36	35	43
Stomach ache	31	35	26	22	35	34	30	26	37
Hot sweats	27	28	26	28	35	23	18	30	31
Trouble sleeping	16	16	17	16	22	14	6	14	29
Lacking energy	16	21	11	16	22	14	9	19	20
Skin dryness	10	14	6	13	9	9	6	7	17
Tiredness	9	11	7	3	17	9	3	9	14
Irritable	7	9	6	3	17	5	6	2	14
Lack of self confidence	6	11	2	3	4	9	12	5	3

were given a set of cards, each naming a separate symptom of illness, and asked to agree on a rank order placing the symptom that 'you yourself would be most worried about' at the top. Our interest was in the ensuing debate, rather than in the results *per se*. However, the ranking was helpful in illustrating the perceived importance of physical as opposed to more ambiguous symptoms. Following this, participants were asked to discuss various sources of help for people with the aforementioned range of symptoms. Finally, they were asked to comment on their likely reaction if they were asked by the clinic receptionist to complete a questionnaire about their health while waiting to see their GP. Having given their initial responses the moderator then distributed an example questionnaire containing the sort of items used for psychiatric case finding.

In the course of dealing with such exercises, participants not only offered views and attitudes about the issues at hand, but also divulged opinions on a wide array of matters relating to the identification and management of common mental disorder. In this chapter, we focus solely on matters that were relevant to the issue of what is and what is not interpreted as a 'real' illness.

What is a real illness?

As one can see from the results presented in Table 9.1. The kinds of symptoms that individuals expressed worry about tended to be physical symptoms rather than psychological ones, or those associated with social behaviour and social functioning (irritability, lacking energy, and so forth). Interestingly, most groups had difficulty deciding upon where to place 'suicidal thoughts' in the rank order. Some people considered such thoughts to be very important whilst others considered such thoughts of little consequence. The overall emphasis on somatic symptoms is noteworthy in the light of claims by anthropologists such as Kleinman (1980) who have often argued that an emphasis on somatic symptoms is a characteristic of Asian (specifically Chinese) rather than of Western cultures. Taken on its own, of course, the results in the table are merely suggestive of a lay viewpoint. To understand the nature of the viewpoint one has to turn to talk (about symptoms) rather than a study of rank order in itself.

As we have indicated, talk about symptoms of illness occurred throughout the focus group meeting. However, two exercises in particular concentrated on discussion of what was and what was not to be regarded as proper illness. One of these was talk generated during the ranking exercise, whilst the other was talk generated by discussion of vignettes. Vignettes were used to prompt people to discuss whether or not there was anything 'the matter with the person' described in the vignette and, if so, then what the person might do to alleviate any problems. As with the ranking of symptoms exercise, it soon became clear that few people regarded lack of self-confidence, feeling that it was 'not worth going on', lack of energy, poor sleep patterns and so forth, as indicative of a medical problem. Rather, these were seen as problems in living (to call upon a notable phrase), and things that ought to be dealt with by oneself rather than by medical specialists.

Thus, in one of the urban groups the following interchange took place in relation to this vignette. (Words in {brackets} contain information inserted by the authors.)

Extract 1. Valleys men 35–45

> Dewi: Well. You know, what can she actually do about . . .? You know, you can't really go to a doctor and say, 'I'm on {welfare} benefits can you help me' can you?
> Ed: I don't think really by looking at that its not really a/
> Dewi: /A doctor's situation./
> Ed: A doctor's situation . . .

This notion that problems relating to mood and social functioning are not indicative of a medical complaint is given further emphasis in the following interchange—revolving as it does around a wider discussion of psychological problems.

Extract 2. Cardiff men 35–45

484 Nick: . . . they don't want to go the doctors, because they don't perceive it as being a medical problem

485 Dale: That's the main thing in' it.

487 Nick: They don't perceive it as a medical problem. Well I haven't got a bad leg, or you know . . . that's not a doctor's problem because it's not a physical injury. They haven't got a broken arm, they haven't got their eye coming out of their socket and they haven't got a cut in the head.

488 Dale: You if you went in there {i.e. to the surgery with the problems indicated in the vignette}, he {i.e. the GP} would think you were a real fool if you walked in there.

Lines 488–9 reference a widely held view that primary care physicians are not particularly interested in anything other than symptoms of physical disorder.

This emphasis on the physical as against the psychological and the social emerged in numerous discussions. Here, for example, are a group or rural women involved in the symptom-ranking exercise. Words contained in [brackets] refer to contributions from people other than the speaker.

Extract 3. Mid-Wales women (aged 65+)

564 Ang: You know I think something like this would be pretty low down. I couldn't see me going to the GP saying 'I've got no self-confidence' [no, no]

Wendy: And we leave physical symptoms here. And we say yeah you don't go to the doctors for these kind of things [laughs, yeah, yeah] because you are being silly. But you go for these because they are real. [Yeah]

569 Rois: So this side is real? {Pointing toward a list of physical symptoms}.

570 {This is confirmed, and the discussion continues}.

597 Ang: You wouldn't go to the doctors with that though the suicidal thoughts. I wouldn't have thought.

598 Chris: It's easier to get help for chest pains than suicidal thoughts [Yes, that's right]

600 Bev: Although its serious you wouldn't go to the doctors though I wouldn't have thought.

Views about the relative unimportance of psychological symptoms or of symptoms relating to social functioning were also evident among much younger women. In the following (edited) extracts two specific issues are underlined. First, physical symptoms (lines 927–8) are necessary before medical help is sought, and that symptoms relating to mood, tiredness, and so forth can be dealt with solely in the lay referral system if not entirely by oneself (lines 929–30 and 934).

Extract 4. 'Valleys' women (35–45)

927 Clare: It's usually physical pains when you go to the doctors, isn't it?

928 Rather than like some of these are like physical things, {pointing to symptoms on the cards} but they're not /

929 Gaynor: You just would deal with them yourself wouldn't you?

930 Hayley: Take a few tablets.

931 Heather: I think there is a tendency to think that a psychiatric problem is not as important as a physical problem.

933 Ela: It is though [Oh yes]

934 Heather: It is. I know that. But you know, you think, pull yourself together sort of thing.

935 Ela: That's what people tell you, you see. That's what people used to say 'come on pull yourself together for God's sake'. There are plenty of people worse off than you [Yeah. Yes]

Extract 5. 'Valleys' women 18–25

166 Kirsty: If you have got something to complain about, a physical symptom, you have got something to show them.
167 Mair: Or even identify it. [yeah]
168 Kirsty: He {i.e. the person in the vignette with psychological problems} might think he doesn't have much of a reason {to attend the GP}, but if you have got a physical complaint it's easier to go {to the GP} I think.

There are in fact three main conclusions that can be drawn on the basis of our data (of which the above extracts are merely illustrative). First, that as far as a real illness is concerned, only physical symptoms count. Second, that psychological symptoms are not appropriate to 'take to the doctor'. Third, that (as far as lay perceptions are concerned) primary care practitioners are not really interested in psychological problems even were a person to present with such problems.

Implications for illness deception

We argued in our introduction that sickness is about performance, and that it involves elements of a contract between patient, doctor, and community. We, of course, have concentrated on what is required for entry into the sick role, rather than on the performance of illness during the phase of liminality, or the exit phase.

Based on our Welsh data, we would suggest that entry into, and performance of the sick role favours the recruitment of unambiguous physical symptoms. We also suggest that psychological symptoms, and symptoms relating to what might be termed social functioning tend to fall far below the horizon of what is regarded as 'proper' and legitimate illness. As a consequence, psychological symptoms are less likely to be used to enforce the social contract that is, according to Parsons, implicit in the playing of the sick role. Indeed, such symptoms are insufficient to gain the official sanction of the community. (Some commentators have argued that the sick role therefore differs for those with psychiatric symptoms compared with those who display only physical symptoms—see, Weiner et al. 1999.)

These conclusions might be peculiar to Wales, but they certainly fit with the findings of other researchers in the United Kingdom, such as Bellaby (1999). In the latter case—based on research into sickness among pottery workers in the English Midlands—it was evident that few members of the workforce were ready to consider episodes of 'the nerves' as a cause for sick leave. Bellaby also notes how false claims to sickness can be sanctioned by both work-mates, doctors and management, but that such sanctioning has to be viewed as part of a wider social contract of the kind that we have spoken of. This emphasis on the social (as opposed to merely individual) performance of sickness is also a point that was emphasized in Prout's (1986) essay on childhood sickness. Indeed sickness, it seems, is an integral part of the moral economy of work and effort. A full understanding of false claims to sickness requires attention to that moral order as much as it does to any individual.

In Act 3 of Le Malade Imaginaire, the central character is required to feign death. Molière himself played that role and died—on stage. Death, of course, ends all performance. Sickness, on the other hand, is nothing but performance. It involves a performance assembled in terms of the cultural precepts of the age. A central question, therefore, is not so much to determine whether this or that person is acting to the social or cultural gallery—for they invariably are. Rather it is to ask whether the act is legitimate in its context. And as we know, issues of legitimacy are rarely resolved by appeal to the facts. More likely, they are resolved by the forceful exercise of social, economic, and political influence.

Acknowledgements

The study referred to was concerned with investigating the disclosure of emotional symptoms in primary care. It was funded by the National Assembly for Wales Research and Development Office. The grant holders were Glyn Lewis, Roisin Pill, and Lindsay Prior. The main researcher for the project was Fiona Wood. The authors wish to record their thanks to Professors Lewis and Pill for permission to use the project data, and to the National Assembly for project funding. Naturally, the views expressed within this chapter are those of the authors alone.

References

Alexander, L. (1982). Illness maintenance and the new American sick role. In *Clinically applied anthropology* (eds N. J. Chrisman and T. W. Maretski). D. Reidel, Dordrecht.

Bellaby, P. (1999). *Sick from work. The body in employment.* Ashgate, Aldershot.

Bloor, M., Frankland, J., Thomas, M., and Robson, K. (2001). *Focus groups in social research.* Sage Publications, London.

Eisenberg, L. (1977). Disease and illness. Distinctions between professional and popular ideas of sickness. *Culture, Medicine and Psychiatry*, **1**, 9–23.

Frankenberg, R. J. (1986). Sickness as cultural performance: drama, trajectory and pilgrimage. Root metaphors and the making social of disease. *International Journal of Health Services*, **16**, 603–26.

Freidson, E. (1970). *Profession of medicine, a study of the sociology of applied knowledge.* Harper and Row, New York, NY.

Goldberg, D. and Huxley, P. (1992). *Common mental disorders: a biopsychosocial approach.* Routledge, London.

Hahn, R. A. (1983). Rethinking 'illness' and 'disease'. *Contributions to Asian Studies*, **18**, 1–23.

Kitzinger, J. (1995). Qualitative research: introducing focus groups. *British Medical Journal*, **311**, 299–302.

Kleinman, A. (1973). Medicine's symbolic reality. On a central problem in the philosophy of medicine. *Inquiry*, **16**, 206–13.

Kleinman, A. (1980). *Patients and healers in a context of culture.* University of California Press, Berkeley, CA.

Lewis, G. (1975). *Knowledge of illness in a Sepik society. A study of the Gnau of New Guinea.* The Athlone Press, London.

Lloyd, K. R., Jacob, K. S., Patel, V., Louis, St., Bhugra, D., and Mann, A. H. (1998). The development of the Short Explanatory model Interview (SEMI) and its use among primary-care attenders with common mental disorders. *Psychological Medicine*, **28**, 1231–7.

Mayou, R. and Sharpe, M. (1995). Diagnosis, disease and illness. *Quarterly Journal of Medicine*, **88**, 827–31.

Morgan, D. L. (1992). Designing focus group research. In *Tools for primary care research* (eds M. Stewart, F. Tudiver, M. Bass, E. Dunn, and P. G. Norton). Sage Publications, London.

Parsons, T. (1951). *The social system.* Routledge & Kegan Paul, London.

Pill, R., Prior, L., and Wood, F. (2001). Lay attitudes to professional consultations for common mental disorder: a sociological perspective. *British Medical Bulletin*, **57**, 207–19.

Pilowsky, I. (1993). Dimensions of illness behaviour as measured by the illness behaviour questionnaire. *Journal of Psychosomatic Research*, **37**(1), 55–62.

Prout, A. (1986). 'Wet children' and 'little actresses': going sick in primary school. *Sociology of Health and Illness*, **8**, 111–36.

Turner, B. S. (1987). *Medical power and social knowledge*. Sage Publications, London.

Turner, V. (1982). Liminal and limnoid in play, flow and ritual: an essay in comparative symbology. *From Ritual to Theatre*. Performing Arts Journal Publications, New York, NY.

van Gennep, A. (1960). *The rites of passage* (Trans. C. K. Vizedom and G. L. Caffee). Routledge & Kegan Paul, London.

Weiner, A., Wessely, S., and Lewis, G. (1999). You don't give me flowers anymore: an analysis of gift giving to medical and psychiatric inpatients. *Social Psychiatry and Psychiatric Epidemiology*, **34**, 136–40.

10 The contemporary cultural context for deception and malingering in Britain

W. Peter Robinson

Abstract

Scene-setting comments address discontinuities between cultural prescriptions about the abstract values of truthfulness and honesty and the particular circumstances where departures from these are expected, condoned, and applauded. Falsifications to protect the feelings of others are approved. In competitive situations, as contrasted with cooperative ones, deceiving opponents can be necessary for winning and success, and in an individualistic competitive society which values wealth, power and status as markers of success, the achieving and retention of these can be expected to take precedence over truthfulness and honesty in relevant situations. Malingering is but one device to be employed to such ends. However, those who exploit this means may well feel a need to justify such conduct to themselves and to others. Two mechanisms for such justification are: engaging in behaviour that yields self-fulfilling prophecies of producing the symptoms of debilitating states, and *ex post facto* self-deluding reconstructions of events. Both are illustrated in respect of Paid Sickness Absence (PSA) and Pensionable Early Retirement (PER).

There are certain sociological conditions that will influence the incidence of malingering. *First*, there needs to be a cultural and legislative framework that recognises the existence of relevant debilities. *Second*, the chances of malingering are enhanced for debilities which are simply social constructions, those with quantitatively varying rather than qualitative symptomatology, and those of uncertain controllability. *Third*, circumstances must be such that authorized gatekeepers find it easier to allow false claims than to deny real ones. *Fourth*, there should be minimal post-decision checking and no sanctions for recoveries. *Fifth*, acceptability of such conduct by sub-cultures will encourage false claims, and acting in the same direction will be a belief that elites and those in authority are feathering their own nests improperly. Since all these conditions can be found in contemporary Britain, it is not surprising that malingering in PSA and PER is widespread.

Introduction

Whilst there are many sub-cultural groupings in Britain, severally characterized by the particular beliefs, values, norms, and life-styles, it is also possible to point to certain cultural commonalities that have developed over the last thousand years. For longer than that, Christianity was the dominant religion, with its prescribed virtues and proscribed sins. It is true that the various denominations were prone to persecute, kill, and make war on other Christians and non-Christians in the name of a set of beliefs that held love and forgiveness to be prime values. Paradoxes and dissociations of such a kind will be a recurring motif of this chapter: discontinuities among beliefs and between verbally expressed beliefs and actions. Perhaps the most common form of discontinuity is where a commitment to a virtue at an abstract and general level seems to disappear in particular contexts. Honesty may be held up as a universal virtue that permits exception when filling in tax forms or making pleas of 'Not guilty' in courts of law.

In the last 50 years, the influence of the pulpit has declined, as has the verbal subscription to religious and metaphysical beliefs underpinning that influence. Other religions have sounded other trumpets, and the invasive mass media have come to be a major carrier of a culture that reminds citizens of their secular values via appeals to certain abstractions that can still evoke near universal verbal assent: freedom and liberty, justice and fairness, care and concern for the weak. In contrast, aspirations for *egalité* and *fraternité* have been more muted since the government of Mrs. Thatcher was elected to office in 1979. Notwithstanding those changes there are generally held and generally followed working assumptions in the population in respect of truthfulness and honesty, trustworthiness, cooperation, and consideration. Both explicitly and implicitly, the media and its voices also endorse the individual right to pursue personal pleasure. Like other social norms, these carry the dual implications; they are simultaneously descriptive of what happens and prescriptive as to what conduct should be.

These commonalities can be invoked in much of everyday societal living and are, but there are also many sub-cultural contexts where they would enjoy no more than lip-service (literally!). In contexts of intergroup and interindividual conflict or competition, they are likely to be subordinated to the goal of *winning*. Enhancing and maintaining personal and ingroup power, wealth, and status remain the sociological constants that they have been since time immemorial. Success or failure in such contexts vary in import for individuals, from the avoidance of death and suffering at one extreme to becoming *numero uno* in some arena of endeavour at the other. In Britain, awards and prizes have proliferated in recent years well beyond the school classroom; 'Best X' of the year can be celebrated by newspapers, magazines, TV channels, radio station, and all manner of associations for a great range of achievements. Many recipients of such awards are selected by means of dubious reliability and validity. The Queen's Honours system, for example, has expanded beyond the credibility of many people. How these awards are achieved is of less concern to those involved than that they are obtained, with only the occasional question being asked about coincidences of awards with donations to political parties. This is of course not new, but each generation pretends to a self-righteousness about its own conduct. When Lloyd George was Prime Minister in the early 1900s, the price of peerages was well known by those with such aspirations. Truth is not just the first casualty of war (Knightley 1975); both it and other forms of trustworthiness are pervasive casualties in competitive activities (Robinson 1996).

Hence, the major thrust of this chapter will be to argue that pretending to illness in the service of gain is but one strategy among many others to be used in 'competitive' contexts. It is a strategy whose incidence can be encouraged or discouraged by the opportunities made available for it in a society and by the cultural norms governing the utilization of such opportunities. Indeed, pretending to illness to maximize pensions may be seen as no more morally objectionable than the writing of one's own excessive pension rights and pay-offs, as practised by members of elites, and probably less so. Why not pretend to be ill to avoid work and watch the sporting events commonly patronised by the rich? (The World Cup for football was clearly going to give rise to so much 'malingering' that churches postponed services, schools were permitted to postpone examinations, and much of industry and commerce let workers off when England were playing.)

The minor thrust will address the motivating thinking processes that individuals can and do use to rationalize and justify taking such actions as excessive Paid Sickness Absence (PSA) and dubious Pensionable Early Retirement (PER). Textbooks of social psychology, and to a lesser extent those of sociology, still present idealized models of human functioning in benign and moral worlds where the norms of virtue are observed by all except 'deviant minorities'. The models of cognition typically assume the existence of forces pushing for consistency among the values, beliefs, and desires within a person and for consistencies between what people say and what they do. Such models may be helpful and even necessary heuristic assumptions for investigative purposes, but they are logically flawed and empirically unreal representations of human experience and conduct. For example, while lying when so named may be condemned, and truthfulness may be generally applauded, our society expects its members to protect the feelings of others. Under the labels of 'consideration', 'altruism', and 'white lies', untruthfulness is expected and endorsed, and it remains socially acceptable and accepted in many situations. Other human cognitive characteristics can initiate *self-fulfilling prophecies* (Merton 1957) that can result in psychosomatic states and conditions; for example, a belief in a particular incapacity can lead to not doing what is necessary to acquire or recover that capacity and hence confirm that belief (see below). Additionally, the cultural climates of societies such as the United Kingdom and the United States seem to encourage the adoption of cognitive activities by individuals which serve to create and sustain *self-serving* delusions (Taylor 1989). The focus will be mainly confined to the ways in which these two mechanisms affect the decisions and actions of those who take excessive PSA and inappropriate PER on health grounds, rather than on those who appear to suffer from extreme psychiatric disorders or accidental industrial injuries.

It is worth noting that there have been and continue to be times and places where one suspects malingering will have been very rare or non-existent, for example, Ancient Rome, Nazi Germany. In both of these, attempts to avoid military service on any grounds were likely to result in punishments as severe as might be encountered on that service. In the British army of 1914–18 even a total collapse of capacity could be labelled as 'malingering' or 'cowardice', and victims could be and were executed. The tragedies of 'shell-shock' in fact served as a stimulus to the development of both psychology and psychiatry, as dramatically illustrated in the portrayal of Rivers' work in Sassoon's diaries (1946). Statistical data confirm that in present-day Britain the pendulum has now swung in the other direction towards exaggeration of symptoms and malingering being common practice (see Chapters 1 and 19).

Just as deceit is parasitic on honesty and lying is parasitic on truth telling, so malingering is parasitic on genuine debility. It is therefore sensible to begin by listing the necessary societal conditions for admitting and administering claims for PSA and PER, where these claims are advanced on grounds of ill-health. Until these are in place, issues of such malingering cannot arise. Once they do exist, their likely consequences will be affected by a number of sociological and social psychological factors, and these will be the main foci of this paper.

Necessary sociological conditions for malingering to be feasible

A legislative framework

There has to be at least a quasi-legal framework that recognises acute ill-health as grounds for PSA and chronic ill-health for PER. The current British framework has three administrative weaknesses, of which the second is empirically inevitable. The first turns around the concept of intention and requires that recipients shall not have intentionally acted to debilitate themselves. How *intentionality* is to be validly inferred has been and will continue to be a continuing difficulty for those administering the apposite legislation (see Chapter 6 by Malle). For some types of ill-health, *variations in severity* will also pose difficulties for those who have to draw administrative lines on quantitative dimensions. Finally, with the continuing emergence of new psychological forms of debility whose aetiology and prognosis remain obscure, there is not only uncertainty about the implications of these conditions, but doubts as to *their existence* (see Chapter 1). In relation to the first, there is no doubt that some people suffer from low back pain, but its occurrence and severity can be induced either unintentionally or intentionally by adopting exacerbating postures and sitting on ill-designed chairs (Noyes 2001). 'Stress' is recognized as a pervasive condition of post-modern existence, but it is evident that the same stressor can be motivating for one person at one time, but debilitating for others and for the same person at other times (Cooper and Robertson 2001). Claims to be suffering from post-traumatic stress disorder (PTSD) and repetitive strain injury (RSI) cover a range of potential causation from the obvious to the highly improbable. Not all the debilitating states of the nineteenth century have survived. Will seasonal affective disorder (SAD) survive? Most of the sets of initials of recent appearance have wide margins for subjective judgement—and disagreement.

Authorized gatekeepers to filter PSA and PER claimants

Given the subjective qualities of some of the conditions referred to, and human fallibility in decision-making, one question arising is in which direction gatekeepers should make their 'errors' when they are in doubt. Given the culture, the current answer has to be it will be judged better to accept false claimants than to reject genuine ones. Pragmatically too, successful false PER claimants are likely to disappear into society, and their employing organizations may well assign higher priority to losing employees than the validity of the grounds of their departure. In contrast, dismissing a claim could lead to litigation and protests from an employer, as well as personally directed charges of callousness.

Minimal post-decision checks on PSAs and PERs

With the establishment of PSAs as a right, and with minimal checks on validity, it is not surprising that the right is abused, as is evidenced by correlations between the amount permitted and the incidence of use across various occupations and by statistical associations between PSAs and reasons why people would want to take days off, particularly for sporting events. In Britain, some PERs are free to work in similar jobs either in Britain or overseas, the latter with no limits on earnings. They are free to work in jobs other than those from which they were pensioned. Some PERs are even allowed to return to their own professions with their original employers, either part-time or even full-time—under certain circumstances. It is noteworthy that Australia has found a reduction in claimants now that it has introduced checks, with potential reversals and reductions of pensions.

The 1980s+

The establishment of the relevant legislation and its executive personnel had been in place for most of the twentieth century, but in Britain in the 1980s, the sociological context of its operation was transformed in two main ways. In the names of over-manning and financial inefficiency, heavy industries were reduced to minimal scales: mining, iron and steel, shipbuilding, cotton and wool, the manufacturing of textiles and shoes, along with much engineering. Fishing was emasculated, and agricultural labour was reduced. With scant warning and re-training rare, whole communities were consigned to the unemployment register, many with little prospect of jobs in the future. This was mainly a blue-collar experience, but white-collar workers did not escape from Thatcherite ideology, particularly in the public sector. In this sector, greater accountability and efficiency were the overt demands, but state education, the National Health Service (NHS), and social welfare agencies were additionally defined as 'bastions of socialism' rather than as organizations staffed by vocationally committed professionals. The government ordered frequent structural changes whose efficacy was neither piloted nor systematically evaluated subsequently; that practice continues. In teaching, new examination qualifications were invented and abandoned, new syllabuses devised and changed, new school governance arrangements implemented, school inspections re-organized. Administrative demands from the centre escalated. Schools and colleges were combined into larger units. Some people had to re-apply for their jobs and more than once. Some were re-deployed and/or offered early retirement deals. Other public services suffered in the same way: frequent unevaluated changes, combined with increasing bureaucratization of job specification. In the cases of social welfare, health care, and education, the salaries of the mainstream professionals remained pegged well below their 1970s' relativities. Banks and insurance companies also changed from being life-long employers to hire-and-fire operations, as short-term demands rose and fell.

In contrast to the mainstream of public sector employees and semi-skilled and unskilled workers, pay levels of higher management soared. By 2000, Chief Executives of the top 100 companies were paid on average £965 000 a year, with share options and bonuses perhaps doubling this figure and retirement benefits geared to half or two-thirds of final salaries. Meanwhile the minimum wage had been raised to £4.10 per hour—£7462 per annum, with a prospective pension equivalent to just over £4000 a year. The differentials exceed 250 and 100, respectively.

These examples are presented early, simply as some reminders of the extent and kind of changes that have influenced the occupational careers of those currently or recently in the workforce. These effects have been either directly or indirectly initiated and sustained by the declared policies and practices of central governments, mainly with appeals to the presumed benefits of individualism, competition, and performance-based financial rewards based on 'free market' forces. In fact these are 'free' only for those in charge of setting salaries and wages; the rest of us have our pay assigned to us. For a large proportion of the workforce, and especially those over 45 years of age and current pensioners, these changes led to considerable 'relative deprivation' and dissatisfaction with their jobs (Runciman 1966).

The cultural context of everyday life

Cultures are not like scientific theories. They are not a consistent set of practices logically deduced from policies which in turn have been deduced from an axiomatic set of principles (values) to form a coherent whole. Any two core values will necessarily come into conflict with each other, for example, liberté and egalité. In fact any society-wide culture is more like a disorderly collage of values and norms which survive in spite of the tensions and paradoxes among them. What can be asserted then about British culture? It might reasonably be claimed that the British presuppose a general 'good faith' among their members and that this is realised through the operation of the principles mentioned in the introductory paragraphs:

1. Truthfulness and honesty are expected and preferred to lies and dishonesty (Gilbert 1991; see also next section).
2. Cooperativeness and helpfulness are expected and preferred to exploitation and unhelpfulness (Lerner 1980; Bierhoff 1996).
3. Authorities should be trustworthy (Dionne 1993; Fukuyama 1995).

These principles hold regardless of divisions of society into its traditional groups by gender, social class, ethnicity, religion, etc. They are weaker between these groupings than within them, and in so far as the groups are in competition with each other for power, wealth, and status, such norms will cease to be prioritised. This is particularly apposite in respect of social class.

In addition, however, and as also mentioned earlier, there are many sub-cultural contexts other than these which are competitive rather than cooperative. In some of these misleading others is a necessary condition of winning. In others, it is conducive to doing so. The now ubiquitous world of national and international sporting activities is founded on the notion of winning; it is the point of the activities. Of course, there are many latent social functions of sporting occasions, The 'taking part' in the rhetoric of the Olympic Games is a significant component, but, as at ancient Olympia, so in the modern games, there is only one pedestal for the gold medal, and people cheat, with performance-enhancing drugs, for example. The days of the amateur individual have been past for some years now. Football and rugby matches at the highest levels in Britain can often seem to be composed mainly of offences and professional fouls, with the victor's outcome dependent on which team has had fewer of these detected by the referees. When did a player last confess to a foul that the referee had missed? Even chess championships are not immune to underhand tactics, regardless of the vaunted 'spirit of the game'. When winning takes precedence, and most especially when large sums of money are involved, cheating becomes prevalent.

Dishonesty and lying reach their climaxes in wars, with vast resources being deployed in espionage, counter-espionage, disinformation, and propaganda. Famous victories in the past have often turned on doing the unexpected in terms of tactics and strategies, from Themistocles at Salamis and Hannibal at Cannae to Hitler's Blitzkrieg. While their armed forces are trying to deceive the enemy, the warring governments are trying to deceive their own forces and citizenry at large—in the interests of victory (Knightley 1975).

The world of business is competitive. Can goods be sold to customers? The good news for buyers is in large print, the bad news in small print or absent entirely. Advertising as persuasion is seldom 'honest, truthful, and decent', and whilst people can enjoy the humorous absurdities, they are seduced by false claims, about which the official watchdogs do little or nothing. Caveat emptor. Between businesses there is both real and phoney competition. The multi-nationals may compete at the margins, but connive at maintaining their profits, with occasional attempts to bankrupt competitors, for example, in the newspaper industry. If money has to change hands to gain contracts, then it changes hands. Numerically, most countries have institutionalized payments to officials from companies wishing to operate in their societies. Britain is not exempt from such 'corruption'. Even for gaining jobs in the business world, empirical studies show that 20–30 per cent of applicants omit or include false information in their written applications (Robinson *et al*. 1998).

It is not just the world of business where deceit is common. Over the last 20 years when schools and universities have been set targets for increasing examination pass rates, these have been achieved year after year. But then it is colleagues in the roles of examiners who mark the examinations! In the universities' Research Assessment Exercise and (Teaching) Quality Assurance, relationships between written reports and reality were not invariably those of valid representation, any more than documentation in schools have been for their inspectors. (Residing in hospital writing this, I have learned more about some of the devices exploited to 'achieve' performance targets in the NHS. If there is a need to reduce expenditure, take in more low-cost long-stay patients requiring minimal medication, but if there is a need to increase turnover, then boost the number of quick in-and-out patients.) The selection and presentation of ingroup-serving statistics have become normative for public sector organizations, and none more so than by the government itself. For example, the definition of 'unemployment' has been changed more than 20 times in the 22 years prior to 1995 (Hutton 1996).

Finally, it may be noted that for many years courts of law have recorded many pleas of 'Not guilty' that have been followed by verdicts of 'Guilty'. Perhaps the major difficulty for jurors is in deciding which set of witnesses has lied more. In various ways and by various means both those who are doing the deceiving in these contexts and the citizenry at large rarely condemn these practices. Efforts are made to preserve these activities from the label of 'lying'; the word itself carries a judgement of condemnation. Other words are preferred, except in accusations in courts of law. Even in those all the lying seems to be forgotten once verdicts have been reached. It is very rare for those on the losing side to be charged subsequently with perjury.

If competitive contexts are acceptable areas for deception, does this acceptance extend to deception of the general public by authorities, and if not, what are the consequences?

Empirical evidence about public beliefs and lying in public

First, however, it may be asked what the British public believes about the trustworthiness and truthfulness of those in authority? Then it can be asked how the public evaluates any lying by authorities? In 1993, Gallup (Gallup Polls 1993, Social Trends 397) reported percentages of a national sample who believed that those in the following positions had high ethical standards (1982 figures are given in parenthesis): government ministers—9 (22), members of parliament—7 (15), civil servants—15 (20), lawyers—37 (48), the police—38 (56), journalists—9 (?). The declines over a decade are substantial. When fewer than 10 per cent of a category are seen as having high standards, their status as role models must be correspondingly weak. How frequently do members of various groups lie? Of four student samples given slightly different lists of organizations and occupations and asked to assess the frequency of lying, the 'very often' category was chosen by high percentages: *The Sun* (with an estimated daily readership of 9 000 000) >90, advertisers >80, governments >80, politicians >60, chief executives >50, police commissioners >50 (see Robinson 1996). For professors, scientists, and archbishops these percentages were lower than 10. When asked to *evaluate* lies by such authorities, for 9 of 13 examples, over 80 per cent of a national sample selected 'wrong' or 'very wrong' from the six categories offered. Cross-tabulations showed statistically significant variations related to gender, socioeconomic status, region of residence, and political affiliation, but the commonality was much more impressive than the intergroup differences.

In an as yet unpublished survey of various occupations such as domestic staff, plumbers, solicitors, and general practitioners, there was also a (surprising) measure of agreement about the appropriateness of levels of pay for various occupations, with little evidence of self-serving biases. The mean differential from the highest to the lowest was 15 to 1. This compares unfavourably with the actuality of 250 to 1 referred to earlier. Various authors have documented the escalating differentials of income and wealth since 1979 (Rubenstein 1981; Wilkinson 1994; Hutton 1996).

It would appear from these various results that untruthfulness and cover-ups are seen as having become normative in the speech and actions of persons occupying social positions in The Establishment. Furthermore, the 'sleaze' of recent Conservative governments and the 'spin' of New Labour have typically been for the benefit of self and fellow-members of elites. There has been no apparent concerted action taken by authorities to correct corruption. The long delayed court proceedings against the British MPs Jeffrey Archer (Crick 1996) and Jonathan Aitken (Harding *et al.* 1999) may be thought to epitomize the system, as did the failure to expose Robert Maxwell (Bower, 1988) while he was still alive. There has been no reform of the libel laws that have protected people like these three (Hooper 2000).

A series of semi-structured and unstructured interviews about these issues with opportunity samples of the adult population approached in shopping malls have led to the following provisional conclusions about the behaviour and attitudes of the public:

1. People have remained as observers of these events and not become participants in them. For example, almost no one had written to MPs or taken any other action in respect of any of the 'scandals' of the last 20 years.
2. They have felt anger and disgust, and impotent (alienated). 'There is nothing we can do.' This is consistent with the recent lowest turnout ever in the British national election of 2000, in which a mere 25 per cent vote for Labour led to a massive majority in seats won.
3. The affairs have entered into their daily talk at home, at work, and in the pubs, and these conversations have performed three main functions: (a) filling silence; (b) phatic communion (Malinowski's term (1923/1949) for the pleasure of chatting with others like oneself); (c) differentiation of the ingroup from the outgroup, with inward self-congratulation and outgroup derogation: *we* are decent folk, *they* are not.

Interpretation of public stance on lying by authorities

There is general disillusion with the conduct of authorities. They are viewed as self-serving, deceitful, and untrustworthy. There is anger that no serious and effectual action is being taken to punish or reduce corruption or to reduce the great increase in income and wealth differentials of the last 20 years. These sentiments, however, find expression only in conversation and an expression of impotence to effect any influence. Given the absence of potent organizations concerned to increase the extent of honesty and fairness, the impotence is a realistic appraisal.

The conduct of the British public

Does the ingroup righteousness of the public match its conduct? Are the public law-abiding and truthful to authorities? To answer these questions with hard data is difficult, and for several areas of activity no more than rhetorical questions and guestimates, and what everyone knows, can be offered (see Chapters 1 and 19 for some more precise data). For car driving, exceeding the speed limits, shooting traffic lights, and drunk driving are all illegal. Not telling the truth in accidents and not informing owners of damage caused to their vehicles in car parks are dishonest. To the casual and not so casual observer, all are normative activities to the extent of being frequent and accepted.

In respect of work, the unpermitted removal and use of employers' items, unsanctioned phone and Internet calls, and abbreviated hours of work are treated as 'perks', but these are all forms of thieving, just as much as taking unwarranted paid sick leave is (see Baron and Poole, Chapter 19). Tax evasion by under-declaring income is almost certainly itself underestimated in the official figure of 10 per cent (an Australian investigation found 70 per cent). The estimate of the market research company Taylor Nelson AGB was a mean of £1140 per person for 1994 (*Financial Times*, 10 June 1995). The poorest fifth was estimated at obtaining 33 per cent of their spending and surplus without declaring it, and the wealthiest fifth 50 per cent. Unlicensed cars and TVs are believed to cost millions in lost taxes, as are value added tax (VAT) and customs and excise evasions. Cigarettes and beer are illegally imported by the truckload across the English Channel. Whatever the 'black economy' amounts to as a percentage of gross national product (GNP), it is high enough to be substantial.

Benefit frauds are estimated at 1 per cent. False or exaggerated claims on insurance have been estimated as running at £10 billion a year (Association of British Insurers 2001). In one of two relevant Bristol undergraduate projects, Mair (1996), 20 per cent of an opportunity sample interviewed at Heathrow had made false travel insurance claims and 30 per cent false home contents claims. In both cases, knowing someone who had got away with it appeared to be an important conducive factor (Sutherland and Cressey 1970—differential association hypothesis), and needing the money the primary motive. Similar conducive factors were cited by burglars in a Nuffield sponsored project (Troy 1997). The burglars had been punished, but the insurance fraudsters not. The implication of observations such as these, and many others that could be cited, is that some of the laws of the land are no longer seen as having moral force. Neither are they enforced.

Without including the full range of possible dishonest, delinquent, and criminal behaviours, and without listing the changes in laws that have provided legal but unjust differentiation to favour wealth accumulation by the richest stratum, it is safe to suggest that in today's Britain *de facto* pragmatism is in the ascendant over truthfulness—within limits. Not everyone shoots the lights invariably, not everyone always evades every tax they can. Most of the people most of the time may be truthful and honest, but given specific situations and circumstances, law-breaking, dishonesty, lying and deception are practised and tolerated—and in some cases admired.

How do such considerations impinge on attitudes and actions in respect of invalid PSA and PER? Merton's (1957) Opportunity Theory provided a classical conceptual framework for comment upon ends/means relationships in society, where 'ends' are the values aspired to and 'means' refer to ways of realizing these values. Applied to jobs in particular the framework yields four immediate possibilities:

1. *Ends and means both available and socially acceptable.* For persons whose work was expected to give satisfaction over and above money received, and who were treating their employment as a vocation, then it would be essential both that their time be spent in caring, nursing, teaching or whatever, and that they could see the benefit of their efforts to those cared for, nursed, or taught. A fair day's pay for a fair day's work would offer a comparable equilibrium, when pay is the primary consideration.

2. *Ends definable, but socially accepted means unavailable.* Merton saw this combination as requiring *innovation*, with delinquent and criminal behaviour being one obvious means of acquiring money, for example. Both PSA and PER could be normative within a sub-culture.

3. *Loss or absence of ends, but the existence of acceptable means.* *Ritual* can take over. Formally the work gets done. The rule-book of procedures is followed. There will be verbal subscription to the institutional values and in the maintenance of the rules, but there will be no personal commitment to the purported functions of their organization.

4. *Absence or loss of both ends and means.* *Rebellion* is an active assertion of the intention to destroy a hated system, *revolution* is rebellion with an aspired to alternative as a replacement. *Retreatism* is the passive mode of coping. Both PSA and PER could qualify as retreating.

It may be useful to consider two hypothetical examples with significant different opportunities arising out of their experiences of employment in the last 20 years: individual workers whose jobs disappeared in the 1980s, and public sector workers. It is difficult to see why industrial workers should have seen taking either excessive PSA or PER on grounds of ill-health as giving rise to moral issues. With authorities being seen as untrustworthy and self-serving, why should industrial workers threatened with redundancies have had scruples about minimizing their losses and optimizing their pleasures. Denied both ends and means, with even strikes and massive publicity proving futile, what were the options? Where such industries were concentrated geographically, whole communities became unemployed. Some redundant workers tried innovatory techniques by moving or re-training. Others waited for re-development schemes. The pragmatic solution was to maximise welfare payments, preferably with the connivance of PER gatekeepers, not so much to gain rewards, but to minimise the chronic losses arising through no fault of their own. If ill-health conditions needed exaggeration or simulated development to enhance payments, why not select these? Certainly these could be residual innovatory tactics. 'Malingering' would seem to be an odd, even if legally accurate, word to apply to such conduct. Neither was such conduct likely to be condemned by peers in the same or similar situations. Those most prone to assume moral positions and condemn the reactions of redundant workers were probably to be found mostly among those who were financially secure, successful, and unable to see that 'society' through its government had betrayed those workers. Get wise, get even.

The stereotypical scripts for vocationally committed professional public sector workers were different. Their work-related values became unattainable as they were obliged into the massive bureaucratization that purported to render its victims accountable and efficient. Change after systemic change was introduced, regardless of feasibility or sense. The means of policing, educating pupils, nursing the sick, rendering life better for the families in difficulties, were all undermined. Stress levels rose, as did PSA. Some escaped by moving overseas or to the private sector (innovation). Many ritualized the means, playing their roles strictly by the rules, until they could afford to escape. Many older and hence more expensive employees were offered government or institution funded enhanced years to supplement their PER. Others were retired on grounds of ill-health. Again, with so many retirees receiving sponsored benefits, and others being unable to continue to work, it is not surprising that some others exaggerated or simulated appropriate symptoms, again with the possible connivance of their line-managers and employers: get wise, get even, get out.

The thrust of these lines of argument is that Britain as a society has become more capitalistic and individualistic, in ways that eliminated many jobs and destroyed the satisfactions to be obtained in others. Given the opportunities created for unchecked PSA and funded PER, excessive PSA could become normative, and advantageous terms for PER a consummation devoutly to be desired. Stigma were not an issue within occupations or their communities. Personal adjustments may have been, but these difficulties could be preferred to the other options available.

Personal adaptations and adjustments

Earlier comments have illustrated the societal opportunities provided for genuine PSA and PER and have indicated cultural pressures and norms encouraging people to take advantage of these. With such a flow of claimants, it is not surprising that they will have included the genuine, the fraudulent,—and those who become drawn in as a result of self-fulfilling prophecies and differential associations. Self-fulfilling prophecies are a widespread phenomenon via which initially invalid expectations of self and others become true as a result of the conduct of those involved. Obvious relevant examples would be people intensifying skeletal pains by adopting dysfunctional exercises and postures, so that little by little the pains could become increasingly difficult to reverse. Likewise, an initial decision that one cannot face a particular class of pupils or a particular home visit can become generalised to all classes and all home visits. The more the sub-culture supports and sympathizes, the greater the probability of the decremental spiral leading to attempts to escape permanently. To distinguish between self-fulfilling prophecies that are unintentional consequences and those which are initiated intentionally is surely impossible, especially in societies which increasingly accept that unconscious motivations and other hidden rationales may underly even an intentional initiation. Both PSA and PER can be increased and sustained by self-filling prophecies.

How do those who have slid into PER adjust to and justify the change? Popular books such as Taylor's *Positive Illusions* (1989) and Sutherland's oddly titled *Irrationality* (1992) offer catalogues of kinds of thinking that can and do enable individuals in Western societies to minimize the potentially debilitating effects of living. Just as Freud's (1946–67) defence mechanisms of the ego were essentially a list of intellectual devices for protecting oneself from shame and blame, so the biases exposed by causal attribution studies (Weiner 1986) attest to the pervasive presence of such reasoning in everyday life. In societies which personalize blame and failure and simultaneously seek scapegoats and demand norm-related success, what are people to do to sustain a positive self-image? Very many empirical studies show the extent to which perceived failures of individuals are attributed to situational factors and misfortune, that is, causes which are external to and beyond the control of the persons. In contrast, personal successes tend to be ascribed to personal competence and effort. Such processes are the norm rather than the exception. They operate for organisations such as governments just as much as they do for individual citizens.

Reminiscing is a constructive process, and if necessary, self-fulfilling prophecies and delusional thinking can combine to ensure happy memories of skrimshanking PSA and justified PER. In the 1960s, President Kennedy offered an injunction that Americans should not ask what America could do for them, but what they could do for America. In the last 20 years of the twentieth century, several million British adults asked what the British government was doing *to* them and *to* their country. Destructive mass unemployment was an initial effect. Destruction of job satisfaction among committed employees was another. The efficiency of the police, the courts, the NHS, State Education, and Social Services has been reduced. Continued low government expenditure on state retirement pensions has been viewed by many as a swindle. Such actions have not encouraged a culture of trust and honesty. Reversing the trends and the cultural norms that support them will not be easy.

References

Bierhoff, H. W. (1998). Prosocial behaviour. In *Introduction to social psychology* (eds M. Hewstone, W. Stroebe, and B. Stephenson), 2nd edn., pp. 375–402. Blackwell, Oxford.

Bower, T. (1988). *Maxwell: the outsider*. Mandarin, London.

Cooper, C. L. and Robertson, I. (eds) (2001). *Well-being in organizations*. Wiley, Chichester.

Crick, M. (1996). *Jeffrey Archer—Stranger than fiction*. Penguin, London.

Dionne, E. J. (1993). *Why Americans hate politics*. Simon and Schuster, New York, NY.

Freud, S. (1946–67). *The ego and the mechanisms of defense*, revised edition. International Universities Press, New York, NY.

Fukuyama, F. (1995). *Trust*. Hamish Hamilton, London.

Gallup Polls. (1993). *Social trends 397*. Gallup, London.

Gilbert, D. T. (1991). How mental systems work. *American Psychologist*, **46**, 107–19.

Harding, L., Leigh, D., and Pallister, D. (1999). *The liar. The fall of Jonathan Aitken. The Guardian*, London.

Hooper, D. (2001). *Reputations under fire*. Warner Books, London.

Hutton, W. (1996). *The state we're in*. Vintage, London.

Knightley, P. (1975). *The first casualty*. Harcourt Brace, New York, NY.

Lerner, J. J. (1980). *The belief in a just world: a fundamental delusion*. Plenum, New York, NY.

Mair, H. (1996). Insurance fraud. BSc thesis, University of Bristol, Bristol.

Malinowski, B. K. (1923–49). The problem of meaning in primitive societies. In *The meaning of meaning* (eds C. K. Ogden and I. A. Richards), 10th edn., pp. 296–336. Routledge, London.

Merton, R. K. (1957). *Social theory and social structure*. Free Press, Glencoe, IL.

Noyes, J. (2001). *Designing for humans*. Psychology Press, London.

Robinson, W. P. (1996). *Deceit, delusion, and detection*. Sage Publications, Thousand Oaks, CA.

Robinson, W. P., Shepherd, A., and Heywood, J. (1998). Truth, equivocation/concealment and lies in job applications and doctor–patient communication. *Journal of Language and Social Psychology*, **17** (2), 149–64.

Rubenstein, W. D. (1981). *Wealth and inequality*. Faber, London.

Runciman, W. G. (1966). *Relative deprivation and social justice*. Routledge, London.

Sassoon, S. (1946). *Siegfried's journey*. Faber & Faber, London.

Sutherland, E. H. and Cressey, D. R. (1970). *Principles of criminology*, 8th edn. Lippincott, Chicago, IL.

Sutherland, S. (1992). *Irrationality*. Penguin, London.

Taylor, S. (1989). *Positive illusions: creative self-delusion and the healthy mind*. Basic Books, New York, NY.

Troy, C. (1997). *How rational are our views on criminal sentencing?* BSc thesis, University of Bristol, Bristol.

Weiner, B. (1986). *An attribution theory of motivation*. Springer-Verlag, New York, NY.

Wilkinson, R. (1994). *Unfair shares*. Barnardos, Ilford.

Section 4

Illness deception and clinical practice

11 Illness falsification in children: pathways to prevention?

Judith A. Libow

Abstract

Illness falsification by young people has received only limited attention although retrospective data on adult patients with factitious disorder suggests that medical deception can begin during adolescence or even earlier. Certainly many children have ambiguous or chronic, undiagnosed medical problems, often categorized generically as psychosomatic or somatoform illness. While it is particularly difficult to assess both intent to deceive and motivation for secondary gain in children, recent reviews have documented a small but intriguing number of cases of intentional medical deception by children as young as 10 years, spanning a wide range of symptoms from rather crudely induced bruises to very elaborately induced infections and other complex medical puzzles.

New case material is presented demonstrating the often complex relationship between illness falsification by children and collusion with parental training or active by proxy abuse. Suggestions as to aetiology and promising areas for early intervention, such as recognizing possible familial patterns, are proposed. An important starting point is the recognition that the physician may greatly enhance treatment effectiveness by considering the possibility that a young patient's symptoms may be under conscious control.

Introduction

In many patients, factitious disorder and other forms of illness deception have origins relatively early in the life cycle, even before they are commonly identified in young adulthood. The fact of early origins is not only intriguing in terms of the possibilities of earlier identification of illness deception, but also in possibly enhancing our understanding of the aetiology of this interesting and disturbing process. Examination of this problem in children and adolescents suggests that even very young people can and do falsify illness intentionally, with nearly as much creativity as adult patients, but children may be more receptive to early intervention (Libow 2000). Given the preliminary findings that early confrontation may more likely result in admission by the child and successful cessation of deception, better exploration of the problem of childhood and adolescent illness falsification may offer our best opportunity for prevention of adult factitious disorder and/or chronic malingering.

The interface of physical and psychological factors in the expression of illness has always posed challenges to clinicians. An understanding of the full range of 'psychosomatic disorders' has been a particularly important goal for both physicians and mental health professionals, given the extensive investigations and treatments consumed by medical patients with symptoms that 'cannot be explained by a general medical condition'. There is the added frustration that treatments often prove ineffective. Over the decades, psychological theories of psychosomatic disorders have moved from a mind–body dualism inspired by psychoanalytic thinking to more interactional theories involving specific organ pathways affected by unconscious conflicts, moving finally to more integrative theories incorporating biological, psychological, and social influences on health (Kenny and Willoughby 2001). Yet despite the growing complexities of our theories, we still face significant challenges when assessing and treating the patient who presents with a puzzling medical problem that has likely psychological factors.

In many ways, all of the psychosomatic disorders and disorders of illness deception pose even greater challenges for clinicians when they manifest in young people. Adult models are not helpful because they generally lack a developmental perspective, and in some cases, even the diagnostic criteria are of questionable applicability to young people. Our diagnostic system for psychosomatic disorders, including fabricated illnesses, found in DSM-IV (American Psychiatric Association 1994) is based on adult cases (Fritz *et al.* 1997) and does not acknowledge the fact that medically unexplained illnesses are common in children. Factitious disorder is defined in DSM-4 as the 'intentional production or feigning of physical or psychological signs and symptoms' with the motivation to assume the sick role, and in the absence of external incentives such as economic gain (American Psychiatric Association 1994). In the case of young people, the descriptive terms 'illness deception' or 'illness falsification' are preferred because most documented cases describe single events or limited background and historical information necessary to clarify issues of motivation and specific gain, and thus, do not necessarily meet the DSM-IV criteria for factitious disorder even though they reflect clearly intentional deception.

Extent of the problem

Within the realm of adult psychosomatic illnesses, factitious disorders are one of the least known and least studied, although descriptions of falsified or exaggerated illness go back several centuries in the medical literature (Eisendrath 1996). Factitious disorders are characterized by the intentional production or feigning of illness in the absence of the clear external incentives that are present for malingerers. In the not uncommon case where there is both an apparent motivation to assume the sick role and external incentives, factitious disorder would be diagnosed when assuming the sick role was judged to be the primary goal. Given the covert nature of disorders involving conscious deception, the true prevalence of falsified illness in the general population is not known, although there are some studies which have attempted to identify the percentage of medical patients within a specific diagnostic group whose symptoms are judged to be factitious in origin (Reich and Gottfried 1983).

Studies of adult patients with various forms of illness deception including malingering and factitious disorder have reported evidence that there may be earlier origins of this behaviour, regardless of the age at which patients are eventually identified. Raymond (1987) reported on a literature search of 186 patients with Munchausen syndrome, the most persistent and chronic form of factitious disorder, which were reported between 1951 through 1985, and where age of onset was indicated. While the average age at diagnosis of Munchausen syndrome was 32 years, the mean age of onset was reported as 21.2 years of age. Significantly, 41 per cent had reportedly developed the syndrome by age 18, and 74 per cent by age 24 years. Many of these patients must have manifested early signs of illness deception in adolescence and perhaps earlier, but remained undetected for years.

Reich and Gottfried's (1983) study of adult factitious disorder reported that all of their patients who were inducing their own infections had commenced this behaviour in adolescence, although they were commonly identified years later. From the number of papers that retrospectively identify earlier origins, it is clear that many patients practice illness deception for many years before a diagnosis is finally established. This raises intriguing questions about the developmental process by which a young person establishes a pattern of deceiving physicians and family, and comes to manifest this behaviour in later life. It also raises questions about the often delayed process of identifying this problem by physicians, and the reasons for a lack of vigilance or reluctance to consider diagnoses of factitious disorder or malingering at the earliest stages in the evolution of the process.

Diagnostic confusion

It is well known that non-specific, non-physiological, and functional problems are significant concerns in paediatric and adolescent practice (Silber 1982) although there is often little diagnostic specificity to the assignment of somatoform diagnoses and surprisingly little consideration of intentional deception. In fact, the terms 'somatoform' or 'psychosomatic' disorder are often used quite loosely to include any medically presented problems with both physical and psychological components.

While data do not exist on the actual prevalence of malingered and/or factitious illness in children, there are some data on other categories of somatoform disorders. For example, Prazar (1987) suggests that the prevalence of conversion symptoms for children and adolescents in primary care settings is between 5 and 13 per cent, appearing as early as 7 or 8 years of age. These children are described as characteristically egocentric, labile, demanding, and attention-seeking. Yet we have no way of knowing whether a small or large number of these patients may actually be deceiving their physicians intentionally because, as in adults, the detection of intentional deception in younger people is difficult. Patients are unlikely to directly admit to deception, leaving the physician in the unpleasant position of having to either 'catch the patient in the act', or having to devise some clever plan that proves the patient can only be intentionally inducing or exacerbating the medical problem. With young children, some physicians have been successful in revealing the child's conscious control of the symptom through making bets or predictions that the child cannot, in fact, control the target symptom. In some cases the youngster will 'win' the bet by proving his or her ability to immediately resolve the problem. While this is clearly not a reliable or definitive method of assessing conscious control, it can prove helpful in these often murky areas.

The concept of a child inducing illness may be particularly aversive or unpalatable to physicians treating children, perhaps contributing to the substantially greater preference for or comfort with identifying 'psychosomatic' disorders in children (Campo and Fritsch 1994). Just as paediatricians treating seemingly devoted mothers often have great difficulty even entertaining the notion that a mother may be harming her child intentionally even when faced with compelling evidence as in many cases of Munchausen by proxy abuse (Schreier and Libow 1993), it seems equally challenging for a paediatrician to believe that an 11- or 14-year old could be successfully deceiving him or her, as opposed to unintentionally enacting unconscious conflicts.

Issues of motivation are as difficult as issues of intentionality when it comes to children, so that distinguishing between malingering and factitious illness becomes equally challenging. Differentiating the nature of the motivation underlying illness deception may be even more problematic for child patients. For adult patients, determining that a patient with a questionable 'illness' is, for example, seeking eligibility for disability payments seems much clearer a motivation than the often more indirect gains achieved by younger patients. Yet the default assumption that neither the child's medical symptoms nor motivations are under conscious control or awareness—a decision often made with little consideration even of the possibility of deception—may preclude important opportunities for accurate identification.

Contributing to the clinician's difficulty in using a diagnostic system based on adult models and diagnoses is the fact that children's lives lack the time frame to provide a context of historical data and established behavioural patterns which are so useful in informing our diagnoses of adults. For example, even children with somatizing patterns of behaviour are unlikely to present with the eight multi-organ symptoms and extensive histories necessary for a somatization diagnosis. Furthermore, children are still in the process of undergoing transformations in their conceptual skills, including their conceptions of illness, comprehension of treatment regimens, coping skills, and relationships with their parents—all factors known to affect their interpretation and management of symptoms, compliance with treatments and illness behaviours (Kenny and Willoughby 2001). These are complex areas to examine and assess in children who may not even be particularly articulate or communicative.

In addition to all of the above difficulties in accurately suspecting as well as assessing intentionality and motivation, there are a number of not uncommon medical problems in young people which can involve varying degrees of intentional falsification yet are rarely classified as such. For these puzzling conditions, the degree of conscious participation may actually shift over time, or vary with different incidents. Examples include pseudo-seizures (Goodyer 1985; Stores 1999) in which a child may have a *bona fide* seizure disorder yet also manifest pseudo-seizures that may or may not be intentionally feigned. Other examples include dermatitis artefacta which may include an element of occasional or frequent exacerbation of a *bona fide* rash or infection. Lyell (1976) describes several adolescent cases of factitious dermatitis artefacta and recommends that the physician remain alert for and suspicious of factitious illness while pointing out that patients may have great difficulty explaining their motives even while aware of their deception. Also in this category is Gardner–Diamond syndrome, which may be factitious (Sheppard *et al.* 1986), as is paradoxical vocal cord motion (Maschka *et al.* 1997) which may also include a combination or a fluctuating mix of intentional and nonintentional vocal cord activity resulting in respiratory difficulty. Such factors as the problem's resolution during sleep, lack of patient cooperation during medical evaluations, poor treatment compliance, and a fascination by the patient with the medical world are suggested as possible clues to illness deception.

Differentiating external incentives in children

The process of assessing the patient's degree of conscious motivation for external gain versus unconscious motivation is difficult even in adult patients. Such factors as obtaining disability income or supporting a lawsuit are among those more commonly identified in adult malingerers, and are generally assessed through observation of the objective gains obtained by the patient in the course of the 'illness' and the degree of calculated behaviours of the patient directed toward these ends. Malingerers are also described as less apparently driven by the desire for medical tests and painful procedures for their own sake than are factitious disorder patients, and are much less cooperative in subjecting themselves to unpleasant procedures unless there are tangible gains to be had.

However, the identification of conscious motivation in the child patient is rather more complicated. Due to their nature as dependents, children with any illness will almost always gain from increased parental attention and solicitousness, and will avoid having to attend school during their period of invalidism. Their illness almost always allows for the avoidance of developmentally appropriate demands on their time (such as homework and peer socialization) which may be rewarding for many children. Many children are showered with gifts from family members during periods of illness (stuffed animals, videogames, etc.). Children from disorganized or impoverished families may find the life of an invalid (e.g. a nurturing hospital environment, playrooms stacked with toys, reliable daily meals) a welcome change from home, regardless of whether they could articulate these incentives. In summary, it is quite a challenging task to rule out external gain for young people in favour of unconscious motivation to assume the sick role, since certain benefits are nearly universal.

Illness falsification in children

Despite the evidence that illness deception can begin prior to adulthood, the phenomenon of illness falsification by children and adolescents has received surprisingly limited attention. A recent literature review by this author (Libow 2000) identified a small but intriguing number of reports describing 42 cases of conscious deception by children as young as 4 and averaging about 14 years of age. Subsequent to that review, 16 additional cases have been located (Sneddon and Sneddon 1975; Stutts and Hickson 1999). While this number may seem quite small, it is important to remember that it represents only cases of active induction of illness and excludes all cases of exaggerated symptoms (e.g. headaches, stomach pain, dizziness, etc.) that may be escaping notice as intentional deception or are being more conservatively grouped within the conversion symptoms, psychosomatic disorders, or one of the many medical problems of unknown origin. In adult illness deception, it is believed that there is significantly more exaggerated symptomatology than actively induced illness, and there is no reason to believe that this is different for younger people. Furthermore, it is difficult to estimate the number of actual cases of illness deception by children based solely on the percentage that have been recognized or reported as such in the literature.

As in adults, the falsifications by children and adolescents span a wide range of symptoms from rather crudely induced bruises to very elaborate manipulations involving induced infections, haemorrhages, and other complex medical puzzles. The most commonly reported conditions include fever of unknown origin, ketoacidosis, purpura, and infections. Not surprisingly, the deceptions of the youngest children tend to be the most concrete and simple, such as warming thermometers with heating pads or sucking on drinking glasses to cause facial rashes. As in adult illness falsifications, some of the deceptions of the older children are quite creative and elaborate, such as ingesting steroids to cause factitious Cushing syndrome (Witt and Ginsberg-Fellner 1981), or introducing egg and other foreign matter into the bladder to cause proteinuria and feculent urine (Reich *et al.* 1977).

The gender ratio for children is remarkably close to the 3 : 1 female to male ratio noted for adult factitious disorder patients (Taylor and Hyler 1993). All 13 of the children under 14 years of age for whom data were available (Libow 2000) actually admitted to or did not deny their intentional deceptions when they were confronted, resulting in a 100 per cent confession rate, while only 55 per cent of the older children admitted to their falsifications when confronted.

Aetiology of illness falsification

A number of explanatory models have been proposed for the development of somatization and/or illness falsification in children. Most obvious is the notion of children's vulnerability to learning, suggestion, and modelling of the somatizing behaviours of a parent (Krener 1994) who him or herself focuses on somatic representations of emotional states. Parents may even more actively reinforce the 'sick role' through their directed attention and caring for the child when ill, and the benefits they provide the child when incapacitated (Eisendrath 1996). O'Shea *et al.* (1984) expand upon this notion, proposing that for some emotionally immature mothers who are unable to relate emotionally to their children, the production of illness allows the mother a meaningful way to interact as caregiver to the youngster, which can become a learned and reinforced behaviour for the child.

The role of 'symptom coaching' by an actively fabricating parent may be quite powerful (Sanders 1995) and unfold in a gradual process of increasing collusion by child with parent which begins with naïve participation and may progress over time through a series of steps to active self-harm. This notion is supported by findings such as McGuire and Feldman's (1989) case studies of several Munchausen by proxy victims who began manifesting conversion disorders in adolescence and the early signs of symptom falsification. Munchausen by proxy abuse involves the intentional exaggeration or falsification of signs of illness in a child by a caregiver for the purpose of assuming the sick role through the child proxy. As in other forms of factitious disorder, the behaviours can range from mild exaggeration to life-threatening medical abuse, but physicians are often deceived into colluding with these deceptions for surprisingly long periods of time before recognizing the true nature of the 'illness' (Schreier and Libow 1993). The Munchausen by proxy literature offers several cases that demonstrate a multi-generational pattern of a parent falsifying her own illnesses in young adulthood, then moving on to Munchausen by proxy abuse, and eventually having a child who develops adult factitious disorder in later life (Palmer and Yoshimura 1984).

There are a number of ambiguous cases of illness falsification in children that have been described in the literature, combining primary falsification by a child with some level of care-giver collusion, or perhaps a prior history of Munchausen by proxy abuse of the child (Libow 2002). These 'blended' cases remind us that the parent's role should always be examined in any child case of suspected illness deception. In addition to the possibilities of modelling and direct reinforcement of deception by the parent, this author's earlier paper suggests that there are other elements of the Munchausen by proxy victimization experience which may promote the development of independent deception by the child. This includes feelings of powerlessness, chronic lack of control, and disappointment with the impotent physician figure who is unable to protect the child from a parent's medical abuse which may eventually foster the development of illness falsification by the young person.

It is also useful to consider the functions of lying for children. While the parent may have originally modelled or reinforced deception by the child, deceiving the physician may also serve some of the functions described in a fascinating paper by Wiley (1998). She points out that lying can serve to protect oneself or others, help a person obtain concrete benefits, promote self-esteem, or gratify an otherwise unobtainable fantasy. It can also promote autonomy/individuation, gratify sadistic wishes, or enhance personal power through devaluing others. A child feeling powerless or destructively enmeshed with a disturbed parent might very well find the act of illness deception a useful means of establishing some autonomy and control, albeit through very destructive means.

Case examples

Case A

Jose was a 6-year old Mexican-American boy who was referred for psychological services by the Neurology Department of a large urban hospital after being seen more than 16 times by specialists for monthly 'attacks' of vomiting, debilitation, and aggression. His mother described these incidents in unusual detail and said they always lasted for 4 days. During these 'attacks' Jose could not walk but was confined to a wheelchair and was absent from school. According to his single mother, a 30-year old woman never married to his abusive father, Jose's symptoms began at about 1 year of age. Despite MRIs, abdominal ultrasounds, and a variety of evaluations by neurology, gastroenterology, and endocrinology, there were no physical findings for his unusual 'attacks'. Nevertheless, Jose was medicated unsuccessfully with seven different medications over the course of 2 years. After his referral for psychological services, Jose was weaned off all medications. The many inconsistencies and incredible details of his illness raised major suspicion of illness deception although Jose would sit convincingly in his wheelchair, groaning in pain, clutching his emesis basin, unable to walk. Eventually, Jose was able to admit privately to his therapist that his mother wanted him to be sick and had encouraged his illness behaviours. However, it took Jose an additional 6 months of supportive psychotherapy before he was able to get up from his wheelchair during an 'attack' and eventually cease these behaviours completely.

Case B

Amy was a 12-year old Caucasian girl who lived alone with her single mother, who had a significant psychiatric history including her own self-admitted illness deception in adolescence. Amy was removed from her mother's care at age 11 after several years of being repeatedly treated for seizures which were never documented, and being over-medicated for headaches. She was noted to have a highly enmeshed relationship with her mother at the time of her removal. She was on several medications including Klonapin and Tegretol, from which she was successfully weaned when she left her mother's home.

The immediate precipitant for Amy's removal from her mother's custody was that she had begun to fabricate sexual abuse reports involving neighbours, which she eventually admitted were entirely false. She also pretended several times to have 'staring spells' after placement in a foster home. She eventually admitted that she was consciously falsifying these staring spells, but was unable to articulate the reasons for this behaviour, except that she had been 'upset' at the time. There was no evidence of maternal involvement in Amy's deceptions after her placement in foster care.

Prospects for early intervention

These cases are consistent with other findings that children manifesting factitious illnesses may be more responsive to direct confrontation than adults engaging in illness deception. For example, Wyllie *et al.* (1991) found that despite the fact that paediatric pseudo-seizure patients tended to have more episodes than adult patients, their psychogenic seizures stopped immediately after diagnosis in 44 per cent of the younger patients, but only in 20 per cent of the adult patients. They suggested that different psychological mechanisms may be relevant at different ages of onset, with anxiety or stress reactions more common for children and adolescent pseudo-seizure patients, while personality disorders may be more common in adults. They also suggested that the longer duration of psychogenic seizures in adults prior to diagnosis may have contributed to greater persistence of the problem.

Recommendations for physicians

As simple as it seems, it would be most useful and productive for the perplexed physician to begin by asking a child directly whether deception might be involved in a persistent medical problem that is otherwise unexplainable. If there is no admission of involvement, it is possible that a playful bet or prediction might result in the child's willingness to relinquish the symptoms. In some cases it might allow a child to save face and escape from a situation of deception that may not have entirely started intentionally (e.g. as in the treatment of a child with oral purpura which initially began innocently from sucking on a drinking glass and progressed to repeated incidents). Of course, the ability to ask or cajole the youngster into a discussion of intentional deception is predicated on the physician's awareness that young people can and do, on occasion, engage in such behaviour. Perhaps the starting point for family physicians is the willingness to question an often automatic assumption that medical complaints without an identifiable physical basis are necessarily unconscious and unintentional.

In addition to carefully exploring the possible benefits to the child of remaining 'sick' and the ongoing reinforcers in the family and medical world, the physician should consider the possible role of familial patterns of illness deception. Specifically, a thorough medical history of the patient should also include a careful medical history of siblings and caregivers which may provide important clues to possible parental factitious disorder, Munchausen by proxy abuse or other forms of collusion. Improbable histories of multiple unusual accidents, diseases or illnesses in a family, at a minimum, warrant further investigation. The physician's willingness to ask uncomfortable questions and entertain alternative explanations may be a critical factor in allowing a youngster to free him or herself from participation or collusion.

There are those in both the medical and mental health professions who feel that the elucidation of a patient's intent to deceive or individual motivations guiding the deceptions are too unscientific or impossible to discern, as they are so often based on inference and behavioural observation. However, it is just these issues of motivation and intent which are so crucial in making the appropriate treatment and placement decisions for the child. The most thorough understanding of the youngster's goals and intentions will help parents and medical caregivers develop a plan to prevent further reinforcement of the illness behaviours by the child's environment. It will also help prevent misattribution of symptoms to other disease entities or diagnoses resulting in further fruitless investigations or harmful treatments. The identification of illness deception in children and adolescents may offer our first and best opportunity to effectively intervene in the problem before it evolves into an increasingly covert adult problem of long duration.

References

American Psychiatric Association (1994). *Diagnostic and Statistical Manual of Mental Disorders*, 4th edn. American Psychiatric Association, Washington, DC.

Campo, J. V. and Fritsch, S. L. (1994). Somatization in children and adolescents. *Journal of the American Academy of Child and Adolescent Psychiatry*, **33**, 1223–35.

Eisendrath, S. J. (1996). Current overview of factitious physical disorders. In *The spectrum of factitious disorders* (eds M. D. Feldman and S. J. Eisendrath), pp. 21–37. American Psychiatric Press, Inc. Washington, DC.

Fritz, G. K., Fritsch, S. L., and Hagino, O. (1997). Somatoform disorders in children and adolescents: a review of the past 10 years. *Journal of the American Academy of Child and Adolescent Psychiatry*, **36**, 1329–38.

Goodyer, I. (1985). Epileptic and pseudoepileptic seizures in childhood and adolescence. *Journal of the American Academy of Child Psychiatry*, **24** (1), 3–9.

Kenny, T. J. and Willoughby, J. (2001). Psychosomatic problems in children. In *Handbook of Clinical Child Psychology, Third Edition* (eds C. E. Walker and M. C. Roberts), pp. 359–72. John Wiley and Sons, New York, NY.

Krener, P. (1994). Factitious disorders and the psychosomatic continuum in children. *Current Opinion in Pediatrics*, **6**, 418–22.

Libow, J. A. (2000). Child and adolescent illness falsification. *Pediatrics*, **105** (2), 336–42.

Libow, J. A. (2002). Beyond collusion: active illness falsification. *Child Abuse and Neglect*, **26**, 525–36.

Lyell, A. (1976). Dermatitis artefacta in relation to the syndrome of contrived disease. *Clinical and Experimental Dermatology*, **1**, 109–26.

Maschka, D. A., Bauman, N. M., McCray, P. B., Jr, Hoffman, H. T., Karnell, M. P., and Smith, R. J. (1997). A classification scheme for paradoxical vocal cord motion. *Laryngoscope*, **107** (11, Pt 1), 1429–35.

McGuire, T. L. and Feldman, K. W. (1989). Psychologic morbidity of children subjected to Munchausen syndrome by proxy. *Pediatrics*, **83** (2), 289–92.

O'Shea, B., McGennis, A., Cahill, M., and Falvey, J. (1984). Munchausen's syndrome. *British Journal of Hospital Medicine*, **31**, 269–74.

Palmer, A. J. and Yoshimura, G. J. (1984). Munchausen syndrome by proxy. *Journal of the American Academy of Child Psychiatry*, **23**, 503–8.

Prazar, G. (1987). Conversion reactions in adolescents. *Pediatrics in Review*, **8** (9), 279–86.

Raymond, C. A. (1987). Munchausen's may occur in younger persons. *Journal of the American Medical Association*, **257** (24), 3332.

Reich, P. and Gottfried, L. A. (1983). Factitious disorders in a teaching hospital. *Annals of Internal Medicine*, **99**, 240–7.

Reich, P., Lazarus, J. M., Kelly, M. J., and Rogers, M. P. (1977). Factitious feculent urine in an adolescent boy. *Journal of the American Medical Association*, **238**, 420–1.

Sanders, M. J. (1995). Symptom coaching: factitious disorder by proxy with older children. *Clinical Psychology Review*, **15**, 423–42.

Schreier, H. A. and Libow, J. A. (1993). *Hurting for love: Munchausen by proxy syndrome*. Guilford Publications, New York, NY.

Sheppard, N. P., O'Loughlin, S., and Malone, J. P. (1986). Psychogenic skin disease: a review of 35 cases. *British Journal of Psychiatry*, **149**, 636–43.

Silber, T. J. (1982). The differential diagnosis of functional symptoms. *Adolescence*, 1982, **17** (68), 769–78.

Sneddon, I. and Sneddon, J. (1975). Self-inflicted injury: a follow-up study of 43 patients. *British Medical Journal*, **3**, 527–30.

Stores, G. (1999). Practitioner review: recognition of pseudoseizures in children and adolescents. *Journal of Child Psychology and Psychiatry and Allied Disciplines*, **40** (6), 851–7.

Stutts, J. F. and Hickson, G. B. (1999). Factitious disorders in children and adolescents. *Ambulatory Child Health*, **5**, 313–21.

Taylor, S. and Hyler, S. E. (1993). Update on factitious disorders. *International Journal of Psychiatry in Medicine*, **23**, 81–94.

Wiley, S. D. (1998). Deception and detection in psychiatric diagnosis. *The Psychiatric Clinics of North America*, **21** (4), 869–93.

Witt, M. E. and Ginsberg-Fellner, F. (1981). Prednisone-induced Munchausen syndrome. *American Journal of Diseases in Children*, **135**, 852–3.

Wyllie, E., Friedman, D., Luders, H., Morris, H., Rothner, D., and Turnbull, J. (1991). Outcome of psychogenic seizures in children and adolescents compared with adults. *Neurology*, **41**, 742–4.

12 Distinguishing malingering from psychiatric disorders

Michael Sharpe

Abstract

Malingering is rarely considered when a person has evidence of definite physical pathology that explains their symptoms. Psychiatric illness offers a special challenge in that few psychiatric diagnoses have associated physical pathology but are diagnosed purely on subjective report. This leaves those with psychiatric illness potentially open to the accusation their illnesses are merely feigned. Theoretically, malingering is distinguished from psychiatric illness by the absence of psychopathology, the identification of 'secondary gain', and a conscious intent to deceive in order to obtain the gain. However, psychopathology is hypothetical, secondary gain is non-specific, and the determination of the extent that intent is conscious probably impossible. Hence, only inconsistency of symptoms as a proxy for lack of psychopathology is objectively demonstrable. It is argued that the answer to a question of 'Is this patient malingering?' should be reframed, as 'Are this patient's symptoms and disability consistent with a psychiatric illness'. The answer should include a summary of the evidence for inconsistency, an opinion about the presence of a relevant psychiatric illness and a clear statement about the limitation of such an opinion. Malingering is not a psychiatric diagnosis and its identification arguably not a medical task.

What is malingering?

To malinger is to pretend, exaggerate, or protract illness in order to escape duty or achieve some other advantage (Gorman 1982). Within the military setting, the gain is most likely to be the avoidance of duty (see Palmer, Chapter 3). In civilian life, the gains a malingerer might seek are more varied and include not only avoiding work and obligations, but also obtaining various benefits including money. The allegation of malingering is serious and pejorative and few would wish to apply it inappropriately. However, the feigning of psychiatric illness does undoubtedly occur. Overwhelming evidence proves it in a small number of cases (Sparr and Pankratz 1983) and it may be suspected in many others. The degree of exaggeration that occurs in routine clinical practice in unknown. Marked deception is however probably relatively rare outside special situations such as medical legal practice. The concept of malingering is a complex one and it may be regarded as having a number of components. All of these components must be present for a judgement of malingering to be appropriate (see Table 12.1). As we shall see, they are all also potentially problematic, especially in relation to psychiatric illness.

Table 12.1 Characteristics of malingering

- Unexplained by disease—symptoms and/or disability are not adequately explained by objectively defined disease
- Gain—there is a tangible external gain from presenting as ill
- Intention—deliberate and conscious intent to deceive the doctor or other persons
- Context and value—a situation where the genuineness of illness is scrutinized.

The symptoms and disability are feigned

The core concept of malingering is that the person is feigning or exaggerating symptoms and/or disability. This, of course, begs the question as to what criteria are used to identify when symptoms are 'genuine'. For medical conditions, this judgement is usually based largely on whether the reported symptoms and disability are consistent with the observed physical pathology. In psychiatry where few diagnoses have any identified physical pathology, this issue is more difficult to address.

The person stands to gain from been regarded as ill

Malingering also implies that the deception is done to obtain personal advantage. The advantage obtained in the external world, such as financial compensation, has been referred to as secondary gain (Fishbain *et al.* 1995) (as opposed to primary gain where the advantage is only to achieve a desired change in the person's internal world). However, many persons, whose symptoms are a clear consequence of disease such as cancer, may appear to obtain gain from being ill. For example, they may obtain compensation for previous exposure to asbestos. Secondary gain is therefore a necessary but by no means a specific feature of malingering.

There is an intention to deceive

Malingering implies not only that the symptoms and impairment are feigned, but also that the person has the conscious and deliberate intent of deceiving others to obtain the secondary gain. Intent is a complex concept however. First, there is probably a continuum from fully conscious to unconscious intention. Second, the intent to exaggerate may have other motivations than the obtaining of secondary gain. For example, patients may exaggerate their symptoms to gain the doctor's attention in order to ensure adequate treatment. Finally, the usual way of determining a person's actual intent is for the patient to express this verbally. Establishing a person's intention, when you have reason to doubt the veracity of what he/she tells you, is deeply problematic (see Malle, Chapter 6).

Malingering is context dependent

Finally, even if all the aforementioned criteria are fulfilled, whether the label of malingering is applied or not depends on the context and the associated value judgements. For example, if a prisoner of war prevented the enemy acquiring sensitive information by feigning mental illness, we would probably regard this as an heroic act rather than as malingering. Whether behaviour receives the pejorative label of malingering depends on the context and whether we approve of their deception or not.

Summary

Malingering is a complex concept with a number of elements. Its basis is that symptoms are exaggerated or made up. In order to determine its presence one has to have reliable criteria to determine what is a genuine psychiatric illness. Given that few psychiatric diagnoses have any identifiable physical pathology, this criterion cannot be used to validate the diagnosis. We must therefore consider further how psychiatric illness is defined, before going on to consider in more detail its distinction from malingering.

What is a psychiatric illness?

Psychiatric illness may be defined in several different ways as listed in Table 12.2.

Subjectively defined illness

Most psychiatric illness is defined in terms of symptoms. In this context, it is important to consider the distinction between 'illness' and 'disease'. Illness is the patient's subjective experience of symptoms; disease is the objectively identifiable pathology (Susser 1990). Psychiatric conditions should therefore be regarded as illnesses, not as diseases (although this distinction is often 'fudged' by calling them 'disorders'). This observation leaves the person with psychiatric illness open to the charge that they do not really have an illness but are merely manifesting a deviant behaviour (Szasz 1991). It is, however, generally accepted that subjectively defined illness represents as genuine an experience of suffering and impairment as those illnesses that are defined by objective pathology. Increasing evidence from functional imaging in patients with psychiatric disorders supports the view that, even if such conditions do not have gross pathology, they are associated with brain states that are distinguishable from normality (Gur 2002).

It is also worth noting that the problems posed by subjectively defined illness are not limited to psychiatry. The so-called medical 'functional somatic syndromes', which make up a large part of medical practice, and include conditions such as chronic fatigue syndrome, irritable bowel syndrome, migraine headache, and various pain complaints (Wessely *et al.* 1999) are also defined only in terms of symptoms. Indeed such patients are also likely to meet criteria for the psychiatric diagnosis of somatoform disorder (American Psychiatric Association 1994).

Hence, if we accept that subjectively defined illness can be real illness, we depend on the honesty of the patient reporting the symptoms. The lack of obvious criteria for validating those reported symptoms objectively make a judgement of possible malingering problematic.

An abnormal mental state or behaviour

Given that psychiatric illness is defined in terms of symptoms and the fact that we all experience symptoms, we must ask when do subjective symptoms and associated behaviour become an illness. The generally accepted answer is when they are unusually severe and persistent. Hence,

Table 12.2 What the label 'psychiatric disorder' may imply?

- A purely subjective or 'mental' illness
- A statistically abnormal state or behaviour
- A condition described in the psychiatric diagnostic classifications
- A manifestation of psychopathology

although we all get depressed, major depression is only diagnosed when the symptoms that define depression have persisted for at least 2 weeks and are associated with 'clinically significant distress or impairment' (American Psychiatric Association 1994). A key feature of the definition of illness therefore is persistence over time and usually across situations. This requirement of consistency may be used to address the question of malingering (see below).

It appears in a diagnostic classification

For symptoms to indicate a psychiatric illness, they must not only be severe and persistent, but they must also match a recognized pattern. The recognized patterns that allow a doctor to diagnose psychiatric illnesses are described in textbooks, shaped by clinical experience, and listed in official diagnostic classifications. The main current classifications of psychiatric disorder are the fourth version of the *Diagnostic and Statistical Manual* (DSM-IV) of the American Psychiatric Association (1994) and the 10th edition of the International Classification of Diseases (ICD-10) of the World Health Organization (1992). These two classifications are both widely used. They are similar but not identical. It is important to note that the definition of psychiatric illness contained in these manuals, although based on scientific research, is ultimately the creation of committees. Hence, psychiatric diagnoses (and arguably all diagnoses) are not based on 'carving nature at the joints' but are ultimately best regarded as constructions for practical purposes (Scadding 1996). As an example of this, diagnostic descriptions can be seen to differ between classifications and between different versions of the same classifications. Neither do the specific diagnostic categories have precise boundaries as it is recognized that even if a patient's symptoms do not clearly fit the diagnostic criteria they may have an 'atypical' form of the condition (Davidson *et al.* 1982).

These classifications are therefore essentially guides to clinical practice and service adminis-tration (Kendell 1975). They are not 'rule books' that reliably and precisely define which illnesses are 'real' or legitimate and which are not (even though they may be misused by the courts and other for this purpose). Once one appreciates these limitations, it can be seen that 'degree of fit' with defined categories is a potentially useful but imperfect way of distinguishing 'genuine' from feigned psychiatric illness.

It is an expression of psychopathology

One approach to the validation of psychiatric illness is the concept of 'psychopathology'. This is based on the supposition that there can be malfunctions or pathology of the mind akin to the physical pathology of the body (Lewis 1953). Psychopathology is quoted by both the current major classifications (World Health Organization 1992; American Psychiatric Association 1994) as a justification for regarding the illnesses described in them as valid. However, psychopatho-logy, unlike physical pathology is a hypothetical concept; we cannot dissect the patient's mind to discover an objectively verifiable lesion. Although recent advances in biological psychiatry provide the beginnings on an objective 'neuropsychopathology' based on observable evidence of dysfunction in brain systems (Gur 2002), at present we have to infer psychopathology from clinical observation. Those observations are first whether the pattern of the patient's symptoms is consistent with recognized psychopathology (i.e. recognized patterns of symptoms) and second whether the symptoms are associated with dysfunction, in practice meaning that they are disad-vantageous to the patient. For example, in order to decide whether a patient's report of inability to drive a motorcar is an expression of psychopathology, we might proceed as follows. First, we could seek evidence of a pattern of symptoms, consistent with recognized descriptions of anxiety, was present so that the psychopathology of anxiety could potentially be inferred. Second, we might judge whether not being able to drive was disadvantageous (rather than advantageous) to the patient to infer dysfunction. If both were present, we might conclude that the disability was a result of psychopathology. Hence, whilst the concept of psychopathology provides some theoretical validity to the concept of psychiatric illness, in practice however, it is of limited value as it still relies on the patient's subjective reports and the clinician's judgement.

Summary

Psychiatric diagnoses have proved to be of considerable utility in enabling clinicians to pool and share information about patients and to define relatively homogenous groups of patients for the purposes of clinical practice and research. They are based mainly on specified patterns of symptoms and behaviours. They do not have precise boundaries and allow atypical forms. They are underpinned by the theoretical concept of psychopathology and whilst the identification of objectively definable abnormalities of brain function, for example on functional imaging scans, offers the promise of an 'objective neuropsychopathology', such methods remain of little practical use at present. How then can we distinguish feigned from 'genuine' psychiatric illness?

Distinguishing malingering from psychiatric illness

As the diagnosis of most psychiatric illnesses is based on reported symptoms, the problem becomes one of how we distinguish a feigned subjective illness from a 'genuine' subjective illness. In other words, if I tell you that 'I feel depressed', how can you judge if I am telling you the truth? Ultimately of course, you cannot, because you cannot know my subjective experience better than I know it myself. But you can make a judgement. I will argue that the core of that judgement is based on the concept of consistency. That is we expect a psychiatric illness to be consistent in a variety of ways. Possible inconsistencies are listed in Table 12.3.

Inconsistency

The first type of consistency to consider is that between the different elements of the history. A history with inconsistent listing of dates of symptoms may reflect illness such as cognitive impairment (Barsky 2002). However, in the absence of other explanations, significant inconsistency in the history may raise doubts about whether the reported symptoms reflect illness. The second sort of inconsistency to consider is that between the described symptoms and the patient's observed behaviour. For example, the patient who says they are depressed but do not behave as if they are. Again, there are other potential explanations for this, such as the concept of 'masked depression' (Fisch 1987) but such an inconsistency may also question the presence of illness. The third type of inconsistency is between the reported symptoms and those described in the diagnostic

Table 12.3 Types of consistency used to support a diagnosis of illness

- Within the history
- Between history and observation of behaviour
- Between symptoms and published diagnostic criteria
- Between history from patient and informant
- Between the patient's history and the medical records
- Over time (between examinations or during admission)
- Between the history and other sources of information (see Table 12.4)

manuals as typical of specific psychiatric illnesses. The value of this must not be overestimated however, given the need to accept atypical cases. However, the failure to report typical symptoms and especially the endorsement of very atypical symptoms may raise doubts about the presence of illness (Jaffe and Sharma 1998). The fourth area of consistency is between the reported history and a variety of other observations that are distinct in time and/or place. Whilst some psychiatric conditions do typically fluctuate over time (panic attacks, for example can be unpredictable potent causes of symptoms) marked inconsistency will also raise doubts about whether the person is ill.

The conscious motivation to deceive

Even if gross inconsistency is observed and the symptoms do not convincingly fit that expected for a psychiatric illness, one cannot necessarily conclude that the person is malingering. That is because the definition of malingering requires a conscious and deliberate intention to deceive. A problem arises if one accepts, as most people do, that motivations can be unconscious to various degrees. Perhaps the most problematic issue in the distinction of psychiatric illness from malingering is represented by the diagnoses of dissociation and conversion disorders. As with malingering, these diagnoses are defined on symptoms with loss of function (such as weakness or loss of memory) that result from unconscious processes (Mai 1995). DSM-IV differentiates conversion disorder from malingering as follows: 'The distinguishing feature of conversion symptoms being the lack of conscious intent in the production of the symptoms.' Psychiatry has conventionally considered unconscious exaggeration of symptoms and disability to be a genuine illness (Ford and Folks 1985). Given that we have no 'intentometer', the judgement about whether deception is conscious or unconscious is difficult if not impossible. Recent attempts to distinguish conversion disorder from feigned symptoms using functional brain imaging are intriguing but far from conclusive (Spence *et al.* 2000).

The nature of the secondary gain

Even illness that is judged both feigned with deliberate and conscious motivation does not necessarily qualify as malingering. The psychiatric classifications define certain gains as indicating illness rather than malingering. Specifically, if illness is feigned with the aim of obtaining medical attention and treatment, rather than some other gain such as money, it is deemed a genuine psychiatric illness, namely factitious disorder (Sutherland and Rodin 1990). DSM-IV differentiates factitious disorder from malingering as follows: 'In contrast [to malingering] in factitious disorder the motivation is a psychological need to assume the sick role as evidenced by the absence of external incentives for their behaviour' and 'Malingering may be considered to be adaptive under certain circumstances (for example in hostage situations) but by a definition a diagnosis of factitious disorder always *implies psychopathology*' (American Psychiatric Association 1994). On the face of it, this means that if a person feigns illness apparently in order get money they are well and if to obtain unnecessary medical attention they must be ill! We see again that the key issue is the theoretical imputation of psychopathology, which is implied by behaviour, and judged maladaptive. In practice, although patients with factitious disorder may be distinguishable by a long history of similar behaviour and associated severe psychopathology, the distinction from malingering may often not be clear (Eisendrath 1996). The distinction has some clinical utility, but its ultimate theoretical basis appears to be questionable.

The context

Even if we believe that the person has fulfilled all the necessary criteria, would we always find it appropriate or helpful to label the behaviour as malingering? Probably not, because in routine clinical practice many doctors, perhaps especially psychiatrists, are unlikely to label their patients as malingerers. That is because in clinical practice, the doctor's primary role is to help his or her patients with their subjectively voiced needs, not to determine their 'genuineness'. Some psychiatrists may even regard malingering as an expression of a psychological need that they should help the patient to address in a way that was more socially acceptable. There are, however, exceptions to this, which are discussed below.

Why is malingering itself not a psychiatric disorder?

In this context, it is interesting to consider why malingering is not generally considered a psychiatric illness. The current psychiatric classifications do not include malingering as a diagnosis but list it in their appendices. DSM-IV refers to malingering as: 'An additional condition that may be a focus on clinical attention' (American Psychiatric Association 1994) and ICD-10 as 'Factors influencing health status and contact with health services' (World Health Organization 1992). On the one hand, it involves the reporting of symptoms, and it is deviant (in that it goes beyond the minor exaggeration for illness for social convenience most people occasionally use). On the other hand, it is judged not to be a manifestation of psychopathology. It is interesting to pursue this question further by asking what we would need to do to successfully argue that malingering should be 'upgraded' from behaviour to a psychiatric disorder. We might, for example, differentiate between successful and unsuccessful malingerers (Edens *et al.* 2001). If a person malingered persistently but unsuccessfully—that is, their behaviour was manifestly dysfunctional, would they then be awarded psychiatric disorder status (perhaps with 'dysfunctional malingering disorder or DMD'). Here we stray into the territory of whether a persistent maladaptive outcome associated with distress should be sufficient to define a behaviour as an illness and consequently to make it a legitimate reason to seek medical attention. This is a contested area that has been frequently debated in relation to the so-called personality disorders, which are regarded as dysfunctional, but not as being associated with psychopathology (Lopez-Ibor 1997). (Also see Chapter 7.)

Summary

We can see from the above that malingering can theoretically be distinguished from psychiatric illness because it violates the theoretical assumptions of psychopathology. However, the distinction is difficult and arguably often impossible in practice. Controversially, one might wish to argue that a persistent unsuccessful malingerer whose life was damaged by his behaviour might, like the alcoholic, be considered to have progressed from simple social deviancy to psychiatric illness. This is not currently an accepted view however.

What can be done in practice?

Given the difficulty in making a positive 'diagnosis' of malingering, what can be realistically done in practice? In the remaining part of this chapter, I shall address how the clinician may address this problem. I will argue that the label of malingering should be applied only with extreme caution, if at all. Rather the clinician should confine him or her self to a judgement about the extent to which he or she is convinced that the patients in question suffer from a relevant psychiatric illness (see Chapter 17). I shall also argue that the key evidence to be sought and upon which to make this judgement is that of consistency (Vanderploeg and Curtiss 2001). Statements about consciousness of motivation and associated gains are, in reality, opinions and should be regarded as such (but see Chapter 6).

In what circumstances is a judgement about 'genuineness' of illness required?

Concern with whether a person has the illness they purport to have arises where the doctor sees himself or herself as having a role in determining that person's eligibility for something. There are two main reasons for this. The first is for the patient's own welfare. An example would be when a treatment is contemplated that may harm the patient (e.g. psychosurgery). This is most likely to be an issue where the exaggeration is related to a factitious disorder. The second is for the general good. This may occur when the doctor has to determine the patient's eligibility to precious shared resources such as state benefits, compensation, or a scarce treatment (e.g. intensive psychotherapy). In such cases, a judgement, however difficult it might be, is arguably required. This judgement is best made based on all the available evidence.

Detecting inconsistency

Research suggests that, at least on the basis of routine medical assessments, doctors are rather poor at detecting when patients are feigning symptoms (Faust 1995). Indeed, the only truly valid means of detection would appear to be when the patient admits that they are doing this, for example, 'Sorry—I was putting it on doc!' In other cases, a decision on whether the patient is genuinely psychiatrically ill or not is a judgement, and one best based on the consistency of the totality of the evidence available as described above. How can the doctor best obtain evidence of such inconsistency?

The context

There are certain contexts where the risk of exaggeration or even feigning of symptoms is likely to be higher. These will include where the patient: (a) stands to gain substantially, or to avoid a negative consequence by claiming to be ill; (b) has a previous history of similar behaviour; and (c) has a history of repeated deception of others or even a diagnosis of psychopathic personality disorder. It is important to note that whilst such factors probably increase the risk of the misleading reporting of symptoms it cannot be assumed. Even liars get sick.

The patient's history

First, it should be obvious that a good quality and appropriately lengthy clinical interview is likely to be a better detector of inconsistency than a cursory one. Allowing the patient the appropriate time to describe their problems exhaustively using predominantly open-ended questions, as opposed to simply requiring that they endorse symptoms from a checklist, is likely to give the doctor a much better idea of the extent to they are describing symptoms that he or she would regard as consistent with the clinical diagnosis. The factors in the history which are often suggested as reasons to doubt the history include an overly dramatic presentation of complaints, symptoms that do not match accepted symptom patterns and internal inconsistency between the aspects of the history.

There is also some evidence that endorsement of long lists of proffered symptoms can identify feigning in experimental paradigms, but in a clinical setting may simply reflect a tendency to agree with a doctor. The history should also address the patient's previous history to seek evidence of persistence and recurrence of specific patterns over time.

The mental state examination

In the mental state examination, the main task is to identify patterns of symptoms that suggest psychiatric illness and to compare it with the usual range of presentations as described in texts. This may best be detected using semi-structured diagnostic interview such as the SCID (Spitzer et al. 1992). The mental state examination also provides an opportunity to compare history and observation; for example, if the person describes severe anxiety or depression, do they manifest this in the interview?

The physical examination

This is of limited value when diagnosing psychiatric disorders. Where there are physical complaints, however, such as in conversion disorder it may be informative. For example, a patient with unexplained back pain who is unable to raise his/her leg straight but is able to sit straight up (Waddell et al. 1984).

Other sources of information

Inconsistency may also be suspected from information obtained from sources other than the patient, for example, covert video surveillance.

History from an informant

The history from an informant may or may not corroborate the patient's story. It should be noted however that an informant may have a stake in proving the patient ill (e.g. if they are a spouse who also stand to gain from a legal settlement) or may be under emotional or other pressure from the patient to concur with his story. Major discrepancies may however cast doubt on the presence of psychiatric illness.

Investigations and psychometric tests

There are very few diagnostic investigations in psychiatry and there are none specific for malingering. Neuropsychological tests may have value in assessing the patient who reports cognitive impairment. Much has been made of tests that seek inconsistency and in particular those that determine whether responses to a task the person can do that is worse than that expected by chance (Slick et al. 1999) (and see Chapter 25 by Frederick). Similarly, extreme or improbable responses on a variety of self-report scales such as the MMPI have been advocated as effective discriminators between genuine illness and feigning (Bagby et al. 2000). However, whilst such a result clearly demonstrates one aspect of inconsistency, it does not establish if the inconsistency is consciously motivated. Investigations and tests are therefore of probably of less value that is sometimes claimed.

Observation over time

Observation of the patient over a period longer than the duration of a typical clinical interview may provide additional information. Such observation may be achieved in one of several ways as listed in Table 12.4.

Table 12.4 Sources of information that allow the testing of consistency across situations

- Observation of the patient by the doctor (e.g. arriving or leaving the consultation)
- Notes recorded by others in the patients records
- Reports of other professionals, for example, a physiotherapist
- An inpatient assessment
- Covert surveillance of the patient by private detectives often recorded on a video camera

Often, the non-medical investigation of covert surveillance by private detectives provides the strongest evidence. In a legal context, it is also the most likely source of information that a lawyer will use to challenge the veracity of patient's reported disability. In some cases, there will be very striking discrepancies between the behaviour observed on the resulting videotape and the portrayal of disability to the clinician. This may be useful in documenting inconsistency when severe disability is being claimed, for example, in complaints of paralysis or severe phobic avoidance. However, for many psychiatric disorders, this is of limited value as conditions such as depression are variable and not easily assessed by surveillance.

Issues arising in relation to specific psychiatric diagnosis

In order to supplement the general suggestions made above I shall consider specific psychiatric diagnoses.

Post-traumatic stress disorder (PTSD)

This psychiatric diagnosis is defined by symptoms that are essentially those of a chronic anxiety disorder with the special characteristic of the re-experiencing in imagination of a traumatic event. This re-experiencing is associated with emotional arousal and a marked tendency to avoid reminders of the event (Davidson and Foa 1991). PTSD is unusual amongst psychiatric illnesses in that the defining phenomena actually encapsulate a specific traumatic event. It therefore makes issues of eligibility for compensation much clearer than for other disorders such as depression. Anecdotally it is suggested that lawyers may focus on the possibility of PTSD and may read out the diagnostic criteria to their clients, thereby schooling patients in how to respond at interview (Sparr 1995). Certainly most psychiatrists experienced in doing medical examinations are sceptical about many cases of alleged PTSD presenting in a context of compensation seeking following very trivial incidents.

PTSD also has features that may assist the examiner seeking evidence of inconsistency. Whilst 'flashbacks' are purely subjective, the behaviour of expression of distress and autonomic arousal associated with recollection of the trauma (observable sweating and shaking) may be less amenable to feigning. The examiner may be suspicious of the patient who recounts the accident in detail with any evidence of such. The tendency to avoid reminders of the trauma also provides a target for subsequent surveillance in order to test the consistency of reported behaviour across situations.

Case example

A 30-year-old man being assessed for compensation said that whilst working as an electrician a water tank had overflowed and led to him suffering an electric shock. He now described avoiding electrical equipment and never going out in the rain because he believed he might be at risk of shock if he got wet. At interview, he described the circumstances of his electrocution in dramatic detail without showing any evidence of distress or autonomic arousal. The examining clinician suspected that the complaints might be exaggerated although his symptoms were in keeping with those listed in the DSM classification. A diagnosis of probable PTSD was made. The doctor was subsequently sent videotape made by a private investigator in which the patient was noted to walk out in the pouring rain to visit a sun bed parlour. This new information cast considerable doubt on the patient's report.

This case illustrates inconsistency across situations and the value of sources of information other than a single interview with a clinician who is predisposed to understanding sympathetically the reports of the patient.

Psychosis

Psychosis is the term for psychiatric illness characterized by delusions and/or hallucinations. The main subtypes are schizophrenia and psychotic mood disorders. Psychosis is more likely to be malingered in a context of avoiding criminal compensation rather than in a case for compensation.

Feigned schizophrenia can be misdiagnosed as genuine schizophrenia as was documented in the much quoted study in which subjects were admitted to psychiatric hospital after reporting (incorrectly) that they were suffering hallucinations (Rosenhan 1973). There has also been a theoretically plausible but contested argument about whether such false reporting can be unconsciously feigned or not. It seems likely that it does, the counter argument being that 'you have to be mad to act mad' (Bishop and Holt 1980).

Case example

A 25-year-old man presented for admission at a psychiatric hospital saying he was frightened because of what he was seeing. He reported distressing experiences including seeing his friend's head rotate through 360° 'like in the Exorcist'. He had a history of poly-drug misuse and was due to appear in court on a drug-related charge. He appeared to be genuinely distressed and did not have evidence of current drug intoxication. His symptoms resolved over several days. It remained unclear whether the psychosis was real, malingered, or 'hysterical' although the presence of apparently genuine distress was thought to favour the latter.

This case illustrates inconsistency with the typical patterns of symptoms. It also emphasized the difficulty in identifying malingering in the apparently psychotic patient.

Somatoform disorders, conversion, dissociation, and functional somatic syndromes

A substantial proportion of attenders at medical clinics have symptoms that are not explained by disease. They are often given a diagnosis of a functional somatic syndrome. The psychiatric classifications offer a parallel scheme in which many patients with such conditions are diagnosed as suffering from somatoform disorders. If there is loss of physical function the diagnosis may be conversion disorder, and if loss of mental function one of dissociative disorder. All these diagnoses require that there is no adequate explanation for the symptoms in terms of physical pathology. The fact that these conditions usually present to medical services, used to patients having diseases, makes an allegation of malingering in such cases much more likely. The diagnosis of conversion or dissociation hangs on the clinician making a judgement that the mechanism is unconscious. Gross inconsistency (e.g. the patients who staggers into the consultation but runs for the bus) is often used to make this distinction, but even that may be inconclusive.

Case example

A 35-year-old woman was seen in the clinic saying that she had 'ME' and requesting a report for the benefits agency. She gave a history of severe disabling fatigue for 5 years following a viral infection. She said that she had not worked and admitted that she had found her previous employment as a teacher very stressful. She was now receiving substantial state benefits and her partner had given up his work to look after her. The mental state and physical examinations were unremarkable. The patient walked very slowly to the waiting room and was collected by her partner who pushed her to the car park in a wheel chair. A diagnosis of chronic fatigue syndrome was made based on the history. Subsequent to the assessment one of the nursing staff reported that she had seen the patient walking out to the shops appearing unaffected by fatigue. When the patient was challenged about this on a future appointment, she said that she had 'good and bad days'. The fluctuation was accepted but the possibility of exaggeration of symptoms noted.

This case illustrates the importance of seeking evidence of inconsistency over time and that the issue of exaggeration is a vexed one in conditions that may fluctuate from day to day.

Further considerations in the detection of malingering

Bias

Given that the judgement is one of opinion it is important that clinicians are aware of the potential biases that may influence them. Perhaps the major potential bias is whether they know, like, and identify with the patient or not. It is probably wise to be aware of the potential for such biases of judgement (whether conscious or unconscious).

Overestimation of presence of illness

A doctor who has developed a relationship with the patients is probably disposed to believing them. Hence, a long-standing family doctor may endorse a patient's claim of disability even when is seems to be based on rather fragile evidence because of his relationship with the patient. Any doctor may see it as his or her prime duty to help patients, not to judge them and may always accept what they say uncritically (see Chapter 15). There is also desire not to make errors and it is generally considered a greater error to miss the diagnosis of an important psychiatric condition than to over diagnose it. For example, treating suspected depression may prevent suicide whilst treating a person who is malingering may not be in the person's best interest but (at least in psychiatry as opposed to surgery) is unlikely to do major harm. Finally, even if patients are thought to be exaggerating this may be sympathetically interpreted as exaggerating to convince the doctor that they are suffering, rather than to deceive them.

Underestimation of illness

The opposite of ignoring exaggerating is excessive scepticism about the veracity of the patient's complaints. This may result from a personal attitude of scepticism toward suffering and disability of patients who have illnesses that are defined only by symptoms. This issue has been especially salient in the controversy over the nature of chronic fatigue syndrome (CFS) (Ware 1992). Doctors employed by defence lawyers to perform independent reports may be also influenced by the lawyers' agenda and be sceptical of the patient's reported disability even when the evidence for it may be strong.

How should doctors address the issue of malingering?

When a doctor is seeking to detect malingering in patients complaining of psychiatric or other subjective disorders he may first wish to ask himself a number of questions.

- *Why do I want to determine the genuineness of this patient's symptoms?* Is it clearly necessary for the patient's welfare? If not should I play the role of detective? In other words, the potential conflict between responsibilities to the lawyer who is paying a fee with the doctor's role as caring physician should be considered. It is important to be clear in ones own mind why one is making a judgement about the patients genuineness.

- *What is your precise aim?* Given that malingering is not a diagnosis, the way to think about and present the findings is not in terms of a diagnosis. To positively 'diagnose' malingering requires that the doctor not only demonstrates inconsistent symptoms or disability, but also that he or she knows the patient's intention and whether it is conscious or not. It is therefore probably more helpful to simply aim to determine whether one is convinced that the evidence is consistent with the patient being genuinely psychiatrically ill.

- *What evidence do I have for inconsistency?* The totality of the evidence should be considered. Probably the most important information is that obtained from sources other than the consultation. Certainly, all medical records should be obtained and read. Where circumstances allow it repeat examination or admission for prolonged observation can be helpful. Where appropriate other non-medical sources of evidence should be obtained.

- *How should I express an opinion?* Where an opinion if offered it should be given as just that. Once the evidence for inconsistency has been presented, it should be made clear that the determination of intention and whether it is conscious or unconscious is not a scientific matter, but simply one of professional opinion.

Conclusions

Malingering describes a form of behaviour in which symptoms and signs of illness are deliberately feigned with the intention of receiving some sort of gain, other than medical care itself. Malingering is not considered a psychiatric diagnosis because, although it may be an extreme form of behaviour, it is judged not to reflect psychopathology. The malingerer is therefore regarded as 'bad not mad'. Doctors are probably poor at detecting malingering in any case. Arguably, the doctor should confine his or her opinion to whether he or she believes that the patient has a relevant psychiatric illness. The most helpful evidence is that of inconsistency. In practice, non-medical evidence is often far more powerful than a medical assessment in determining inconsistency between the patient's reported disability and that that observed in his or her day-to-day life. There is no particular reason to expect a doctor to be better than others at determining either the patient's intent, or indeed the degree to which that intent is conscious. To see oneself as an arbiter of social justice is seductive, but potentially dangerous. The consideration of whether and why patients' complaints may appear inconsistent is an important medical task; the detection of malingering is arguably not.

References

American Psychiatric Association (1994). *Diagnostic and Statistical Manual of Mental Disorders*, 4th edn. American Psychiatric Association, Washington, DC.

Bagby, R. M., Nicholson, R. A., Buis, T., and Bacchiochi J. R. (2000). Can the MMPI-2 validity scales detect depression feigned by experts? *Assessment*, **7**, 55–62.

Barsky, A. J. Forgetting, fabricating, and telescoping: the instability of the medical history. *Archives of Internal Medicine*, **162**, 981–4.

Bishop, E. R., Jr and Holt, A. R. (1980). Pseudopsychosis: a reexamination of the concept of hysterical psychosis. *Comprehensive Psychiatry*, **21**, 150–61.

Davidson, J. R. T. and Foa, E. B. (1991). Diagnostic issues in post traumatic stress disorder: considerations for DSM-IV. *Journal of Abnormal Psychology*, **100**, 346–55.

Davidson, J. R. T., Miller, R. D., Turnbull, C. D., and Sullivan, J. L. (1982). Atypical depression. *Archives of General Psychiatry*, **39**, 527–34.

Edens, J. F., Guy, L. S., Otto, R. K., Buffington, J. K., Tomicic, T. L., and Poythress, N. G. (2001). Factors differentiating successful versus unsuccessful malingerers. *Journal of Personality Assessment*, **77**, 333–8.

Eisendrath, S. J. (1996). When Munchausen becomes malingering: factitious disorders that penetrate the legal system. *Bulletin of the American Academy of Psychiatry and the Law*, **24**, 471–81.

Faust, D. (1995). The detection of deception. *Neurology Clinics*, **13**, 255–65.

Fisch, R. Z. (1987). Masked depression: its interrelations with somatization, hypochondriasis and conversion. *International Journal of Psychiatry in Medicine*, **17**, 367–79.

Fishbain, D. A., Rosomoff, H. L., Cutler, R. B., and Rosomoff, R. S. (1995). Secondary gain concept: a review of the scientific evidence. *Clinical Journal of Pain*, **11**, 6–21.

Ford, C. V. and Folks, D. G. (1985). Conversion disorders: an overview. *Psychosomatics*, **26**, 371–3.

Gorman, W. F. (1982). Defining malingering. *Journal of Forensic Sciences*, **27**, 401–7.

Gur, R. E. (2002). Functional imaging is fulfilling some promises. *American Journal of Psychiatry*, **159**, 693–4.

Jaffe, M. E. and Sharma, K. K. (1998). Malingering uncommon psychiatric symptoms among defendants charged under California's 'three strikes and you're out' law. *Journal of Forensic Sciences*, **43**, 549–55.

Kendell, R. E. (1975). *The role of diagnosis in psychiatry*. Blackwell Scientific, Oxford.

Lewis, A. (1953). Health as a social concept. *British Journal of Sociology*, **4**, 109–24.

Lopez-Ibor, J. J., Jr (1997). The concept and boundaries of personality disorders. *American Journal of Psychiatry*, **154**, 20–5.

Mai, F. M. (1995). 'Hysteria' in clinical neurology. *Canadian Journal of Neurological Sciences*, **22**, 101–10.

Rosenhan, D. (1973). *Science*, **172**, 250–8.

Scadding, G. (1996). Essentialism and nominalism in medicine: logic of diagnosis in disease terminology. *Lancet*, **348**, 594–6.

Slick, D. J., Sherman, E. M., and Iverson, G. L. (1999). Diagnostic criteria for malingered neurocognitive dysfunction: proposed standards for clinical practice and research. *Clinical Neuropsychology*, **13**, 545–61.

Sparr, L. and Pankratz, L. D. (1983). Factitious posttraumatic stress disorder. *American Journal of Psychiatry*, **140**, 1016–19.

Sparr, L. F. (1995). Post-traumatic stress disorder. Does it exist? *Neurology Clinics*, **13**, 413–29.

Spence, S. A., Crimlisk, H. L., Cope, H., Ron, M. A., and Grasby, P. M. (2000). Discrete neurophysiological correlates in prefrontal cortex during hysterical and feigned disorder of movement. *Lancet*, **355**, 1243–4.

Spitzer, R. L., Williams, J. B. W., Gibbon, M., and First, M. B. (1992). The structured clinical interview for, DSM-III-R (SCID) 1: History, rationale and description. *Archives of General Psychiatry*, **49**, 624–9.

Susser, M. (1990). Disease, illness, sickness: impairment, disability and handicap. *Psychological Medicine*, **20**, 471–3.

Sutherland, A. J. and Rodin, G. M. (1990). Factitious disorders in a general hospital setting: clinical features and a review of the literature. *Psychosomatics*, **31**, 392–9.

Szasz, T. (1991). Diagnoses are not diseases. *Lancet*, **338**, 1574–5.

Vanderploeg, R. D. and Curtiss, G. (2001). Malingering assessment: evaluation of validity of performance. *Neurological Rehabilitation*, **16**, 245–51.

Waddell, G., Bircher, M., Finlayson, D., and Main, C. J. (1984). Symptoms and signs: physical disease or illness behaviour? *British Medical Journal*, **289**, 739–41.

Ware, N. C. (1992). Suffering and the social construction of illness: the deligitimation of illness experience in chronic fatigue syndrome. *Medical Anthropology Quarterly*, **6**, 347–61.

Wessely, S., Nimnuan, C., and Sharpe, M. (1999). Functional somatic syndromes: one or many? *Lancet*, **354**, 936–9.

World Health Organization (1992). *The ICD-10 Classification of Mental and Behavioural Disorders*. World Health Organization, Geneva.

13 The nature of chronic pain: a clinical and legal challenge

Chris J. Main

Abstract

In cases of personal injury, in which litigation is involved, claimants need to *prove* they have been injured. In cases of chronic pain, this can be particularly problematic since pain is a subjective sensation. Pain may be claimed in terms of self-report or may be inferred on the basis of observation of pain behaviour, but its legitimacy may be challenged. Given the difficulties of pursuing litigation it seems probable that *total* fabrication is rare, but the issue of exaggeration is frequently raised, particularly if there is considered to be a mismatch between the nature of the injury and the presenting symptoms or if the pain-associated disability is considered to be 'excessive'. Unfortunately scientific studies have demonstrated a relatively weak relationship among these parameters, even in non-litigants and a degree of inconsistency in symptom presentation is not uncommon, particularly in distressed patients. Identification and interpretation of exaggeration therefore is particularly difficult and requires careful and systematic assessment of both clinical history and presenting symptomatology, including consideration of *intent*. Allegation of deception should be made only on the basis of compelling evidence. Detection of malingering or fraud as such is a matter for the court not the expert witness.

Introduction

In cases of chronic pain, there are frequently disagreements among orthopaedic and neurological specialists about the reasons for continued incapacity. Pain, as a sensation, is essentially subjective and can only be inferred from observation or from self-report. In routine clinical practice, there is seldom need to doubt the patient's veracity but in the context of medicolegal assessment of pain-associated disability there may be reason to doubt the claimant. Allegations of malingering and even fraud may arise. From a narrow perspective, malingering can be viewed in simple terms as either present or absent. More often the issue is more complicated. The claimant may not be able to give a clear picture of the precise nature of their incapacity; their pain may be variable in its effects and the claimant's *perception* of their limitations may not be commensurate with the physical findings determined on medical examination. Claimants may have been told that their pain is imaginary or 'psychological'. They may feel compelled to demonstrate the extent of their incapacity and convince their assessor of their 'genuineness'. In so doing they may exaggerate. They may or may not be aware of their inconsistency. In this chapter it will be argued that the concept of malingering in the context of personal injury needs to be viewed in a broad rather than a narrow context, and seen as part of a spectrum of exaggeration ranging on the one hand from mild inconsistency in symptom presentation of which the claimant may be unaware, to deliberate fraud as a conscious and deliberate act on the other. Prior to discussion therefore of the context of malingering per se in the context of assessment of chronic pain, it is necessary to understand both the *context* in which the appraisal is taking place, and also have familiarity with clinical assessment and management.

The nature of expertise in the context of medicolegal assessment

The role of the expert in the context of a medicolegal assessment is different from that of the treating clinician. They are asked to give an opinion of the evidence presented to them. The 'evidence' may include a wide range of materials, such as clinical records, occupational records, and videotaped evidence over and above the symptoms presented by the claimant. The relationship between the client and the medicolegal assessor is therefore radically different from that between patient and doctor. In chronic pain cases in which the evidence of physical injury is not considered sufficient to explain the extent or persistence of the claimant's symptoms, a psychological opinion may be of crucial importance. The opinion has to be both authoritative and credible.

The task confronting the expert witness therefore is a complex and highly technical one, yet the basis of the opinion, of course, is clinical. The basis of a witness's expertise lies not only in the elucidation of 'facts' to support his/her opinion, but also in the authority with which the opinion can be located within his/her familiarity with similar injuries and with the usual variation in responses to treatment. Determination of feigned symptoms or exaggeration has to be understood in this context.

A clinical perspective on pain and disability

Much of the fascination in understanding chronic pain and in the challenge to the assessor of the chronic pain claimant lies in the fact that pain is first and foremost a subjective phenomenon. We can only rely on the claimant's self-report or observe their behaviour. Issues of exaggeration and malingering arise when there appears to be a mismatch between the nature of the injuries sustained and the extent of the claimed incapacities. Questions of exaggeration, deception and malingering in the context of chronic pain can only be understood adequately from an understanding of the varied impact of pain, psychological adaptation, and resulting disability.

The nature of pain and disability

Since the formulation of the Gate-Control theory of pain (Melzack and Wall 1965), it has been recognized that severity of pain does not bear a simple relationship to the degree of tissue damage. The experience of pain is influenced not only by the amount of tissue damage but also by the way the information is processed when it reaches the brain. A range of psychological factors have been shown to influence the perception of pain. Furthermore, studies of disability (Waddell *et al.* 1984) have demonstrated that disability, or limitation in function, is explained by both physical and psychological factors. The later development of the *biopsychosocial* model of disability (Waddell 1987; Turk 1996) acknowledged the complicated interplay between medical, psychological, and social factors. These scientific developments in the clinical field have begun to influence appraisal of pain and incapacity in the legal context.

Psychologically mediated pain-associated incapacity is now being considered as a possible consequence of injury.

At the heart of the biopsychosocial model is the assumption of an on-going sensation that is nociceptive in origin or which is perceived by the sufferer as being painful. The patient's cognitions, that is, what they think and understand about this sensation, however, will influence their emotional reaction to it. The behaviour demonstrated by the individual at any point in time will be a product of their beliefs and the emotional response to the pain and may in turn be influenced (reinforced or modulated) by the social environment in which the behaviour takes place. The model offers a radically different way of understanding the nature of pain-associated incapacity. It is important therefore to have an understanding of the influence of psychological factors on perception of pain and development of disability.

Nature of psychological factors

Much of the early literature, although illuminating, was not supported by scientific research. During the last 15 years, however, a considerable quantity of research into the psychology of pain and pain-associated incapacity has been published. There are a number of useful sources for detail regarding the nature of psychological factors on pain perception and response to treatment (Gatchel and Turk 1996; Morley *et al.* 1999; Linton 2000; Main and Spanswick 2000).

The self-report of the patient, whether in terms of beliefs, emotions, or report of symptoms (and disability) is the cornerstone of clinical assessment. In eliciting such information, a structured interview approach should be complemented by the use of some of the many well-validated assessment tools.

It is convenient to conceptualize psychological factors into three main types: emotional; cognitive, and behavioural; some examples of which are shown in Table 13.1.

In chronic pain patients, distress of various sorts frequently accompanies symptom presentation. Of its many variants depressive symptoms and heightened concern about symptoms in general are particularly important (Main *et al.* 1992). A wide range of cognitive factors are associated with the perception of pain and response to disability. It is particularly important to assess specific beliefs about pain or treatment (DeGood and Tait 2001; Lackner *et al.* 1996) and pain coping strategies (Jensen *et al.* 1991; Keefe *et al* 1997). A brief description of such features and utility in a medicolegal context is presented elsewhere (Main 1999).

Table 13.1 Types of psychological features

Emotional (distress)
Symptom awareness and concern
Depressive reactions; helplessness
Anger & hostility

Cognitive (beliefs about pain and disability)
Significance; controllability
Fears and misunderstanding about pain

Behavioural (pain behaviour and coping strategies)
Guarded movements and avoidance patterns
Coping styles and strategies

Pain behaviour: identification of the behavioural component

Interpretation of pain behaviour in the chronic pain patient is not straightforward. It is important to emphasize that pain behaviours cannot be understood in isolation. Formal assessment of the emotional and cognitive components is normally undertaken by a psychological specialist, but most controversy arises in the interpretation of pain behaviour; and in particular in apparent differences between claimed and observed levels of incapacity. There are many different examples of pain behaviour, ranging from the simple to the complex (Fordyce 1976; Keefe and Block 1982). Many such behaviours are crucial in the interaction between patients and doctors or therapists during treatment. Patients may communicate pain both verbally and non-verbally. Their expressions of pain in turn may produce a range of reactions from the treating professionals. Since the turn of the century (Collie 1913) responses to examination that were considered excessive or not entirely consistent with the physical findings were frequently taken *de facto* as evidence of malingering . Initially such assessments were carried out for evaluation of compensation. Although in later years behavioural signs came to form part of clinical assessment, the assessments often were impressionistic and unstandardized. Then Waddell *et al.* (1980) developed a standardized assessment of behavioural responses to examination, originally known as 'non-organic' signs. The presence of such responses to examination suggests that the patient does not have a straightforward physical problem and that a more careful psychosocial assessment is required. Such responses are predictive of poor response to 'straightforward' physical treatment. They have been widely used in medicolegal settings as indicators of malingering, a use for which they have never been intended or validated. A more detailed description and guide to their interpretation is presented elsewhere (Main and Waddell 1998).

Pain behaviour: the interpretation of chronic pain (or pain behaviour) syndromes

Many chronic pain patients are characterised not by isolated or specific indicators of pain behaviour but by an entire pattern of invalidism. Terms such as 'functional overlay' or 'illness behaviour' are sometimes used to describe the symptomatic presentation of patients whose chronic pain syndrome is not apparently explained by the physical findings. Unfortunately such categorizations are frequently 'diagnoses by exclusion' made on by the identification of explanatory psychological mechanisms, but on the basis of absence of 'adequate' physical findings. Ambiguities in the use of such terminology are addressed more fully elsewhere (Main and Spanswick 1995).

It has been suggested that chronic pain syndromes in which psychological features are prominent may be more usefully described as *psychologically mediated chronic pain syndromes*. The syndrome is described more fully in Main (1999, pp. 138–9) as is the content of a typical psychological report (pp. 139–40).

In conclusion, chronic pain patients can display widespread changes in behaviour following injury. Pain behaviour can be *described* but it cannot be interpreted or understood without appropriate evaluation of emotional responses, beliefs, and appraisals. In assessment of pain-associated disability, it should be recognized that guarded movements and patterns of avoidance may be fear-mediated and influenced by concerns about further injury. Furthermore, it should be remembered that specific beliefs and emotional responses may be influenced not only by nature and intensity of pain, but also by previous treatment and assessment. Pain behaviour therefore can only be fully understood in terms of its *social context*. Pain may affect a wide range of activities and displays of pain behaviour can produce marked and unpredictable reactions of others. Medicolegal assessment needs to be understood in this context.

The nature of psychological and psychiatric opinion in the context of personal injury (PI) litigation

The nature of psychological and psychiatric opinion

In the majority of cases of PI, such as road traffic accidents, liability for the original accident may not be in dispute; but the key issue may be one of extended causation, that is, the extent to which a *chronic* pain syndrome can be considered to be attributable to the accident in question. In such an evaluation issues both of independent causation and the claimant's credibility may arise. The extent to which a psychologically mediated chronic pain syndrome should be classified as a psychiatric injury or not has been the subject of some debate. In considering such issues, it is important to consider the objectives for a medicolegal assessment. These are shown in Table 13.2.

Difficulties in clinical diagnostics can lead to problems in assessment of 'condition' in medicolegal contexts. Historically, 'psychological injury' was defined in terms of identifiable psychiatric disorder, and although 'pain and suffering' were explicitly identified in terms of grounds for compensation, they were not recognized as an injury as such. The DSM-IV recommends differentiation of *somatoform disorder* from *pain disorder* and states:

> An additional diagnosis of Pain Disorder should be considered only if the pain is an independent focus of clinical attention, leads to clinically significant distress or impairment and is in excess of that usually associated with the other mental disorder.
>
> (DSM-IV 1994, p. 461).

Most PI claimants on which an expert psychological opinion is sought would be considered to have a *pain disorder* rather than a non-pain related mental illness.

According to Shapiro and Teasell (1998) there already exists a diagnosis in DSM-IV which is not considered as a mental disorder but is consistent with a biopsychosocial conceptualization of chronic pain, that is, *psychological factors affecting a general medical condition* the criteria of which are shown in Table 13.3.

In summary, psychiatric diagnostic criteria are not particularly helpful in elucidating the psychological features associated with chronic pain. However this problem is of more than academic significance. If chronic pain and pain-associated incapacity cannot be explained in terms of physical signs or structural damage; and if the presenting problem is a chronic pain syndrome rather than

Table 13.2 Purpose of evaluation

- Detection of specific psychological injury (such as a diagnosable psychiatric disorder (e.g. DSM-IV)
- Determination of a psychologically mediated pain syndrome
- Evaluation of the genuineness or veracity of the client

Table 13.3 DSM-IV criteria for psychological factors affecting a general medical condition

A general medical condition is present
Psychological factors adversely affect the medical condition in one of the following ways:

- The factors have influenced the course of the general medical condition as shown by a close temporal association between the psychological factors and the development or exacerbation of, or delayed recovery from, the general medical condition
- The factors interfere with the treatment of the general medical condition
- The factors constitute additional health risks for the individual
- Stress-related physiologic responses precipitate or exacerbate symptoms of the general medical condition

Reproduced from Shapiro and Teasell (1998, p. 26).

a diagnosable mental illness, it could be argued that the claimant has not sustained a recognized injury and therefore is not entitled to be compensated. If, on the other hand, it is accepted that chronic pain is a genuine medical condition, characterized primarily by psychological and behavioural dysfunction, and frequently with equivocal physical signs, then assessment of injury by a psychologically competent pain specialist becomes the appropriate basis for the medicolegal case.

Arriving at a psychological opinion therefore is a complex task involving the integration of a number of different clinical dimensions. The major focus may rest less on the origin of the pain (which in the case of specific accidents may be relatively unambiguous), but more on the nature of the injury and the components of the resultant incapacity. In arriving at an overall opinion, it is necessary therefore to integrate a range of perspectives. Each component of the psychological opinion should if possible be clearly appraised before any attempt is made to integrate the opinion. Although at times problematic in terms of quantification of 'injury', in a proportion of patients, the litigation process itself can have a significant influence on the manner and content of symptom presentation.

Medicolegal assessment of malingering, faking (illness deception), and exaggeration

Probabilistic opinions and the 'burden of proof'

It has been argued that a competent medicolegal assessment must be founded on familiarity with the condition and on careful clinical appraisal. Ziskin (1995), however, offers a powerful critique of expert clinical judgement, in terms of subjective distortions and bias. Although many of his specific concerns relate to forensic issues his analysis contains much of relevance to psychological opinion in the context of PI. Judgement appears to be affected by both intellectual and emotional biases. In the context of medicolegal assessment, reliance on systematic assessment of the specific psychological features (as outlined above) may serve as a partial safeguard against bias, but the 'evidential base' of judgements of malingering or exaggeration appears to be even more problematic. It should be remembered, however, that the standards of proof differ in scientific and in legal contexts. The expert witness is charged with providing an opinion only 'on the balance of probabilities', that is, more probable than not'. This allows for much less certainty than is usually required in scientific medicine.

Nonetheless, in chronic pain cases, in which there is not strong support either for structural damage or identifiable psychiatric illness, the legitimacy of the claimant's pain and pain-associated complaints may become the major focus of the legal battle. In the absence of 'no-fault' compensation, the burden of proof lies with the claimant, that is, they have to prove on the balance of probabilities that they have sustained an injury as a consequence of the negligent act. Furthermore, defendants have a right to challenge their evidence. In cases of chronic pain syndrome, the attack may be directed not only at the clinical validity of their symptoms, but at the truthfulness of their self-report. It is necessary therefore to consider issues of exaggeration, illness deception, and malingering as facets of symptom presentation and pain-associated disability.

The nature of malingering

It is possible to consider malingering from both a broad and a narrow perspective. In the context of chronic pain, malingering in the narrow sense would be equivalent to complete fabrication of symptoms, that is, feigned pain. A broader view of malingering would be to understand it continuum of exaggeration ranging from mild inconsistency in pain report or pain behaviour at one end to deliberate and wilful illness deception amounting to fraud at the other. Although the incidence of total fabrication is unknown, it seems improbable that most such claimants would be likely to proceed far in the medicolegal system. As Mendelson (1995) points out,

> when malingering rather than a medical diagnosis proper is raised in a legal context, it becomes an allegation of fact and . . . in determining whether the allegation of malingering is or is not sustainable, the court will consider legal facts rather than opinions formed by a medical witness. (p. 434)
>
> For the medicolegal expert therefore, the issue is more likely to be one of exaggeration (whether deliberate or not). However 'the line between exaggeration and fraudulent pretence of illness, disability or disease is very fine indeed
>
> (Mendelson 1995, p. 429)

In summary, in chronic pain assessment consideration of 'malingering' should be concerned primarily not with the detection of fraud as such nor with the identification of primary diagnosable psychiatric disorder but with an appraisal of the extent to which there is evidence of *exaggeration* in the presentation of symptoms. There are difficulties both in identification and in interpretation.

Difficulties in the identification of exaggeration in the context of chronic pain

There are three general difficulties for the medicolegal assessors in the assessment of exaggeration.

1. There are wide variations in symptoms, disability, and work compromise which cannot be accurately predicted from injury or supposed damage.
2. Disability and work compromise are multiply determined.
3. Psychosocial factors are far more important than physical factors in the development of chronic disability.

A competent assessment of all these facets would seem to be beyond the competence of most medicolegal assessors, but the law requires a medical opinion nonetheless. It may be helpful therefore to consider the problem of exaggeration from a slightly different perspective in terms of firstly the problem of 'mismatch'. Legally, the term 'exaggeration' does not imply *intent* as such; but some sort of mismatch is implied.

What is known about the extent of mismatch? Attribution of mismatch however implies an underlying set of fundamental equivalences as shown in Table 13.4.

Clinical research, however, has demonstrated a wide range of variation amongst these facets of illness and dysfunction. Indeed, arguably, one of the most important factors in the move from the pathology-based medical model to the biopsychosocial model of illness was recognition of the poor correlation between symptoms, signs and the development of pain-associated disability (Waddell 1998).

Table 13.4 Assumed equivalences in the judgement of 'mismatch'

Accident and injury
Injury and damage, 'that is, physical signs'
Signs and symptoms
Symptoms and limitations (disability)
Disability and work compromise

Difficulties in the interpretation of exaggeration

A particularly difficult feature of clinical assessment is the ascription of motive to the claimant. It is trivially true that all claimants in prosecuting a claim have an interest in outcome, whether financial or in terms of redress for a perceived injustice. In a minority of cases, the prime mover behind litigation appears to be a third party, such as a relative or representative. If there appears to be evidence of exaggeration, however defined, the first question is whether or not the exaggeration is intended or deliberate. It is not possible at this juncture to enter into extended debate about conscious or unconscious processes, but it would certainly seem to be the case that a proportion of claimants are unaware that they have been inconsistent in their self-report, and that deliberate exaggeration may be offered as an explanation for this inconsistency.

Viewed simplistically, mismatch might be taken *de facto* as evidence of exaggeration. Usually exaggeration would be considered to require a component of *intent*, although as discussed by Malle and Knobe (1997) and Malle (see Chapter 6), the interpretation of intentionality has to take into account four different components as shown in Table 13.5.

There are not as yet sufficiently developed assessment tools for the assessment of intentionality in medicolegal contexts. There are, however, a number of important issues which need to be addressed. They are shown in Table 13.6.

Deliberate exaggeration

What then do we make of deliberate exaggeration? Is it simply a clinical correlate of malingering? Claimants may exaggerate for different reasons. Taking a robust view, all such deliberate exaggeration might be viewed as deceit. A distinction can, however, be made between 'exaggeration with the intent to convince' and 'exaggeration with the intent to deceive'. In what circumstances might the former arise? As for example when the claimant is convinced that they are not being believed, whether as a consequence of the reaction of family, of work-mates, of health care personnel or of previous medicolegal assessors. In extreme cases, they may discover they have been the subject of videotape surveillance. *If* they perceive themselves as having a genuinely disabling chronic condition, they may believe they have to exaggerate to convince the assessor of their genuineness. It could be argued of course that deliberate exaggeration of whatever nature is deceitful and casts

Table 13.5 Four components of intentionality (Malle and Knobe 1997)

1	Desire for an outcome
2	Beliefs about an action that leads to that outcome
3	Intention to perform the action
4	Awareness of fulfilling the intention when performing the action

Table 13.6 Key questions in interpretation of exaggeration

Is it deliberate?
  If so, what is the intent?
  Is it with the intent to deceive?
    If so, properly a judicial not a 'clinical matter';
  Is it with intent to convince?
    More likely if iatrogenic distress/confusion
Is it 'unconscious' (non-deliberate)
  If so, what is the evidence?
    Is it mediated by distress?
    Is it based on misunderstandings about pain, hurt and harming?
    Is it part of a 'learned behaviour pattern'?

trenchant doubt on the entire claim. On the other hand, it is easy to understand how in the morass of medicolegal assessment a claimant can become confused and make errors of judgement. Should deliberate exaggeration be established, however, it is a matter for the court rather than the expert witness to take a view on it.

Unconscious exaggeration

It may be difficult to explain inconsistency in terms of genuine variation in clinical symptomatology. Clinically, chronic pain patients frequently present as distressed, disaffected or confused, and may appear to exaggerate. They may be bemused also not only at the persistence of their pain, but also at the medicolegal process itself.

Perhaps 'unconscious exaggeration' is a contradiction in terms and the term 'over-reaction' would be preferable (although use of this term also carries a danger of ascribing motive rather than just describing mismatch or inconsistency). In a medicolegal assessment, the assessor should consider whether the 'over-reaction is mediated by distress, is based on misunderstandings about pain, hurt and harming or has become part of a 'learned behaviour pattern'? (In arriving at such an assessment the assessor may be guided by standardized psychometric assessment in addition to clinical history and symptom presentation.)

Conclusion

In the context of chronic pain assessment it seems appropriate to take a broad rather than a narrow definition of malingering and approach the task of medicolegal assessment by viewing malingering as one end of a spectrum of exaggeration, the nature of which requires careful clinical appraisal.

Improved decision making: towards development of a 'gold standard'

The clinical and legal challenge: the need for improved decision making

We do not as yet have tools of sufficient sensitivity and specificity for medicolegal use in claimants with chronic pain. We can present our view on the available evidence, but we can do no more than this. In offering ourselves as clinical experts we must be careful not to find ourselves in the role of 'thought police' or moral adjudicators. That is the role for the law acting on behalf of society. Insofar as we give a view on exaggeration, our ground must be clearly stated, in terms of both identification and interpretation. We must be clearer about the boundaries of clinical expertise. What about specific expertise in illness deception and exaggeration? Is there any? Are our measures robust enough for medicolegal use? Faust (1995) has recommended the establishment of a 'gold standard', but what sort of scientific gold standard? It is not even clear what *types* of information should be adduced.

Challenges in the development of a gold standard

There are a number of major problems in the development of a 'Gold standard' (see Chapter 8). First, there is only a legal judgement in an extremely small proportion of cases. Most cases are settled by lawyers prior to a judgement in court. Only potentially expensive cases are fought. Clinicians do not usually receive specific feedback from lawyers on specific strengths or weaknesses of their reports or critical issues. Finally, in negotiating settlement, there is a lot of poker playing (and bluff).

Faust (1995) has recommended the development of psychometric instruments *specifically* validated for the detection of deception. A recent review of evidence on this topic is presented in a previous publication (Main 1999). My view remains that: 'There is an inherent attractiveness in being able to detect faking or malingering, using a psychometric assessment such as the MMPI', but I concluded 'it is clear that the research supporting the use of the "faking scales" is based on shaky foundations' (Main 1999, p. 143). Furthermore, the process of validation remains problematic. In summary, although at this time there are well-established clinically focused assessment tools, there are no assessment tools of sufficient sensitivity and specificity to permit both the identification and interpretation or exaggeration or deception in chronic pain syndromes.

Symptom validity testing (Pankratz 1988) has been developed to investigate misrepresentation of neuropsychological symptoms. According to Faust (1995) the test has limited sensitivity, even in that context. It has not to my knowledge been validated for the assessment of chronic pain. Indeed, in a later edition of the book, Pankratz acknowledges the influence of *context* on clinical decision making. (Pankratz and Binder 1997, pp. 235–6).

Psychometric approaches involving integrity testing have been used in personnel selection (Iacono and Patrick 1997). They identify a number of different instruments. Having reviewed the available evidence, however, they conclude 'Although on balance overt integrity tests appear to have some validity, these tests account for considerably less than 20% of the variance in criterion measures ... the low validity and many problems inherent to these tests makes it difficult to use them in a setting where assessment of a single person is important ... hence it would be imprudent for clinicians to place much stock in individual scores' (Iacono and Patrick 1997, p. 281). Insofar as I am aware, the position remains unchanged, and certainly I know of no data validating the use of such approaches in the assessment of chronic pain.

The structured interview remains the bedrock of clinical judgement and ought to remain so, since the patients' presenting characteristics remain the key cornerstone of clinical judgement . Given Ziskin's pessimism about our ability to arrive at reliable clinical judgements, however, it may be desirable not only to develop a standardized and validated interview format but to supplement the information where possible by standardized clinical psychometric assessment, and wherever possible corroborative information. As previously discussed, behavioural measures such as the Behavioural Signs Test (or Waddell signs) (Waddell *et al.* 1980), although widely used, are also widely misused (Main and Waddell 1998). It is at best a screening measure, insufficient in itself as a measure for the identification or interpretation of exaggeration (or deception). More recent research into non-verbal communication would appear hold some potential, but Craig *et al.* (1999) identify a number of difficulties in the identification of malingering, including requirement of evidence of conscious intent, complexity in judgement of subjective experiences and absence of single or unique markers for deception.

A recent detailed review of psychophysiological approaches to deception using polygraphy (the so-called 'lie-detector' test), is reviewed elsewhere (Iacono and Patrick 1997). In fact, there have been long-standing scientific (and ethical) concerns about the validity of such procedures for assessing veracity (Gale 1988; Levey 1988) such that its use was considered legally inadmissible in the United Kingdom; and in fact similar concerns have previously been raised in the United States (Brooks 1985). Iacono and Patrick (1997, p. 263) conclude 'psychologists should be wary of polygraph testing ... many problems associated with reliance on polygraph techniques in clinical or forensic settings include (1) Inadequate research addressing their validity, (2) the lack of polygraph training forcing psychologists to rely on the opinion of polygraphers who are inadequately trained in psychophysiology and psychometrics, and (3) the dearth of information available on the use of these procedures with clinical populations'.

The field of sports medicine has offered systems of human performance measurement, appraised in responses to equipment calibrated according to various degrees of physical challenge. In addition to specific assessment of the range of motion and strength, systems of *Functional Capacity Evaluation* (Isernhagen 1995) have been developed. Such assessments offer a set of performance characteristics which can be compared with normative data. Such data would appear to be useful in pre-employment screening or in determination of initial performance level prior to tailored rehabilitation, but are sometimes also used to give an appraisal of *effort*. As such they would appear to be of potential use in a medicolegal context. Mayer (2000), however, advocates caution:

> It must be recognised that the term *effort* must be used guardedly, since its use implies a voluntary aspect to low test performance. Unconscious barriers such as pain, stress, or joint/muscle inhibition may be the primary factors producing 'low' effort. Consequently, the recognition of performance limitations in most patients is not well suited to single evaluations for determining faking or malingering.
>
> Mayer (2000, p. 556)

The same qualifications in terms of identification and interpretation as outlined above with reference to behavioural tests are relevant to performance tests. At present they are not sufficiently validated in terms of sensitivity or specificity for the detection of deception in medicolegal settings and require specific validation for medicolegal assessment.

Conclusions

Undoubtedly we need better models of injury. We now know that the mechanisms of injury are different from mechanisms of chronicity. We need to consider injury and pain from a biopsychosocial perspective. However, there is still a lot we do not know about the nature and content of symptom presentation. The role of *intentionality* (Malle, Chapter 6) would seem to be fundamental but its specific relevance to medicolegal assessment still represents a formidable intellectual and practical challenge. A number of other 'cautions' are expressed by Craig *et al.* (1999, p. 55).

Implications for medicolegal assessment

The clinician's role as an expert witness is not to rescue or destroy the claimant. 'Hired guns' fit better into the old type of legislation than the new one. The prime responsibility of the expert witness is to the *Court*. Indeed, it was always so. A view on inconsistency, illness deception or exaggeration may be asked of an expert witness, but we need to strive for a better evidence-base from which to make our judgements. Such evidence must be derived from sound theoretically based assessments of psychological processes which have been subjected to careful validation in terms of sensitivity and specificity in medicolegal settings. New directions in experimental psychology may offer new ways of identifying and addressing issues of feigned symptoms and exaggeration. Use of the term malingering in the narrow sense (denoting wilful fraud) should be a judgement for the court and not for the expert witness. At this time, when offering medicolegal opinion on claimants with chronic pain, we need to adopt a broad rather than a narrow definition. We need to focus not on malingering but on the identification and interpretation of exaggeration. In the evaluation of chronic pain syndrome, we may reasonably offer a view on exaggeration, supported by a competent and systematic clinical and psychological appraisal, but should be willing to identify illness deception only on the strongest of evidence. Malingering or fraud is matter for the court.

References

Brooks, J. (1985). Polygraph testing: thoughts of a sceptical legislator. *American Psychologist*, **40**, 348–54.

Collie, J. (1913). *Malingering and feigned sickness*. Edward Arnold, London.

Craig, K. D., Hill, M. L., and McMurtry, B. W. (1999). Detecting deception and malingering. In *Handbook of pain syndromes: biopsychosocial perspectives* (eds A. R. Block, E. F. Kramer, and E. Fernandez), Chap. 3, pp. 41–58. Lawrence Irlbaum Assoc, Mahwah, NJ.

DeGood, D. E. and Tait, R. C. (2001). Assessment of pain beliefs and pain coping. In, *Handbook of pain assessment*, 2nd Edition (eds. D. C. Turk and R. Melzack), The Guilford Press, New York, NY.

Diagnostic and statistical manual of mental disorders (DSM-IV) (1994). (4th edn). American Psychiatric Association, Washington, DC.

Faust, D. (1995). The detection of deception. In *Neurologic clinics, malingering and conversion reactions* (ed. M. Weintraub), pp. 255–65. Saunders, Philadelphia, PA.

Fordyce, W. E. (1976). *Behavioural methods for chronic pain and illness*. CV Mosby, St. Louis, MO.

Gale, A. G. (1988). *The polygraph test: lies, truth and science*. Sage, London.

Gatchel, R. J. and Turk, D. C. (eds). (1996). *Psychological approaches to pain management: a practitioner's handbook*. The Guilford Press, New York, NY.

Iacono, W. G. and Patrick, C. J. (1997). Malingering in intellectual and neuropsychological assessment. In *Clinical assessment of malingering and deception* (ed. R. Rogers), 2nd edn, pp. 223–36. The Guilford Press, New York, NY.

Isernhagen, S. (1995). *The comprehensive guide to work injury management*. Aspen Publishers, Gaithersburg, MD.

Jensen, M. P., Turner, J. A., Romano, J. M., and Karoly, P. (1991). Coping with chronic pain: a critical review of the literature. *Pain*, **47**, 249–83.

Keefe, F. J., Affleck, G., Lefebvre, J., Starr, K., Caldwell, D. S., and Tennen, H. (1997). Pain coping strategies and pain efficacy in rheumatoid arthritis: a daily process analysis. *Pain*, **69**, 35–42.

Keefe, F. J. and Block, A. R. (1982). Development of an observational method for assessing pain behavior in chronic low back pain patients. *Behavior Therapy*, **13**, 363–75.

Lackner, J. M., Carosella, A. M., and Feuerstein, M. (1996). Pain expectancies, pain and functional expectancies as determinants of disability in patients with chronic low back disorders. *Journal of Consulting and Clinical Psychology*, **64**, 212–20.

Levey, A. B. (1988). *Polygraphy:an evaluative review*. HMSO, London.

Linton, S. J. (2000). A review of psychological risk factors in back pain and neck pain. *Spine*, **25**, 1148–56.

Main, C. J. (1999). Medicolegal aspects of pain: the nature of psychological opinion in cases of personal injury. In *Psychosocial aspects of pain* (eds R. J. Gatchel and D. C. Turk), pp. 132–47. Guilford Press, New York, NY.

Main, C. J., and Spanswick, C. C. (1995). Functional overlay and illness behaviour in chronic pain: distress or malingering? Conceptual difficulties in medico-legal assessment of personal injury claims. *Journal of Psychosomatic Research*, **39**, 737–53.

Main, C. J., and Spanswick, C. C. (2000). *Pain management: an interdisciplinary approach*. Churchill-Livingstone, Edinburgh.

Main, C. J. and Waddell, G. (1998). Behavioural responses to examination: a re-appraisal of the interpretation of 'non-organic signs'. *Spine*, **23**, 2367–71.

Main, C. J., Wood, P. L. R., Hollis, S., Spanswick, C. C., and Waddell, G. (1992). The distress risk assessement method: a simple patient classification to identify distress and evaluate risk of poor outcome. *Spine*, **17**, 42–50.

Malle, B. F. and Knobe, J. (1997). The folk concept of intentionality. *Journal of Experimental and Social Psychology*, **33**, 101–21.

Mayer, T. (2000). Quantitative physical and functional capacity assessment. In *Occupational musculoskeletal disorders: functions, outcomes and evidence* (eds T. G. Mayer, R. J. Gatchel, and P. B. Polatin), pp. 547–60. Lippincott, Williams & Wilkins, Philadelphia, PA.

Melzack, R. and Wall, P. D. (1965). Pain mechanisms: a new theory. *Science*, **150**, 971–9.

Mendelson, D. (1995). The expert deposes, but the court disposes: the concept of *malingering* and the function of a medical expert witness in the forensic process. *International Journal of Law and Psychiatry*, **18**, 425–36.

Morley, S., Eccleston, C., and Williams, A. (1999). Systematic review and meta-analysis of randomized controlled trials of cognitive behaviour therapy and behaviour therapy for chronic pain in adults excluding headache. *Pain*, **80**, 1–13.

Pankratz, L. (1988). Malingering in intellectual and neuropsychological assessment. In *Clinical assessment of malingering and deception* (ed. R. Rogers), pp. 169–92. The Guilford Press, New York, NY.

Pankratz, L. and Binder, L. M. (1997). Polygraphy and integrity testing. In *Clinical assessment of malingering and deception* (ed. R. Rogers), 2nd edn, pp. 252–81. The Guilford Press, New York, NY.

Shapiro, A. P. and Teasell, R. W. (1998). Misdiagnosis of chronic pain as hysteria and malingering. *Current Review of Pain*, **2**, 19–28.

Turk, D. C. (1996). Biopsychosocial perspective on chronic pain. In *Psychological approaches to pain management: a practitioner's handbook* (eds R. J. Gatchel and D. C. Turk), pp. 3–32. The Guilford Press, New York, NY.

Waddell, G. (1987). A new clinical model for the treatment of low back pain. *Spine*, **12**, 632–44.

Waddell, G. (1998). *The back pain revolution*. Churchill-Livingstone, Edinburgh.

Waddell, G., Bircher, M., Finlayson, D., and Main, C. J. (1984). Symptoms and signs: physical disease or illness behaviour? *British Medical Journal*, **289**, 739–41.

Waddell, G., McCulloch, J. A., Kummell, E., and Venner, R. M. (1980). Nonorganic physical signs in low back pain, *Spine*, **5**, 117–25.

Waddell, G. and Main C. J. (1998). Illness behaviour. In *The back pain revolution* (ed. G. Waddell), pp. 155–72. Churchill Livingstone, Edinburgh.

Ziskin, J. (ed.) (1995). *Coping with psychiatric and psychological testimony* (5th Edition). Law and Psychology Press, Los Angeles, CA.

14 The misadventures of wanderers and victims of trauma

Loren Pankratz

Nor did these impostors have much difficulty in imposing on him, because he met them above half way.

Brodelon. *A history of the ridiculous extravagancies of Monsieur Oufle*. 1711

Abstract

This chapter addresses the problems created by two categories of patients: wanderers and victims of trauma. Both present a risk when they engage in deception—wanderers usually because they withhold information about their history and victims of trauma when they distort their history, manufacture a history, or make false attributions about the cause of their symptoms. All of these patients are successful in deceiving clinicians because they weave false stories into the fabric of their lives so seamlessly. This chapter reviews the texture of their clinical presentation, some current research, and the implications of their successful deceptions on the health care system.

Introduction

In this chapter I discuss the problems created by two categories of patients: wanderers and victims of trauma. Both patient groups present risk when they engage in deception—wanderers typically because they withhold information about their history and victims of trauma usually because they distort their history, manufacture a history, or make false attributions about the cause of their symptoms. I began encountering patients in these categories over 20 years ago, but it took several years before I could find convincing evidence that they present a much larger problem than has been generally recognized. Their deceptions were effectively hidden because they wove their lies into their own personal styles. The costs of missing these problem patients include wasted resources, misdirected treatment, and the appearance of professional incompetence. For the management of wanderers, more collaboration is needed among clinicians, risk managers, and administrators. Research has yet to show that therapists can help even ordinary people who have truly been victims of trauma.

Part 1: wandering patients

In the early 1970s, I noticed how difficult it was to solve the problems of patients admitted to our new psychiatric ward from outside the catchment area of the Veterans Administration (VA)

Medical Center where I worked. These patients came to my attention because some research had shown that hospital staff were not good at predicting how well a patient would manage after discharge. Patients might easily adjust to the therapeutic milieu of a hospital ward but fail when sent home. Therefore, I was intent on working with families to help patients successfully return to their own home setting. But attempts to apply this therapeutic strategy served only to underscore the difficulty in dealing with those from outside our catchment area.

Who were these patients? I designed a prospective study to identify all the patients who wandered into our ward from far away, the results of which were published in an article we sub-titled 'Summering in Oregon' (Pankratz and Lipkin 1978). To qualify as a wanderer in this study, the patient could not have lived in the medical centre catchment area for more than 1 month. Further, the patient could not have a prior residence or a significant social relationship in the catchment area. The target group, therefore, was a highly specific group with no personal ties or social support system available and hence no apparent reason to be in this location.

In 1 year, 14 patients met these strict criteria. Although this number was small, these patients emerged through a highly selective screening process. Because only 30 beds were available, every effort was made to avoid unnecessary and inappropriate admissions. Nevertheless, these wanderers gained access to the ward at the rate of about one a month. In the United States, patients can merely present themselves to a hospital emergency department for an admission; in the United Kingdom, in contrast, individuals are generally referred by a primary care physician for psychiatric services. Thus, our subjects employed a variety of strategies to ensure their admission such as arriving during evening hours and on weekends when fewer referral options were available. Further, during irregular hours, less experienced staff were on duty who were more likely to be influenced by social pressure and less attentive to the underlying psychiatric disorder. Many accentuated their admission demands with suicidal threats or violence. One patient went to an intensive care unit and threatened the staff. He was dragged directly to the psychiatry ward by the police, thus avoiding the inevitable wait in the admission area. Some patients appeared quite psychotic or disturbed in the emergency department but appeared much more normal once they were safely on the ward.

One man who had flown in from Hawaii was brought to our medical centre by airport police because he was seriously confused and suicidal. Once admitted, however, he put his belongings in his footlocker, walked to the dayroom, and asked 'Will the Notre Dame–USC football game be televised in this region tomorrow?' Upon hearing this question, the intern who admitted the patient came to my office and sheepishly announced that he had found another patient for my study.

Once these patients were on the ward, I was able to interview them in a style quite different from that of the staff who had official responsibilities for admitting notes, daily charting, and treatment plans. Instead, I used an 'off-the-record' approach to find out where they had travelled, what problems they feared, and who had been helpful to them. They gave surprisingly candid responses. From this information, I gathered records from previous hospitalizations, checked on hunches about where else they might have been admitted, and called to verify whatever claims they made.

At the end of a year, I identified the following four categories of wanderers, excluding two patients we considered rehabilitated.

- *Disappearing strangers.* Four subjects (28 per cent) in the study disappeared a day or so after they were admitted. Their goal may have been merely to get off the street for a night, but it is even more likely that they became concerned when the staff attempted to confront their problems directly. Before anyone had a chance to address their needs, they were gone, usually AWOL.
- *Charming people.* Two subjects (15 per cent) who adapted to our ward with a low-key and cooperative style were successful because the staff was less likely to pressure those who caused

no problems. Indeed, hospitals that used the therapeutic community model, which was popular in those earlier years, were likely to keep cooperative and helpful patients much longer (Herg 1972). Because no one considered a diagnosis of malingering in these relatively charming people, we never had a clue about their past hospitalizations where they no doubt had learned how to live successfully on a psychiatric ward.

- *Lost souls.* Two patients (15 per cent) were not so much psychiatrically disturbed as socially inadequate. They had no homes, no jobs, no money, and no sense of personal self-worth. It was difficult to discharge them because they had no place to go and seemingly no way to survive. One of these patients had received five different diagnostic labels ranging from inadequate personality disorder to schizophrenia. The records from the beginning of his travels through hospitals suggested that he had good insight and judgement, but gradually his discharge summaries began to describe poor insight and little concern about his problems. This change may have reflected his progressive psychiatric deterioration, but it is equally likely that he learned the role of helpless patient. He was a 'lost soul' whom staff were reluctant to discharge into a world where he had little apparent chance to survive. He continued to stay until we eventually realized that we could not change him or keep him forever. Thus, we discharged him with the resigned expectation that he would simply find his way to yet another hospital.

- *Disturbed and disturbing.* Four wanderers (28 per cent) caused the staff extraordinary confusion and grief. Although their behaviour was severely disturbed, none responded to neuroleptic medication, which caused the staff to speculate endlessly about the diagnosis and treatment strategy. Whereas most patients participated in designing their treatment programs, these patients contributed nothing, avoided therapy, and tested limits. The staff expended all the effort while the patients remained passive. Esoteric diagnostic possibilities were discussed at length. Were they mad or bad? Or both? We seemed unable to discharge these patients because there was always some staff member who had another idea, or another medication, to try. Eventually, however, we were obliged to discharge these treatment failures to the street from whence they came.

Economic burden of wandering patients

Perhaps these wandering patients were more confusing because they had no family that we could consult. Otherwise, we seldom thought of them as different from any of our other patients. However, a review of their previously undisclosed records provided a clearer view of reality. What distinguished these wanderers, as I eventually learned through persistent investigation, was that all had been treatment failures in other hospitals. In contrast, the two individuals that we considered rehabilitated by their stay had no prior hospital admissions. The remainder were only passing through, as they had passed through other hospitals before and would continue to do elsewhere. All of this history was hidden, however, which resulted in our senseless repetition of treatment strategies that others had tried without success. Further, all of these patients, with perhaps one exception, had problems with drugs or alcohol, which was not evident to us at the time.

This experience bent the twig of my professional career. As I moved into other medical settings, these same lessons were repeated. I found wandering and deception associated with factitious post-traumatic stress disorder (PTSD) (Sparr and Pankratz 1983), drug seeking (Pankratz *et al.* 1989), brain injury (Pankratz and Lezak 1987), Munchausen syndrome patients (Pankratz 1981; Pankratz and McCarthy 1986), and a variety of other hospital scams (Pankratz 1989).

Whereas mentally disordered patients seeking psychiatric admissions often created a crisis, the approach of deceptive wanderers seeking medical treatment was usually more subtle. Medical wanderers typically claimed that they had come to town to visit an aunt or because they were on a long-haul truck job. Untangling the histories of these dissembling patients was a complex, time-consuming task. Then, in the early 1990s, I discovered a crystal ball that allowed me to look into the past with sparkling clarity. For many years, the Department of Veterans Affairs had required all of its facilities to submit extensive information on every patient contact to the Data Processing Center in Austin, Texas. It thus became possible, using modem connection, to access that administrative data from the computer on my desk. The administrative information was invaluable for preventing clinical errors. Additionally, it gave promise of providing a window to a larger landscape. Was wandering merely a problem of 'snow birds' and visitors to the Pacific Northwest?

To explore the scope of the problem, we searched for patients with admissions to four or more *different* VA medical centres within 1 year, looking specifically at the 5 years from 1988 through 1992 (Pankratz and Jackson 1994). In each year, we found between 729 and 1013 patients who fit the criteria for wanderer. Each year about 20–25 per cent of the wanderers continued their peripatetic behaviour for a second year. Only 35 patients (about 3 per cent) of the original 1013 wanderers maintained this pattern for all 5 years of the study, but these 'habitual wanderers' created some impressive statistics. For example, using conservative cost values in 1992 dollars, we estimated that these 35 patients consumed more than $6.5 million worth of medical care.

The startling results of our study were filled with clinical, economic, and political implications. In 1991, for example, 810 wanderers accumulated 6266 inpatient admissions, about the same number as the Baltimore and the Cincinnati VA medical centres admitted that year. Some patients went only to psychiatric services and some went only to medical/surgical services, but most utilized both. The majority of admissions were to medical/surgical services, but even so, these 810 wanderers accounted for 2.8 per cent of all acute psychiatric admissions in the VA system. Not only were the admissions found throughout all medical sub-specialties within hospitals, 44 medical centres across the nation admitted one of these 810 patients on an average of once a week. Even more, some of these individuals were discovered using private hospital services through Medicare. (Using our search strategy, a Medicare administrator found a startling number of wandering patients in his database, completely contrary to his expectations.)

The services to these 810 patients were not necessarily inappropriate or based on deceptive presentations. However, the conclusions were inescapable. The 84 254 bed days and 22 600 out-patient visits accumulated by those patients wasted thousands of hours of thousands of clinicians. The fragmented care resulted in duplication of services, diagnostic confusion, and iatrogenic treatment. Furthermore, over 30 per cent of the admissions terminated in irregular discharges, illustrating the tendency toward costly but inconsequential medical care.

Is there an optimum way of managing wandering patients?

How might wanderers be managed more successfully? Our medical centre developed several administrative committees and clinical programs to manage a spectrum of dangerous, drug-seeking, and difficult patients (Drummond *et al.* 1989; Pankratz *et al.* 1989; Starker *et al.* 1991; Sparr *et al.* 1992). We placed a record flag advisory on the electronic records of patients at risk to help busy clinicians manage these patients safely. Physicians acted with more confidence because they knew that administrative and clinical backup was available if necessary. However, these programs did not fully address the larger problem of wandering nor of deception. Therefore, I proposed a national case-management system that would ignore geographical boundaries and provide consultation to all hospital services. The focus was the creation and management of an up-to-date problem list such that the patient's history would be immediately available whenever and wherever the patient was admitted. Although I left before a source of funding could be found, the Portland VA medical centre administrators assigned Shirley Toth, RN, to develop a compre-hensive programme for tracking and coordinating the care of wandering and difficult patients in all VA medical centres of the four-state Pacific Northwest region. Ms Toth has had extensive clinical experience as a nurse in the Emergency Department and as a Quality Management Spe-cialist. Further, she helped establish the patient management programmes pioneered in Portland.

Many hospitals are following this project with interest, and over 100 VA medical centres have shown interest in a similar programme.

More stringent admission standards nationally (for medical, surgical, and psychiatric services) have reduced the total number of hospital admissions. Many inappropriate hospital intrusions, such as created by patients escaping social conflict and failure, have been reduced as well. The remaining high utilization patients are probably more seriously disturbed and chronically maladjusted. Most likely, they have high incidence and prevalence of untreated dental conditions, hypertension, diabetes, dermatological disorders, tuberculosis, and neurological defects, all of which they can manipulate for admission to medical or psychiatric wards (Buckley and Bigelow 1992). As a result, they stretch the diagnostic skills of clinicians because they distort and withhold critical information. The solution is not to deny service but to provide assistance that has some meaningful effect. Unfortunately, psychotherapeutic interventions on their behalf can easily produce iatrogenic results by fostering increased dependence and chronicity (Green and Koprawski 1981). Nevertheless, the medical and economic problems they cause can be reduced if administrators, risk managers, and clinicians work together (Pankratz, 1998).

Part 2: factitious post-traumatic stress disorder

My experiences with wandering patients made me sensitive to the possibility of impostors, and I regularly checked the validity of unusual claims. So my skepticism about the trauma of war had nothing to do with my political opinion about Vietnam or with psychological theory about the effects of toxic events. I merely wanted to make certain that the patient was treated for the right problem. I was also sensitive to the possibility of false claims of personal loss because I had encountered several instances of feigned bereavement, those fabricators who usually present dramatic and heartrending details about the deaths of close relatives (Simpson 1978).

The diagnosis of PTSD first appeared in the third edition of the psychiatric diagnostic manual (DSM-III) in 1980. Soon after, psychiatrist Landy Sparr and I were the first to publish a paper describing the imitators of this disorder (Sparr and Pankratz 1983).[1] We described five men who said they had been traumatized in the Vietnam War; three said they were former prisoners of war. In fact, none had been prisoners of war, four had never been in Vietnam, and two had never been in the military.

Just as there were different styles of wandering, so these pretenders wove their stories into their own personality styles. For example, one man was brought to the medical centre by his wife who had discovered that he was selling her jewellery while pretending to be studying to become a physician's assistant. When his scam was discovered, the patient was contrite and said that he 'needed help'. He had told his wife and in-laws that he had difficulties coping because of atrocities he had witnessed in Vietnam. He told them of buddies being killed and maimed, sudden ambushes, and unbearable conditions. All of his stories sounded authentic because they were principally derived from the book *A Rumor of War* by Philip Caputo. However, we discovered that this man was in the military from 1975 to 1978, after the Vietnam War was over.

A 34-year-old man appeared in the emergency department complaining of left knee and thigh pain secondary to an old shrapnel wound received in combat. He stated that he was a former prisoner of war and was on the verge of 'going crazy'. He said that he needed to be in the hospital or else he might go out of control and hurt someone. He related these feelings to the

---

[1] The earliest report of factitious PTSD is probably found in the epic poem of Robert Copeland, *The highway to the spital-house [hospital]*, 1535. (See AJ Judges (1930). *The Elizabethan underworld*. Routledge, London.) Wandering beggars dressed in military garb (combat fatigues?) glibly described the battles they had fought and the wounds they had suffered. They wandered from hospital to hospital, crowding out the needy and stealing whatever they could.

aggressive behaviour that he learned in Vietnam, and he hinted that he had recently 'wasted' some people with a submachine gun while visiting the Philippines. He described a preoccupation with violence, intrusive thoughts of combat, nightmares, and detachment from others since leaving Vietnam, which he claimed resulted in his 90 per cent service-connected disability for a 'nervous condition'. After admission to an alcohol and drug treatment unit, it was learned that he had been fired 2 years previously from his employment at a state prison where he had learned about VA entitlements. In reality, the patient and his father had the same name, and his father had a service-connected disability from the Second World War. This patient was using his father's eligibility to support his imposture, even though he himself had never been in the service.

These two case examples merely hint at the broad spectrum of psychopathology from which the false stories emerged. The following year, our colleagues at the Reno VA confirmed that veterans pretending battle trauma had also invaded their wards (Lynn and Belza 1984). I was convinced that factitious PTSD was more common than even the most cynical observer would guess, especially after the VA made it known that disability pensions would be available to those with the disorder. I was impressed with the variety of individuals who were able to weave bogus claims so seamlessly into their lives. However, in hindsight it is now apparent that social, psychological, and political factors also obscured the ability of clinicians to see these deceptions clearly.

The scandal of PTSD following the Vietnam War

The old diagnostic concepts associated with war—combat fatigue, shell shock, and war neurosis—carry a notion that after a certain extended period of combat, the weaker soldiers might break down. Compared to other modern wars, there were relatively minor rates of battle injuries and psychiatric casualties in Vietnam (Jones and Wessely 2001). However, the concept of PTSD was developed and adopted in the context of an unpopular war, and there was an implicit assumption, especially by anti-war activists, that anyone who participated in this conflict would have subsequent psychological problems (Lifton 1985). The diagnostic manual suggests that the symptoms of PTSD emerge from an *event*, a stressor that would evoke 'significant symptoms of distress in *most people*', and the onset of symptoms might be *delayed* (emphasis added, American Psychiatric Association 1980, p. 236).

This subtle but non-trivial shift in the conceptualization of the effects of trauma created a new niche for patients. Hacking (1998) described a similar situation in the early 1800s when deserting one's military responsibilities or wandering away from home became viewed as a psychiatric problem caused by a fugue state. Thus began an epidemic of fugue-state wandering or perhaps more precisely an epidemic of *diagnosing* fugue-state wandering. Hacking noted that whereas some mental disorders bear a stigma, a disorder conceptualized as a misfortune that occurs to basically 'decent' souls will attract patients and clinicians. Hacking suggested that PTSD, which has provided psychological camouflage for a wide range of individuals, should probably be removed from the diagnostic manual.

Hacking's dark but unlikely recommendation can be considered in the context of two important works. The first is a book on trauma by Canadian psychologist Marilyn Bowman, and the second is a book about Vietnam veterans by Dallas stockbroker B. J. Burkett.

Two re-conceptualizations of the effects of trauma

In 1997, Marilyn Bowman carefully reviewed the world literature on response to trauma. She concluded that 'toxic events are not reliably powerful in yielding a chronic, event-focused clinical disorder such as PTSD' (Bowman 1997, p. 16). Indeed, most people do not respond to toxic events with persistent symptoms that would rise to the level of a diagnosable disorder, like PTSD. Individuals that do are characterized by pre-existing factors such as long-standing personality traits of emotionality and personal vulnerability, suggesting that their pre-event factors contribute more to serious distress disorders than the toxic event. Children, as well, seem amazingly resilient to trauma and unfavourable environments (Masten 2001).

Because these conclusions seem so far from the clinical practice of most mental health professionals, Bowman devoted a full chapter to consideration of why clinicians are reluctant to look for causes of distress beyond an event. The insight and wisdom of this chapter are compelling. Therapists have fallen for easy explanations, readily blaming others and the environment for the patient's distress. We have confused the acute symptoms of trauma with chronic disability or, even worse, created victims by reinforcing the idea that one's behaviour is attributable to situational events in instances where that is not true.

One could make a case from Bowman's book that mental health professionals were insufficiently prepared to understand the new diagnosis of PTSD. As a result, clinicians were easy marks for those veterans who spun false stories about how their lives were ruined by war. At the same time, we were also buffeted by social and political winds that blew us away from the harbours of psychological science. Perhaps the person most explicit in describing how far we have drifted off course is Dallas stockbroker, B. G. Burkett. Because he has armed himself with military records, when Burkett talks, historians listen.

Colonel Harry Summers Jr. (then retired but now deceased) was a distinguished fellow at the Army War College and editor of *Vietnam* magazine. In the August 1992 issue, Summers wrote that the magazine's review board was scrupulous about keeping inaccurate history out of the magazine. 'Not one of our almost two hundred authors has ever sold us a bill of goods,' he wrote, adding that he and his editors could tell phonies in the 'first three sentences' (Burkett and Whitley 1998, p. 439). That bit of self-confident bragging prompted Burkett to write a response to Summers. In the previous issue, Burkett proclaimed, *Vietnam* had unknowingly *reprinted* a false war story. Furthermore, Burkett told Summers that the senior editor of his magazine, Shelby Stanton, was a pretender. 'Not only can't you or anyone else tell a phony in the "first three sentences," neither you, nor I, can tell in the first three decades of personal contact.'

Summers was shocked at the brash letter from Burkett, insisting that he was wrong. Everyone considered Stanton the authoritative historian of the Vietnam War. He had served 6 years in Vietnam as a paratrooper platoon leader and a Special Forces long-range reconnaissance team commander with multiple covert combat operations that resulted in wounds that had forced him into retirement. At least that is what everyone believed, including Summers. However, Burkett had obtained Stanton's military records, which showed that Stanton had never been in Vietnam, Laos, or Cambodia where he claimed he had conducted combat missions. Instead, the records showed that he had been assigned to a desk job in Thailand, far from the war zones. He had been medically retired for asthma. After Summers confronted Stanton, Stanton's name was removed from the *Vietnam* masthead.

Summers was only one in a long line of writers, publishers, and historians that Burkett set straight. In fact, Burkett makes the case that much of what we believe about the Vietnam War is false because of the media, Rambo movies, and political agendas. Because of the meticulous documentation, *Stolen Valor* won the William E. Colby Award at Norwich University for outstanding military book in the year 2000. The selection committee, called the Colby Circle, included several leading historians. The book has been reviewed favourably by almost all the US and British military journals and is currently being used at military academies and the Naval War College. Burkett was invited to speak at the national convention of the Society of Military Historians when Dennis Showalter, Chairman of the Department of History at West Point, was president of the organization, and Burkett has lectured at prestigious universities.

Given all this attention by historians and military scholars, it is interesting to note that Burkett's barbs directed at the mental health profession have been met with stony silence that could easily be interpreted as massive denial. If Burkett is correct, then much of the research conducted on PTSD is based on misinformation, and we must face the clinical implications.

In 1983, Congress mandated that the Research Triangle Institute in North Carolina investigate the problems of emotional disturbance among Vietnam veterans. The National Vietnam Veteran Readjustment Study (NVVRS) was released after 4 years of study and at a cost of $9 million—facts extolled on the book's dust jacket (Kulka *et al.* 1988). Senator Allan Cranston, then chairman of the Senate Veterans' Affairs Committee, found the results 'shocking'. According to the NVVRS, 15.2 per cent of male Vietnam theatre veterans were currently suffering from PTSD. An additional 11 per cent of veterans were currently suffering 'partial' PTSD, which brought the total number at the time of the study to 830 000 or about 26 per cent of all Vietnam veterans.

Even more amazing was the 'lifetime' prevalence, namely the number who suffered from PTSD sometime during their lives. When lifetime prevalence was added to current PTSD, the study concluded that more than half (53.4 per cent) of male theatre veterans and nearly half (48.1 per cent) of the female veterans had experienced clinically significant stress-reaction symptoms.

This study helped convince Congress to continue funding the Vet Centers that had been established in 1979 as a short-term programme for the temporary needs of readjusting veterans. By 1994, the cost of administering PTSD programmes was $47 million a year, and the 201 Vet Center programmes cost an additional $58 million a year. Yet, if Bowman's interpretation of the effects of trauma is correct, the number of veterans with symptoms from exposure to combat should not be anywhere near this high. Burkett's analysis is more direct: These VA programmes do not cure PTSD; they teach it. Patients move through the Vet Center programmes into service-connected disability status. 'VA hospitals and PTSD programs are havens for malingerers who manipulate the system for their own psychological and financial ends and will ultimately cost taxpayers billions' (p. 233).

Is this just rhetoric? Burkett provides readers with painful and embarrassing examples of veterans deceiving gullible mental health professionals, often naming names. But his argument does not rest on single case studies of therapist incompetence. Burkett attacked the very foundation of the NVVRS report, and thus all the studies that rely on self-reporting.

Burkett wrote a long critique of the NVVRS research methodology, which he sent to me because he thought that he must have misunderstood something. For example, interviewers in this project were told to ask repeatedly the same questions from different angles until they got responses they expected in the belief that Vietnam veterans would be reluctant to talk about their experiences. But subjects give researchers the answers they expect (Orne 1962), even without pummelling their subjects, and such simple variables as the wording and format of questions can have an enormous impact on the outcome (Schwarz 1999). After reading Burkett's critique and the original documents, I concluded that his criticisms of the study were valid. I suggested that perhaps he was the only person who had actually read the methodology of this research. Another troubling possibility was that professionals are willing to forgive methodologic errors in papers they like, but not in papers that are unimportant or unpopular (Wilson *et al.* 1993).

Some of Burkett's criticisms, like the interview strategy, would be obvious to any social scientist—or lay person. However, some of his observations would be evident only to someone with intimate knowledge of the Vietnam War. For example, he pointed out that fewer than 15 per cent of the 3.3 million men who served in the Vietnam theatre of operation were in direct line combat units, a figure that stayed consistent throughout the war. There were periodic terrorist or rocket attacks on these support bases; however, with the exception of the Viet Cong terrorist campaign of 1965 and the Tet offensive in 1968, most rear areas were relatively free from attack.

If only 15 per cent were in combat, how can the NVVRS claim that 50 per cent of Vietnam veterans have experienced PTSD? In fact, most Vietnam veterans have had good adjustment following their service. Despite popular belief, Burkett provides compelling evidence that Vietnam veterans are better educated, have a lower suicide rate, have a higher employment record, are under-represented in prison populations, and have a lower homelessness rate than those who did not serve. All of this is consistent with Bowman's interpretation of the expected long-term outcome. Burkett also noticed that NVVRS subjects reported three times more Purple Hearts than expected in the sample. He concluded:

> Either the study's creators placed a heavy emphasis on choosing those who were wounded and the most likely to be traumatized, or they had a high ratio of liars. I would guess the latter. (p. 227)

Similarly, the NVVRS sample included several hundred women, most of whom served as nurses. Six women in the study claimed that their stress was caused by being a prisoner of war. Not one of the many researchers involved in the study apparently realized that no American military woman ever became a prisoner of war in Vietnam.

No one checked the military records of any subject! Whatever a subject said was taken as fact. Burkett asked the authors for an opportunity to review the military archives of those in their study, even a sample, but they refused. One official told him that the PTSD rates were probably even higher and that while liars could be a problem for researchers, 'skilled clinicians and counselors can weed out the fakes' (p. 231). However, unlike Colonel Summers, mental health professionals seem unwilling to check the facts. Burkett's criticisms have had little apparent effect on the VA, although his book has been quietly discussed.

Some serious implications

Bowman's conclusions and Burkett's accusations have serious implications, beginning with the collection of research data. As a manuscript reviewer of PTSD articles for the past 18 years, I have repeatedly requested that authors supply even the most simple evidence that their subjects experienced the trauma they claim. Rather than comply, these authors sent their papers to other journals. In one review, I supplied the name and phone number of the designated person who could verify the military information on their subjects. But the authors did not take this obvious step, I believe because their data contained several improbable results suggesting that their subjects had lied about their military experiences. Their huge government-funded research project was now expended, and their results were meaningless.

There are now two decades of PTSD research based on veterans' dubious self-reported experiences. Unfortunately, the problems with PTSD revealed in more recent research suggest even greater complexity. In a prospective study, Southwick et al. (1997) showed that Operation Desert Storm veterans were highly inconsistent over 2 years of time, even in their ability to recall very specific traumatic events. One month after the war, 46 per cent of subjects reported one or more traumatic events that they did not recall 2 years later. More disturbingly, 2 years after the war, 70 per cent of the subjects recalled traumatic events that they had not reported 1 month after the event. Subjects with more symptoms appeared to amplify their memory of combat trauma, perhaps as a way of explaining their current distress. The authors concluded that 'If memories of combat are inconsistent over time, then the relationship between PTSD and combat exposure would be a tenuous one' (p. 174).

Burkett used military records to show, for example, that a veteran could not have been engaged in the battles he described because he was assigned to a motor pool in a non-combat zone. But the Southwick study suggests, further, that memories are so plastic that veterans are likely to construct events that did not occur, especially if they had symptoms that begged for an explanation.

The additional use of psychological tests, surveys, and screening instruments is equally worthless without prior verification of the underlying experiences. These tests are easily manipulated by simulators and malingerers (Lees-Haley and Dunn 1994; Calhoun *et al*. 2000), and they provide no indication about the cause of symptoms the individual is experiencing. The symptoms of PTSD must arise directly from a toxic event, a relationship that is difficult to confirm even over an extended period of evaluation. Patients and doctors are often strongly attached to wrong attribution of symptoms, and these misunderstandings are difficult to modify (Pankratz 2002*a*).

Lifetime risk for exposure to potentially traumatizing events is extremely high, ranging from 60 to 90 per cent in the general population. Yet few will subsequently develop PTSD. The National Comorbidity Survey estimated that approximately 8 per cent of the individuals exposed to serious traumatic events had PTSD at some point in their lives (Kessler *et al*. 1995). Even lower numbers, as low as 1 per cent, were found in British combat soldiers individually assessed by clinicians (Simon Wessely, personal communication). Yet the VA continues to award disability status without examination of the full military records. Applicants who are rejected can reapply after reviewing the diagnostic manual, consulting websites, hiring an adjudication expert, or purchasing a manual that trains applicants to aim for 100 per cent disability (Hill 1995). Or, they can concoct an entirely different trauma story and reapply in an adjacent geographical region.

It is my understanding that a small task force of Inspector General agents is trying to identify veterans receiving money on the basis of falsely claimed POW status, but the complexity and expense of adjudicating deceptive claims appears to be an overwhelming task. It will be extremely difficult to reverse the errors of the mental health professionals whose reports provided the basis for these pensions. Further, patients who never experienced trauma or whose symptoms do not arise directly from trauma are not likely to respond to PTSD treatment strategies. Even for those individuals who truly suffered disabling symptoms because of trauma, the labelling process itself may enable them to assume a sick role. Further, it is difficult to conceive of any psychological theory to support monthly payments to patients who maintain symptoms, the costs of which may now be near $2 billion a year. This wholesale distribution of the PTSD diagnosis to veterans may rank as one of the biggest blunders of twentieth century psychiatry.

We must now face the fact that a whole body of research on PTSD, perhaps even studies whose subjects experienced truly terrible combat, may be worthless. An editorial that appeared in the *American Journal of Psychiatry* concurrently with the Southwick article flatly admitted that no one now knows what PTSD really is (Hales and Zatzick 1997). And it is precisely that assumption with which researchers must start when collecting data. Much of the existing PTSD research appears to be an exercise in gathering data that confirms the investigators' hypotheses. But good science and clinical practice seek to challenge existing beliefs through healthy skepticism that demands the consideration of alternative explanations and influences. As a start, Harvard psychologist Richard McNally has expended extensive effort to obtain approval for retrieving archival records from St. Louis for 37 PTSD research subjects that he used in some information processing experiments. McNally has arranged for Burkett to identify any fabricators so that their data can be removed from the study. This small step may have enormous significance for many other studies, but self-correcting strategies are hallmarks of science.

Surprisingly, despite enormous amounts of money spent on treatment, Shalev *et al*. (1996) concluded that remission is rarely achieved in therapy. Perhaps clinicians should focus more on early intervention, assisting those in acute grief and disrupting their slide into chronic symptoms. Yet, even here there is insufficient evidence to support intervention following trauma, and some evidence suggests that intervention may even exacerbate symptoms.

Bowman's (1997) review of treatment provides impressive examples of how intervention can make problems worse. Primarily, there is the risk that outside intrusion of help will be directed away from what individuals actually want or need. For example, Ugandan victims of rape in war were most interested in organizing economic development projects, not in discussing their experiences of rape. Even worse, outside intervention can be actively harmful by depriving community members of the opportunity to struggle together, thereby strengthening their own bonds of enduring support.

Victims' expression of satisfaction or appreciation of service are no indication that an intervention has in fact reduced the intensity or duration of symptoms (McDermott 1996; Litz *et al.* 2002). The emotional spark that occurs between therapist and patient is so powerful that both parties often disdain research, viewing it as irrelevant or contrived (Pankratz 2002*b*).

Litz *et al.* (2002) reviewed six recent PTSD outcome studies that they judged as having sound methodology. In all instances, the psychological debriefing failed to promote change to a greater degree than no intervention at all, and in two of the studies the symptoms of victims became worse over time. Litz and colleagues recommended that psychological debriefing not be provided to individuals immediately after trauma, although they did state that offering comfort and humanitarian assistance is acceptable. In another review, Arendt and Elklit (2001) also suggested that debriefing does not prevent psychiatric disorders or mitigate the effects of traumatic stress.

If early treatment has risks, so does early assessment. Predicting low base-rate responses is always difficult, but a greater problem is the possibility of iatrogenic effects. For example, the term 'shell shock' was officially banned in England in 1917 because it was known to suggest disability (Leys 2000). Belief systems can have such a profound effect on the production of symptoms that clinicians must be mindful of their responsibility in the task of information gathering. Also, clinicians, attorneys, and others can inflame symptoms by the possibility of monetary compensation (Aronson *et al.* 2001).

Conclusions

Twenty years ago there was great enthusiasm for helping the victims of trauma. Training programmes proliferated and treatment strategies were taught with confidence. An army of mental health specialists now make their services available. Communities assume that when disaster strikes, specialized teams of professionals must be brought in to help survivors. Media coverage often focuses on individuals overwhelmed with emotions, implying that these people need help to recover. However, research shows that professionals are sometimes part of the problem. As a result, the PTSD niche is now an admixture of individuals: patients suffering from the traumas of life, impostors, those who have stumbled into PTSD to avoid other labels, and patients directed into PTSD by well-meaning but mistaken professionals. Research, diagnosis, and treatment are meaningful only if you know which path the patient has travelled.

References

American Psychiatric Association (1980). *Diagnostic and statistical manual of mental disorders*, 3rd edn. American Psychiatric Association, Washington, DC.

Arendt, M. and Elklit, A. (2001). Effectiveness of psychological debriefing. *Acta Psychiatrica Scandinavica*, **104**, 423–7.

Aronson, B. H., Rosenwald, L., and Rosen, G. M. (2001). Attorney–client confidentiality and the assessment of claimants who allege posttraumatic stress disorder. *Washington Law Review*, **76**, 313–47.

Bowman, M. (1997). *Individual differences in posttraumatic response*. Erlbaum, Mahwah, NJ.

Buckley, R. and Bigelow, D. A. (1992). The multi-service network: reaching the unserved multiproblem individual. *Community Mental Health Journal*, **28**, 43–50.

Burkett, B. G. and Whitley, G. (1998). *Stolen valor*. Verity Press, Dallas, TX.

Calhoun, P. S., Karnst, K. S., and Tucker, D. D. (2000). Feigning combat-related posttraumatic stress disorder on the Personality Assessment Inventory. *Journal of Personality Assessment*, **75**, 338–50.

Drummond, D. J., Sparr, L. F., and Gordon, G. H. (1989). Hospital violence reduction among high-risk patients. *Journal of the American Medical Association*, **261**, 2531–4.

Green, R. S. and Koprowski, P. F. (1981). The chronic patient with a nonpsychotic diagnosis. *Hospital and Community Psychiatry*, **12**, 479–81.

Hacking, I. (1998). *Mad travelers: reflections on the reality of transient mental illnesses*. University Press of Virginia, Charlottesville, VA.

Hales, R. E. and Zatzick, D. F. (1997). What is PTSD? *American Journal of Psychiatry*, **154**, 143–4.

Herg, M. I. (1972). The therapeutic community: a critique. *Hospital and Community Psychiatry*, **23**, 69–72.

Hill, R. (1995). *How to apply for 100% total disability rating*. Privately Published, Lee's Summit, MO.

Jones, E. and Wessely, S. (2001). Psychiatric battle casualties: An intra- and interwar comparison. *British Journal of Psychiatry*, **178**, 242–7.

Kessler, R. C., Sonnega, A., Bromet, E., Hughes, M., and Nelson, C. B. (1995). Posttraumatic stress disorder in the National Comorbidity Survey. *Archives of General Psychiatry*, **52**, 1048–60.

Kulka, R. A., Schlenger W. E., Fairbank, J. A., Hough, R. L., Jordan, B. K., Marmar, C. R., and Weiss, D. S. (1988). *Trauma and the Vietnam War generation*. Brunner/Mazel, New York, NY.

Lees-Haley, P. R. and Dunn, J. T. (1994). The ability of naïve subjects to report symptoms of mild brain injury, post-traumatic stress disorder, major depression, and generalized anxiety disorder. *Journal of Clinical Psychology*, **50**, 252–6.

Leys, R. (2000). *Trauma: a genealogy*. University of Chicago Press, Chicago, IL.

Lifton, R. J. (1985). *Home from the war*. Basic Books, New York, NY.

Litz, B. T., Gray, M., Bryant, R., and Adler, A. (2002). Early intervention for trauma: current status and future directions. *Clinical Psychology: Science and Practice*, **9**, 112–34.

Lynn, E. J. and Belza, M. (1984). Factitious post-traumatic stress disorder: the veteran who never got to Vietnam. *Hospital and Community Psychiatry*, **35**, 697–701.

Masten, A. (2001). Ordinary magic: resilience processes in development. *American Psychologist*, **56**, 227–38.

McDermott, B. (1996). Sutherland bushfire trauma project: a randomized controlled treatment trail. Paper presented at the meeting of the American Psychological Association, Toronto.

Orne, M. T. (1962). On the social psychology of the psychological experiment: with particular reference to demand characteristics and their implications. *American Psychologist*, **17**, 776–83.

Pankratz, L. (1981). A review of the Munchausen Syndrome. *Clinical Psychology Review*, **1**, 65–78.

Pankratz, L. (1989). Patient deception as a healthcare risk. *Perspectives in Healthcare Risk Management*, **9** (2), 5–8.

Pankratz, L. (1998). *Patients who deceive: assessment and management of risk in providing benefits and care*. Charles C. Thomas, Springfield, IL.

Pankratz, L. (2002a). Hard times, dancing manias, and multiple chemical sensitivity. *Scientific Review of Mental Health*, **1**, 62–75.

Pankratz, L. (2002b). Demand characteristics and the development of dual, false belief systems. *Prevention and Treatment*.

Pankratz, L., Hickam, D., and Toth, S. (1989). The identification and management of drug-seeking behavior in a medical center. *Drug and Alcohol Dependence*, **24**, 115–18.

Pankratz, L. and Jackson, J. (1994). Habitually wandering patients. *New England Journal of Medicine*, **331**, 1752–5.

Pankratz, L. and Lezak, M. D. (1987). Cerebral dysfunction in the Munchausen syndrome. *Hillside Journal of Clinical Psychiatry*, **9**, 195–206.

Pankratz, L. and Lipkin, J. (1978). The transient patient in a psychiatric ward: Summering in Oregon. *Journal of Operational Psychiatry*, **9**, 42–7.

Pankratz, L. and McCarthy, G. (1986). The ten least wanted patients. *Southern Medical Journal*, **79**, 613–20.

Schwarz, N. (1999). How the questions shape the answers. *American Psychologist*, **54**, 93–105.

Shalev, A. Y., Bonne, O., and Eth, S. (1996). Treatment of posttraumatic stress disorder: a review. *Psychosomatic Medicine*, **58**, 165–82.

Simpson, M. A. (1978). Pseudo-bereavement in the Munchausen syndrome. *British Journal of Psychiatry*, **133**, 382.

Southwick, S. M., Morgan, C. A., Nicolaou, A. L., and Charney, D. S. (1997). Consistency of memory for combat-related traumatic events in veterans of Operation Desert Storm. *American Journal of Psychiatry*, **154**, 173–7.

Sparr, L. and Pankratz, L. (1983). Factitious posttraumatic stress disorder. *American Journal of Psychiatry*, **140**, 1016–9.

Sparr, F. Rogers, J. L., Beahrs, O., and Mazur, D. J. (1992). Disruptive medical patients: forensically informed decision making. *Western Journal of Medicine*, **156**, 501–6.

Starker, S., Baker, L., Drummond, D., and Pankratz, L. (1991). Management of the 'difficult' medical patient: organizational strategies. *VA Practitioner*, **8** (6), 91–7.

Wilson, T. D., DePaulo, B. M., Mook, D. G., and Klaren, K. J. (1993). Scientists' evaluation of research: the biasing effects of the importance of the topic. *Psychological Science*, **4**, 322–5.

15 When the quantity of mercy is strained: US physicians' deception of insurers for patients

Matthew K. Wynia*

Abstract

Physicians sometimes are faced with patients needing care that may not be covered by health insurers. This chapter reviews physicians' deception of insurers to help their patients obtain coverage for these services. Recent studies show that the great majority of US physicians do not believe that 'gaming the system' for patients is generally ethical. Still, more than one-third of American physicians report exaggerating patients' severity of illness, miscoding diagnoses, and/or recording signs or symptoms that patients do not actually have in order to provide necessary but uncovered care to their patients. Studies suggest that some available policies might reduce how often physicians resort to the use of deception, but other common policies actually encourage physicians to use deception in service to their patients. Solutions should entail adopting a systems-level approach with two aims. First, to reduce the perceived need to use deception to provide high quality patient care, such as by making the appeals process more user-friendly. And second, to build the legitimacy of coverage decisions by making them more fair and transparent for both patients and physicians.

Introduction

> . . . in the course of justice, none of us should see salvation:
> we do pray for mercy; and that same prayer
> doth teach us all to render the deeds of mercy.
>
> Portia, from *The Merchant of Venice*, Act IV, scene I

Physicians stand uneasily at the junction between the demands and desires of their patients and the demands and desires of the insurers who largely pay for the care their patients receive. Whether or not the insurer is a state-sponsored programme or, as is common in the United States, a private company, mediating these conflicting demands can be challenging. On the one hand, both ethics and legal rules call for honesty and fair dealings with all parties involved in the health care system. On the other hand, ethical and legal rules also suggest that the physician's primary obligation,

---

* The views and opinions contained in this chapter are those of the author and should in no way be construed as representing official policies of the American Medical Association.

over and above any social role, is to advocate for services that will be of medical benefit to his or her patient. In this chapter, I explore the phenomenon of physicians in the United States who feel pressed into making choices between strict adherence to insurance company coverage rules or, instead, doing what they believe is best for their patients and bending or breaking these rules—and why some physicians demonstrably will choose the latter course despite the legal and ethical risks involved. I will first summarize data proving the existence of the phenomenon of 'gaming the system' (Morreim 1991), using as an example, deception for the benefit of patients. Next, I will discuss why physicians may feel compelled to use this sort of strategy, as well as reasons why the use of deception is generally a poor choice. Finally, I will mention a few ways in which the pressures that lead to physicians' use of deception can be reduced. The reader will note that discussing the use of deception to benefit the physician (e.g. billing fraud) is not the aim of this chapter. Billing for services not rendered, or patients not seen, is always unethical and therefore poses different—less morally nuanced—moral dilemmas, which are not directly addressed by the studies under review.

Studies of physicians' use of deception to benefit their patients

Investigations into physicians' use of deception to benefit patients probably originated in studies of physicians withholding from patients cancer diagnoses, or even lying to patients about diagnosis and prognosis. Ostensibly, withholding this information was done—in a rather dramatic display of paternalism—to benefit patients who were thought not 'strong enough' to handle it. Regardless of this motivation and whether or not it was appropriate, the totality of the change in US attitudes in this regard is what is interesting today. In 1961, 90 per cent of US physicians in one survey reported that they preferred not to tell patients of a cancer diagnosis. By 1977, a mere 16 years later, this proportion had been completely reversed and 97 per cent of physicians answering the same survey questions reported a preference for telling cancer patients their diagnosis (Novack *et al.* 1979). (This strong sense of an obligation of truth-telling to patients will reappear at the end of this chapter, when it will be seen, appropriately, to limit physicians' options when patients need services that are not covered.)

Subsequent studies have begun to explore physicians' willingness to use deception in other ways that are intended to help patients. For instance, a number of physicians have expressed willingness to use deception to help their patients protect confidential medical information (Novack *et al.* 1989; Serkes 2001) to keep a marital infidelity hidden (e.g. one spouse presents for treatment of a venereal disease and requests that the other be treated under a false diagnosis), and for other reasons (Novack *et al.* 1989). Recently, two studies have specifically examined US physicians' willingness to use deception to help their patients obtain medical services that might not otherwise be paid for by health insurers. First, Freeman and colleagues used six clinical case vignettes, describing services ranging in severity from potentially life saving procedures to cosmetic rhinoplasty (i.e. a 'nose job'), to examine whether physicians would endorse the use of deception to help patients obtain coverage for each service (Freeman *et al.* 1999). Each scenario presupposed that the condition under consideration was a 'pre-existing condition', that coverage for the service would therefore be denied, and that it was not possible for the patient to pay for the care from their own funds.[1] Of the 169 physicians responding to the survey, 58 per cent would sanction deception of the insurer to help a patient obtain coverage for a potentially life saving coronary artery bypass graft and 56 per cent would do so to potentially salvage a patient's limb through an arterial revascularization procedure. On the other hand, only 2.5 per cent

---

[1] Health insurance plans in the United States commonly do not cover treatment of conditions that were known to exist at the time the patient enrolled in the insurance plan. Since US patients may change insurers once a year or even more often, sometimes without being given a choice, it is conceivable that the scenarios posed to physicians in this study could arise in practice, though how often this occurs is not known.

would sanction deception to help a patient obtain coverage for cosmetic rhinoplasty. Interestingly, physicians were generally more likely to sanction the use of deception if they worked in areas where more patients were covered through managed care health insurance plans (managed care plans often have tighter reimbursement rules and they may also share financial risk with physicians).

In the second recent study, my colleagues and I asked physicians to reveal whether they had, in fact, manipulated insurance company reimbursement rules to help their patients obtain what they considered to be 'needed care' (Wynia *et al.* 2000). Thus, rather than asking about *sanctioning* deception, we asked how often, if ever, in the last year the physician had actually *used* deception by: (a) exaggerating the severity of a patient's condition; (b) altering a patients billing diagnosis, or (c) reporting signs or symptoms that a patient did not have. Each question was predicated on the physicians' belief that the patient needed a service that would not be covered, though the type of service was not specified nor was the reason for non-coverage. We also did not preclude reporting the use of other options instead of deception, such as making an appeal to the health insurer for coverage, asking the patient to pay for the service out of their own funds, providing the service for free, or providing some alternative service that would have been covered. Of the 720 respondents to the survey, 28 per cent reported having exaggerated patients' severity of illness (responding with 'sometimes', 'often', or 'very often' to the question), 23 per cent had altered a billing report, and 10 per cent had written into the medical record signs or symptoms that patients did not have. Of the 39 per cent who said they used one or more of these three tactics, 54 per cent said they had used these tactics more often in the last year than they had 5 years ago.

Why use deception?

At first, it may seem obvious that physicians have a simple pecuniary interest in manipulating reimbursement rules to help patients obtain coverage—after all, physicians are reimbursed for the care they deliver. But the actual picture emerging is considerably more complex. In our study, we examined how physicians were paid, their income, whether they felt increasingly financially strapped, and several other financial variables— but none of these variables were significantly associated with using deception to help patients obtain coverage (Wynia *et al.* 2000). A likely reason for this is that, in practice, scenarios in which deception is used probably only rarely involve any direct financial benefit to the physician. Every one of the six clinical vignettes that Freeman and colleagues used to examine deception represented a general internal medicine physician helping a patient to obtain coverage for subspecialty care (such as a surgical intervention). Such referrals do not entail any direct financial benefit to the physician making the referral [indeed, suck 'kickbacks' are both unethical and illegal (Council on Ethical and Judicial Affairs 2002b)]. Similarly, if a physician exaggerates a patient's symptoms to obtain an off-formulary medication, or to obtain coverage for a diagnostic test (such as an MRI scan), there is no direct financial reward to the physician for doing so.

But even if there is no direct financial reward to physicians, there may still be indirect benefits to physicians who 'game the system' for their patients. Using deception might enable physicians to maintain cordial relations with patients. A large minority (37 per cent) of US physicians report that patients sometimes ask them to lie to insurers, and these physicians are about twice as likely to report using deception to help patients obtain coverage (Wynia *et al.* 2000). Since turning down a patient's request is uncomfortable, time consuming, and risks alienating (and losing) the patient, it is not surprising that pressures from patients are important. Moreover, these pressures might be expected to be increasing, as direct-to-consumer advertising of medical services in the

United States is raising patient awareness of specific therapies, some of which will not be covered or will be covered only in limited circumstances (Landers 2001).

Physicians also report that some alternatives to the use of deception are unattractive (Werner *et al.* 2002). In particular, appealing adverse coverage decisions (asking the insurer to reconsider) is time consuming and a hassle (Grumet 1989; Goold *et al.* 1994). Not only is time spent on appeals not regularly reimbursed, but mounting too many appeals risks being labelled a troublemaker and losing one's contract with the health plan (Fielder 1995; Orentlicher 1995; Liner 1997; Hilzenrath 1998). Reflecting this, we found that physicians who feel more pressed for time are more likely to resort to deception to help patients obtain coverage (Wynia *et al.* 2000). Whether physicians who are more fearful of being terminated by a health plan are less likely to mount appeals, or more likely to use deception, has not been reported.

The potential legal and ethical risks of failing to provide an equal standard of care to all patients, regardless of their ability to pay, also weighs on US physicians. Recent case law suggests that US physicians are legally accountable for providing needed care to their patients and that they do not derive immunity from this obligation when they agree to accept insurance coverage rules (Hall 1994; Manuel 1995). Ethically, providing the same high quality of care to all patients is a clear professional aspiration for physicians even if, as in the United States, it is far from being realized (Council on Ethical and Judicial Affairs 1994). On the other hand, it should be obvious that failure to adhere closely to the language of insurance contracts also poses legal and ethical risks. In the legal realm, there has recently been a crackdown in the United States on medical fraud and abuse (Kalb 1999). In this regard, however, it is interesting that although the majority of respondents to our survey (57 per cent) were somewhat worried about prosecution for fraud, in a multivariate model being worried was *not* significantly associated with deciding *not* to use deception (Wynia *et al.* 2000). In the ethical realm, nearly 85 per cent of respondents did not believe it was ethical to 'game the system for your patient's benefit', including a majority of those who reported doing so (Wynia *et al.* 2000)! Incidentally, these findings suggest that neither further crackdowns on fraud and abuse nor simple reiteration of the ethical impropriety of 'gaming the system' will be very effective in curbing this activity.

What seems to drive physicians most into using deception is a simple belief that 'it is *necessary* to game the system to provide high quality care' (Wynia *et al.* 2000). That physicians recognize 'gaming the system' as unethical, but do it when they perceive it to be necessary, suggests that physicians recognize and weigh their conflicting obligations and often come down on the side of advocacy for their patients rather than enforcing insurance company contracts. This may not, in every case, be unethical. While contractual justice calls for all participants to adhere to agreed upon contracts (Veatch 1972), health care has many features that suggest that it is not merely contractually based (Light 1992). The US health system leans strongly towards a market oriented emphasis on value for money and free choice in health care—allowing patients with good information and options to make choices and then 'get what they pay for' but not more. But it is clear that many patients are not good health care 'consumers' (Hibbard and Weeks 1987; Hibbard *et al.* 1997) and they may unwittingly agree to, or be assigned to, health care coverage rules that do not fully meet their medical needs. For physicians, taking on the role of 'enforcer' of such contracts may not be merely uncomfortable, it may be unprofessional. Professional ethics call for physicians to act as quasi-fiduciaries to their patients, striving to provide the same high quality care to all, regardless what patients can afford to pay (Council on Ethical and Judicial Affairs 1994). Bending, or even breaking, the rules may be seen as an act of beneficence, or mercy, which is also ethically compelling (Beauchamp and Childress 1994)—sometimes even more compelling then acting according to strict justice. As Portia notes in the famous 'quality of mercy' speech from the *Merchant of Venice*, excerpted at the beginning of this chapter, we all sometimes unwisely enter into agreements from which we wish to be excused, and we may pray for mercy from those whom we owe.

In this prayer we demonstrate the high value of compassion and mercy even in the face of a binding contract.

Gaming, and the rules of the game

Even more than an ethical challenge for individual physicians, recent commentators have suggested that the use of deception by physicians may represent a natural consequence of promoting the rules of the marketplace in the US health care system. Patricia Illingworth has provocatively described the use of 'bluffing, puffing, and spinning' in the advertisements and other public statements of US health plans attempting to attract customers (Illingworth 2000). In one case Aetna, a large US health insurer, successfully fought an advertising fraud lawsuit by conceding in court that 'its advertising claims that it was committed to "maintaining and improving quality health care" were "mere puffery" ' (American Health Line 2000). Illingworth suggests that when health plans puff up the quality of care and services they will provide, and gloss over their deficiencies, this leads patients, with doctors as their advocates, to exaggerate their own needs—the rules of the game actually encourage this. She further notes with concern that appropriate health care, unlike many business relations, relies on strict truth-telling, especially between patients and physicians, which could erode under this evolving system.

With this in mind, it is perhaps especially remarkable that physicians' deception of insurers to help patients obtain coverage appears to be socially sanctioned in the United States (Alexander *et al.* 2003). The two studies described above each received extensive coverage in the US popular media and I am aware of only one media interviewer who took a negative outlook towards physicians deceiving insurers—and this was an interviewer from the BBC. He alone asked whether Americans were not concerned that physicians (who are, after all, 'agents of society', he said) were bending and breaking social rules? For the American media, however, this question seemed almost nonsensical; after all, physicians are *not* agents of society, they are agents of their patients, especially when fighting the rules of the widely reviled US managed care industry.

In the end, physicians' use of deception may be most commonly justified by a widespread and general sense that health insurance coverage rules are not fair and are not fairly implemented. The fairness of insurance rules has been questioned on the basis of lack of choice [patients in the United States often do not select their own insurance plans, but rely instead on plans their employers select for them (Gawande *et al.* 1998; Dickey and McMenamin 1999)] as well as on the criteria used to make the coverage decisions (Daniels and Sabin 1998). The US public appears to believe that some coverage decisions are not medically appropriate or are based more on cost than on effectiveness and managed care organizations rank at the very bottom of the trust scale in recent polls (Horowitz 2002). Patients and physicians also understand that the US health care system is not financially 'closed', such that all money in the system must be spent on patient care (Morreim 1995a)—as a result, they may believe that any money saved by adhering closely to coverage restrictions will not go to more deserving patients, but instead will go toward executive salaries, stockholder profits, or other 'inappropriate' uses. This perception is fed by an emphasis among insurers and their investors on the 'medical loss ratio', a measure of the fraction of insurer revenues expended on the actual care of patients (Cook 2000). Insurers with higher medical 'losses' often are punished by dropping stock prices. The best-known example of this is the $1 billion dollars in shareholder value lost by US Healthcare (a publicly held health insurer) over only two bleak days in April 1995, when it 'announced that it would raise doctors' pay in an effort to upgrade the quality of its medical networks [and] ... Angry investors figured that the company's medical loss ratio was going to rise' (Anders 1996).

Why not use deception?

Overall, arguments against the legitimacy of coverage decisions in the United States are rather strong (Daniels and Sabin 1998), and physicians appear to believe that sometimes deception is warranted to get their patients needed care (Wynia *et al.* 2000). So what are the arguments (apart from legal risks) *against* the use of deception by physicians? The question itself will strike some readers as unusual. Truth-telling is an obvious good, yet deception within the US health care system is occurring and appears to hold some public support, so a few comments in defence of truth telling in health care seem appropriate (Bok 1978). First, how long will patients be appreciative before they begin to realize the potential implications of having a willing liar for a doctor? After all, if physicians are willing to lie *for* patients, might they also lie *to* them? Patients might recognize that the use of deception, even for a good cause, could become a bad habit that, once established, is not easily broken. Second, though the health care system is not closed, it also is not fully open (Morreim 1995*a*). That is, although money saved on one patient's care may or may not go to other patients, money that is spent on one patient cannot be used for another. That is, using deception to obtain coverage for one patient's care means that other patients cannot access these same resources. The most egregious example of this would be the manipulation of the organ distribution system by exaggerating one patient's illness, which could deprive a more-deserving patient of a life saving and scarce resource. Third, since the deceptions involved often necessitate documentation, there is a risk that false or misleading information will be entered into a medical record, with harm to the patient as a result. The most dramatic incident of this sort involved Robert Stafford and his wife Pauline. In 1984, Pauline was diagnosed with lung cancer and underwent what appeared to be successful surgery. She had a CT scan of her head to ensure that she did not have metastases to her brain. The scan was read as negative but, unfortunately, the neurologist reading the CT scan had learned through prior experience that Pauline's insurer would not cover a CT scan to 'rule-out' metastases. He therefore instructed his staff to write 'brain tumour' as her diagnosis on the billing form. When Pauline received her copy of this bill, she became despondent. On 14 January 1985, after cooking breakfast and cleaning up around the house, she hanged herself (Stafford vs. Neurological Medicine 1987).

Finally, using deception is, in most instances, socially irresponsible. Fighting openly against adverse coverage decisions, unlike deception, brings an opportunity to change the system for all patients. Conversely, showing compassion by quietly subverting the system may be merciful to an individual patient, but it is destructive to the health care system as a whole. One way to understand this is to consider what would happen if all physicians were to pretend to agree to allocation rules, but then skirt them for their own patients. Such a system would break down rapidly. Moreover, pretending to agree with a system that is unfair would tend to perpetuate the same bad system right up until the moment of its collapse; it does nothing to improve it. Because deceiving insurers can provide individual patients with what they need, it is a quick choice that seems easy to justify; but since it fails to improve the system over time and for others, this is a false economy.

Alternatives to deceiving insurers

Physicians who are convinced that a patient will be denied coverage for necessary care do have some options—though for any individual they will be limited. In some instances, for example, services can be provided for free. This option is limited, however, when the services entail hospitalization, laboratory testing, prescribing medications, or involving other health professionals. Appealing to the insurer for coverage may also be effective, despite the problems of appeals noted previously. Certainly, US physicians today must recognize a professional duty to some-times appeal for coverage, and recognize that this obligation is part and parcel of providing high quality care (Council on Ethical and Judicial Affaris 1995). The amount of time and energy that any one physician must devote to appeals to satisfy this duty is a matter of ongoing debate (Morreim 1995*b*). Physicians might also help patients to obtain coverage elsewhere, such as through a charity organization, or they might ask the patient to pay for the care out of their own funds. Sometimes there will be an equally effective service (or one that is acceptably close to equally effective) that could be substituted and that would be covered. Any of these options, and there are others that may work in certain circumstances (Morreim 1995*a*), would seem generally preferable to the use of deception.

Two related, and highly unattractive, options deserve separate mention. First, physicians might decide simply not to raise the possibility of obtaining services that would be useful but that are not covered. Second, physicians might choose to couch the decision not to pursue an uncovered service in clinical terms, such as by claiming that the service would not be of benefit (Aaron and Schwartz 1984). Using either of these options would run directly counter to well-established ethical standards, which call for physicians to 'assure the disclosure of medically appropriate treatment alternatives, regardless of cost' to their patients (Council on Ethical and Judicial Affairs 2002*a*). They would also be highly destructive to patient trust. Since patient trust is vital to good medical care (Pearson and Raeke 2000), using these options should be avoided. In any event, as was noted at the beginning of this chapter, deception of patients has, fortunately, fallen out of favour among US physicians, as it also has among physicians in the British National Health Service (Klein 2001).

Conclusion: improving the situation

It is unfortunate that as pressures to control health care costs increase, US physicians' use of deception in dealing with health insurers may be expected to increase in parallel. Efforts to more tightly control utilization appear to increase physicians' perceived need to manipulate reimburse-ment rules to provide high-quality care (Wynia *et al.* 2000). Rising pressures on physicians to see more patients in less time will increase time shortages, which also are related to using deception to obtain favourable coverage decisions quickly (Wynia *et al.* 2000). At the same time, the growth of advertising and other means of increasing patient awareness of health care options may lead to increased patient requests for uncovered services (Landers 2001). And, of course, many of the pressures facing US physicians exist in other countries as well; there is little reason to believe that physicians outside the United States will not also respond to these pressures by sometimes manipulating reimbursement systems to help their patients, suggesting that this problem may be widespread and rising both outside and within the United States.

Addressing the mounting pressures that are stimulating physicians to use deception will not be easy. Simply making physicians more fearful of fraud enforcement does not appear to alter this behaviour (Wynia *et al.* 2000). And reiterating ethical prohibitions against 'gam-ing the system' for patients will not be very effective in reducing this activity, since most physicians already concede that it is generally unethical (Wynia *et al.* 2000). In addition, a strong moral case can sometimes be made in support of compassion and mercy, even at the cost of breaking a contractual agreement. But such individual cases do not generalize well. The parable of the father stealing a loaf of bread for his starving child is recognized as mor-ally understandable, and most believe it warrants a softer form of justice; but simple passive acceptance of parental thievery would hardly be an appropriate social policy to address child hunger. Similarly, building a health care system that is full of holes, and assuming that physicians will be willing to use deception to help their patients avoid these holes, is also not wise public policy.

In the end, the problem of physicians' use of deception for the benefit of their patients does not reflect so much a problem of moral decay among many individual physicians as it does a problem at the level of health care systems. Systematic policy decisions create the pressures that lead to physicians' adoption of deception as an undesired, but seemingly least-bad, option. Addressing this problem will therefore require a systemic approach, focused on two related goals. First, health care systems should aim to alleviate the perceived need of physicians to deceive insurers to obtain needed care for their patients. Second, health care systems must aim to improve the fairness and legitimacy of the coverage decisions they seek to impose.

To alleviate the perceived need to use deception, several steps make sense. Appeals protocols should be streamlined and there should be protection from retribution against physicians who choose to mount appeals. Ideally, physicians would be reimbursed for the time they spend in pursuing appeals (with exceptions for those few appeals from which the physician will derive a direct financial benefit if the appeal is successful). Coverage decisions and appeals should be monitored closely, so that the services that are covered can be adjusted from time to time, to meet evolving medical demands. Time pressures also need to be addressed. Doing so may even be cost-effective, if it can ensure adequate time to allow physicians the opportunity to educate patients who request inappropriate services. Advertising restrictions ought to prevent the over-hyping of medical goods and services and should be strictly enforced. Patients, physicians, and health insurers all are harmed when patients are misled into the belief that a cure-all exists but that health plans and physicians are holding it back.

The second goal is at least as important as the first. Where health care coverage decisions are perceived to be driven by inappropriate criteria—to be arbitrary, capricious, manipulated by others, driven by greed, or the like—then patients and their physicians will be unlikely to feel morally bound to adhere to them. To improve the fairness and legitimacy of health insurance coverage decisions, the processes for making these decisions should be made as transparent as possible. The criteria for coverage should be clear, open to critique, and ultimately should rest on principles that most people would view as appropriate (such as medical effectiveness). There should be real opportunity for input from all stakeholders. Coverage decisions should be monitored by panels of physicians and patients (while protecting patient privacy), to ensure continued buy-in on the part of these important groups. Patients should be given meaningful choice in obtaining supplemental coverage for marginal services or for greater convenience. The trade-offs involved in making coverage decisions should be made clear (Wynia *et al.* 2002). And as far as possible the health care system should be closed, so that unused funds go back into health services for others. All of these steps aim to foster a sense of community within health care. Through steps such as these, one can hope that patients and physicians will come to recognize that, even in the United States, health insurance is primarily a social good, where physicians are the stewards of shared resources that must be used for the benefit of all.

References

Aaron, H. J. and Schwartz, W. B. (1984). *The painful prescription: rationing hospital care.* Brookings Institution, Washington, DC.

Alexander, G. C., Werner, R. M., Fagerlin, A. and Ubel, P. A. (2003). Support for physician deception of insurance companies among a sample of Philadelphia residents. *Annals of Internal Medicine,* **138(6)**, 472–5.

American Health Line (2000). HMO lawsuit: court dismisses suit claiming Aetna 'fraud'. *American Health Line,* 14 August, Article number 8.

Anders, G. (1996). *Health against wealth*. Houghton Mifflin Company, Boston, MA.

Beauchamp, T. L. and Childress J. F. (1994). *Principles of biomedical ethics*, 4th edn. Oxford University Press, New York, NY.

Bok, S. (1978). *Lying: moral choices in public and private life*. Pantheon, New York, NY.

Cook, B. (2000). United up, others down in HMO earnings: increases in market share and growth in its third-party administrative business account for United Health Group's high earnings, say analysts. *American Medical News*, 21 August, p. 1.

Council on Ethical and Judicial Affairs of the American Medical Association (1994). Ethical issues in health care system reform: the provision of adequate health care. *Journal of the American Medical Association*, **272**, 1056–62.

Council on Ethical and Judicial Affairs of the American Medical Association (1995). Ethical issues in managed care. *Journal of the American Medical Association*, **273**, 330–5.

Council on Ethical and Judicial Affairs of the American Medical Association (2002*a*). Opinion 8.132: Referral of patients: disclosure of limitations. In *Code of medical ethics: current opinions with annotations*. American Medical Association, Chicago, IL.

Council on Ethical and Judicial Affairs of the American Medical Association (2002*b*). Opinon 6.02: Fee splitting. In *Code of medical ethics: current opinions with annotations*. American Medical Association, Chicago, IL.

Daniels, N. and Sabin, J. (1998). The ethics of accountability in managed care reform. *Health Affairs (Millwood)*, **17**, 50–64.

Dickey, N. W. and McMenamin, P. (1999). Putting power into patient choice. *New England Journal of Medicine*, **341**, 1305–8.

Fielder, J. H. (1995). Disposable doctors: economic incentives to abuse physician peer review. *Journal of Clinical Ethics*, **6**, 327–32.

Freeman, V. G., Rathore, S. S., Weinfurt, K. P., Schulman, K. A., and Sulmasy, D. P. (1999). Lying for patients: physician deception of third party payers. *Archives of Internal Medicine*, **159**, 2263–70.

Gawande, A. A., Blendon, R., Brodie, M., Benson, J. M., Levitt, L., and Hugick, L. (1998). Does dissatisfaction with health plans stem from having no choices? *Health Affairs*, **17**, 184–94.

Goold, S. D., Hofer, T., Zimmerman, M., and Hayward, R. A. (1994). Measuring physician attitudes towards cost, uncertainty, malpractice, and utilization review. *Journal of General Internal Medicine*, **9**, 544–9.

Grumet, G. W. (1989). Health care rationing through inconvenience: the third party's secret weapon. *New England Journal of Medicine*, **321**, 607–11.

Hall, R. C. W. (1994). Legal precedents affecting managed care: the physician's responsibilites to patients. *Psychosomatics*, **35**, 105–17.

Hibbard, J. H., Slovic, P., and Jewett, J. J. (1997). Informing consumer decisions in health care: implications from decision-making research. *Milbank Quarterly*, **75**, 395–414.

Hibbard, J. H. and Weeks, E. C. (1987). Consumerism in health care. *Medical Care*, **25**, 1019–32.

Hilzenrath, D. S. (1998). Healing vs. honesty: for doctors, managed care's cost controls pose moral dilemma. *Washington Post*, Sunday, 15 March, H6.

Horowitz, B. (2002) Trust: Americans have great faith in each other, but their trust in CEOs, big business, priests and HMOs is slipping away. *USA Today*, Tuesday 16 July, A1–2.

Illingworth, P. (2000). Bluffing, puffing and spinning in managed care organizations. *Journal of Medical Philosophy*, **25**, 62–76.

Kalb, P. E. (1999). Health care fraud and abuse. *Journal of the American Medical Association*, **282**, 1163–8.

Klein, R. (2001). What's happening to Britain's National Health Service? *New England Journal of Medicine*, **345**, 305–8.

Landers S. J. (2001). Studies show pharmaceutical ads piquing patient interest: spending on consumer advertising has soared, especially for the newest and most costly drugs. *American Medical News*, 24–31 December, p. 1.

Light, D. W. (1992). Equity and efficiency in health care. *Social Science Medicine*, **35**, 465–9.

Liner, R. S. (1997). Physician deselection: the dynamics of a new threat to the physician–patient relationship. *American Journal of Law and Medicine*, **23**, 511–37.

Manuel, B. M. (1995). Physician liability: new areas of concern under managed care. *Bullentin of the American College of Surgeons*, **80**, 23–6.

Morreim, E. H. (1991). Gaming the system. Dodging the rules, ruling the dodgers. *Archive of Internal Medicine*, **151**, 443–7.

Morreim, E. H. (1995*a*). *Balancing act: the new medical ethics of medicine's new economics.* Georgetown University Press, Washington, DC.

Morreim, E. H. (1995*b*). From advocacy to tenacity: finding the limits. *Journal of the American Geriatrics Society*, **43**, 1170–2.

Novack, D. H., Detering, B. J., Arnold, R., Forrow, L., Ladinsky, M., and Pezzullo, J. C. (1989). Physicians' attitudes towards using deception to resolve difficult ethical problems. *Journal of the American Medical Association*, **261**, 2980–5.

Novack, D. H., Plumer, R., Smith, R. L., Ochitill, H., Morrow, G. R. and Bennet, J. M. (1979). Changes in physicians' attitudes toward telling the cancer patient. *Journal of the American Medical Association*, **241**, 897–900.

Orentlicher, D. (1995). Physician advocacy for patients under managed care. *Journal of Clinical Ethics*, **6**, 333.

Pearson, S. D. and Raeke, L. H. (2000). Patients' trust in physicians: many theories, few measures, and little data. *Journal of General Internal Medicine*, **15**, 509–13.

Serkes, K. (2001). New poll: doctors lie to protect patient privacy. Association of American Physician and Surgeons press release, 31 July, available at http://www.aapsonline.org/. Accessed on 23 July 2002.

Stafford vs. Neurological Medicine, Inc. (1987). 811 F2d 470; 1987 AS App LEXIS 2026.

Veatch, R. M. (1972). Models for ethical medicine in a revolutionary age. *Hastings Center Report*, **2**, 5–7.

Werner, R. M., Alexander, G. C., Fagerlin, A., Ubel, P. A. (2002). The "Hassle Factor": What motivates physicians to manipulate reimbursement rules? *Archive of Internal Medicine* 2002, **162(10)**, 1134–9.

Wynia, M. K., Cummins, D. S., VanGeest, J. B., and Wilson, I. B. (2000). Physician manipulation of reimbursement rules for patients: between a rock and a hard place. *Journal of the American Medical Association*, **283**, 1858–65.

Wynia, M. K., Orr, A., and Cummins, D. S., for the Ethical Force Program Oversight Body (2002). *Draft report: improving fairness in coverage decisions: a discussion report on five content areas for performance measure development.* The Institute for Ethics at the American Medical Association, Chicago, IL.

Section 5

Medicolegal and occupational perspectives

16 Law, lies, and videotape: malingering as a legal phenomenon

Michael A. Jones

Abstract

In the context of the civil law, although malingering may not be uncommon, it is rarely necessary for a court to reach a positive finding that an individual is malingering, given the manner in which the forensic process deals with the evidence when making findings of 'fact'. A conclusion that a claimant is malingering effectively involves an allegation of fraud, which could have potentially serious consequences for the claimant beyond failing in the immediate claim. It is not simply a question of resolving a dispute between medical experts as to whether the claimant's symptoms are genuine or feigned. In many instances, it may be almost impossible for a court or tribunal to conclude that the claimant is malingering without wholly convincing evidence, such as video observation of the claimant over a period of time. Although the standard of proof in civil cases is based on a balance of probabilities, this tends to conceal the fact that the cogency of the evidence required to satisfy this test varies with the issues at stake. It is more difficult to establish fraudulent than negligent conduct. Nonetheless, there remain questions of causation and the assessment of the extent of the claimant's symptoms. The question of whether the claimant is malingering can simply be 'hidden' behind the burden of proof and standard of proof on these issues. Thus, malingering is occasionally central but often marginal, if not irrelevant, to the court's decision-making process.

Introduction

Malingering is not a distinct legal concept, although lawyers are very familiar with the notion of malingering in practice. Within the legal system the term tends to be given its ordinary meaning of the deliberate, conscious feigning of symptoms for an ulterior purpose. The only specific definition that can be found in legislation occurs in the context of military law,[1] and covers: (a) falsely pretending to be suffering from sickness or disability; (b) injuring oneself with intent to avoid service; and (c) doing or failing to do anything to produce, or prolong or aggravate, any sickness or disability, with intent to avoid service.[2] There are no reported cases in which this

---

[1] See Palmer, Chapter 3.
[2] Air Force Act 1955, s. 42; Army Act 1955, s. 42; Naval Discipline Act 1957, s. 27(1). The punishment is imprisonment for a term not exceeding 2 years or any less punishment authorized by the Act.

definition has been considered by a court. The clearest common law statement of what constitutes malingering can be seen in *Jeffries* v. *Home Office*,[3] where it was said that:

> A malingerer is one who deliberately and consciously adopts the sick role, if necessary deceiving his medical advisers to persuade them that his complaints are true.

Sometimes the court will address the issue from the opposite perspective, by saying who is not a malingerer. Thus, in *Bell* v. *Department of Health and Social Security*,[4] the judge said:

> No-one has suggested that this plaintiff is a malingerer. In my judgment she does suffer from a genuine functional overlay. She has pain for which there is no organic cause but she feels it nonetheless.

The question which a hypothetical objective observer might ask of this statement is simply: how can we tell? In other words, if there is no demonstrable organic cause for an individual's expression of pain, how can anyone, doctor, lawyer or judge, have confidence in the individual's assertion that he experiences that pain. It is worth bearing in mind that doctors dealing with the individual in the clinical context do not have to worry too much about whether the patient is exaggerating or even faking. The fact that someone is prepared to fake symptoms in order to obtain medical treatment may itself be a factor in reaching an appropriate diagnosis. In the forensic context, however, the question of 'genuine', 'exaggerated', or 'faked' is crucial since large sums of money may or may not change hands depending upon the answer to the question.[5] That context, which clearly creates different pressures and expectations, is very different from the clinical setting.

This is not to suggest that symptoms attributable to a psychiatric condition are not real. Presumably, it is possible consciously or subconsciously to exaggerate even psychiatric symptoms—as it is also possible to fake the symptoms—which is why for more than a century lawyers have approached the discipline of psychiatry with a certain degree of scepticism. The assumption was that it was easier to fake psychiatric symptoms than physical ones—or at least with physical symptoms there are some objective measures. With psychiatry there are fewer objective measures. Much depends on the history. There are a number of cases where the doctors have examined claimants for medicolegal purposes where they have been fooled by the apparent honesty of the history, and the lying has become apparent from subsequent events.

The question of whether the claimant's symptoms are 'genuine', 'exaggerated', or 'faked' is one that lawyers often ask expert medical witnesses to comment upon, but arguably it is not the function of a medical expert to take a view on the claimant's honesty,[6] and it is certainly very rarely necessary. The function of an expert medical witness in these cases is usually to give an opinion

---

[3] Unreported, 26 March 1999, QBD. 'A malingerer is a person who is not ill and pretends that he is. If he bona fide thinks he is ill he is not guilty of that pretence': per Buckley LJ in *Higgs & Hill Ltd* v. *Unicume* [1913] 1 KB 595, 599. For the purpose of benefit claims the Department of Social Security defined malingering as 'the fraudulent imitation or exaggeration of symptoms with the intention of gaining financial or other rewards or material benefits. It is this obvious external gain that distinguishes malingering from factitious disorder.' *Stress Related Illness—A Report for DSS Policy Group: Part II*, 1998, DSS, para. 19.11.1.   [4] *The Times*, 13 June 1989.

[5] This can be the difference between an award of damages of less than £5000 for a few weeks' pain and loss of earnings, and awards of several hundred thousand pounds where it is alleged that the claimant will never be able to work again. Psychiatrists may be used to the idea, but it still comes as something of a shock to lawyers that relatively trivial physical injury (e.g. low speed whiplash) can result in PTSD, resulting in a claim for in excess of £340 000 on the basis that the claimant will never work again, and that this should be laid at the door of a defendant and his insurers (see, e.g. *Ludlow* v. *National Power plc* (2000) unreported, CA—the trial judge awarded only £3000). Lawyers, and even lay people, may be entitled to express a degree of scepticism about the reality of what is going on in such cases. In *Ludlow*, no psychiatric damage was originally diagnosed or pleaded. The diagnosis of PTSD and its link to the accident was first made 8 years after the accident, and 5 years after proceedings had been issued. (Note that all unreported cases referred to in this chapter have been taken from one of two standard electronic legal databases 'Lexis' or 'Westlaw'.)

[6] 'Doctors are sensibly reluctant to say whether exaggeration is conscious or unconscious. That is a matter for the judge on an appreciation of all the evidence, not least the truthfulness of the plaintiff': *Subrata Mukherjee* v. *Turner* (1995) unreported, CA, per Stuart-Smith L.J.

about the aetiology of the medical symptoms. If there is no medical explanation, whether organic or psychiatric, that is as far as the expert need go. It is then up to the judge to decide whether to take the further step and draw the inference that the claimant is malingering. Ultimately, all judgments about what is genuine and what is faked have to be based upon *evidence* and it is in an appreciation of the way in which courts and tribunals approach the evaluation of evidence that an understanding of malingering as a legal phenomenon is to be found.

In practice, it is comparatively rare for a court to be confronted with the stark choice between whether the claimant is a malingerer or whether he/she should be compensated in full. Why, it might be asked, does malingering not feature more prominently in the law reports? There are a number of factors which could explain this. It is partly because of the seriousness of an allegation of malingering, which effectively requires proof of fraud, but more importantly because it is possible to determine most cases without resorting to such a drastic allegation. It is rarely necessary for the defendant to prove the claimant's intention in order to resist a claim for compensation. This is a product of: (a) the burden of proof; (b) standards of proof; and (c) the law's approach to fact-finding. I will say a little about each of these issues, before considering some of the cases in which malingering has featured and the courts' reaction to the allegation.

The forensic process

Burdens of proof

The burden of proof in civil claims almost invariably lies with the claimant: 'he who asserts must prove'. Thus, a person claiming damages must prove the elements of the 'wrong' which he alleges the defendant committed, and, normally, that the wrong caused him damage. If a defendant asserts that he has a substantive defence, then the burden of proof with respect to that defence lies with the defendant. A substantive defence is where all the elements of the 'wrong' are present, but the defendant claims that he is nonetheless not liable because the defence (such as exclusion of liability, or contributory negligence—a partial defence) applies. If the defendant states simply that he did not commit the wrong (e.g. where there is a claim in negligence, he says that he was not careless or his conduct did not cause the claimant's damage) then, although in a sense this is a 'defence', in that if it turns out to be correct the claimant's action will fail, it is simply a denial of the claimant's assertions and it remains for the claimant to prove those assertions.

Standards of proof

The standard of proof in civil claims is 'the balance of probabilities'. If something is more probable than not then it is treated as proved. The burden of proof in criminal cases is 'beyond reasonable doubt' which means that the court must be 'sure' that the defendant is guilty of the offence with which he is charged. The civil standard of proof, the balance of probabilities, tends to conceal the fact that the *cogency* of the evidence required to satisfy the test varies with the issues at stake.[7] For example, 'professional negligence' can be more difficult to prove than an allegation of negligence in the context of a road traffic accident.[8] Similarly, it is more difficult to establish fraudulent than negligent conduct, in that the court will require more compelling evidence before concluding that person has acted fraudulently.[9] Thus, an allegation of fraud in civil proceedings is treated with a considerable degree of circumspection, since it requires proof of the defendant's intention

---

[7] See, e.g. Pattenden (1988) 7 CJQ 220.

[8] *Dwyer* v. *Roderick* (1983) 127 SJ 806.

[9] *Hornal* v. *Neuberger Products Ltd* [1957] 1 QB 247.

to deceive, or a high degree of recklessness as to the truthfulness of his representations.[10] An allegation of malingering is a charge of fraud and requires positive evidence from the defendants to be put to any witness affected.[11] This is a significant disincentive for the lawyers involved in a case to pursue an allegation of malingering, particularly where: (a) the question of whether someone is exaggerating symptoms may be both a subjective judgment and a question of degree; and (b) the fact-finding process will often render the issue irrelevant.

Findings of fact

Courts and tribunals make findings of fact to which legal rules are then applied. Findings of fact must be based on the evidence available to the court or tribunal. Where evidence is conflicting it must be decided which evidence is accepted and which is rejected, giving reasons. It is important to appreciate that a decision to accept certain evidence, which might entail rejecting conflicting evidence, does not necessarily mean that the court is suggesting that the witness whose evidence has been rejected was lying. If that were the case, then giving evidence on oath would be a dangerous business, since all witnesses whose evidence was rejected would be potentially open to prosecution for perjury. A witness's memory may be flawed; or he/she may be mistaken, but honest. The claimant may subjectively experience his or her injury or illness more severely than any objective evidence might suggest. Thus, rejection of the claimant's evidence, or of evidence given on the claimant's behalf, does not necessarily lead to the conclusion that the claimant was either lying or exaggerating. This truism, that rejected evidence is not necessarily dishonest evidence, is equally relevant to the evidence of expert witnesses. It is not usually suggested that an expert witness whose views have been rejected by the court in favour of other expert evidence was being dishonest or deceitful. The rejection or acceptance of certain pieces of evidence is simply part of the forensic fact-finding process.

Conversely, a finding that the claimant was not malingering is not the same as a finding that the symptoms or disability of which he complains are attributable, as a matter of causation, to the relevant events. The claimant may genuinely believe that his symptoms are due to a specific event, but the evidence, on the balance of probabilities, may indicate otherwise. By the same token even a proven malingerer may have a genuine case, hidden beneath the exaggerated or false behaviour. It is not exclusively honest people who suffer accidental injury. A lie about X does not prove that a statement about Y was also false, although it would go to the overall credibility of the person making the statement, since if the witness was prepared to lie about X, then *maybe* he is lying about Y.[12] Thus, in *Knapman* v. *Charman*,[13] the judge described the claimant as 'an inveterate liar and wholly unaffected by taking the oath'. Nonetheless, 'though a liar the medical evidence did not suggest that he was a malingerer'.

---

[10] The General Council of the Bar advises barristers that they should not draft any pleading containing an allegation of fraud without clear instructions and reasonably credible evidence establishing a *prima facie* case of fraud. It is 'improper conduct' for a barrister to allow a document that he or she has drafted containing allegations of fraud to be served without having seen such evidence. The Guidance is available at www.barcouncil.org.uk (under Rules & Guidance). In *Medcalf* v. *Mardell* [2002] UKHL 27; [2002] 3 WLR 172, the House of Lords held that at a court hearing counsel could not properly make or persist in an allegation of fraud that was not supported by *admissible* evidence, though when preparing a case before trial it was sufficient if he had material of such a character as to lead responsible counsel objectively to conclude that serious allegations could properly be based on it. Credible evidence, even if inadmissible as hearsay, would suffice. [11] *Stojalowski* v. *Imperial Smelting Corp (NSC)* (1977) 121 SJ 118, CA, Waller L.J.

[12] In *Owens* v. *Redpath Offshore (South) Ltd* (1998) unreported (CA) the judge said: 'It is obviously a matter of significance when it becomes clear that a witness has lied on important matters. The simple fact that it has happened does not entitle a court to reject a claim out of hand; accidents caused by the negligence of others happen to both the truthful and the untruthful.' In *Cottrell* v. *Redbridge NHS Trust* (2001) 61 BMLR 72, 91, where there had been an outright conspiracy amongst the witnesses fraudulently to inflate the value of the claim, the judge observed that the fact that the witnesses had given evidence known to be false in support of a wholly bogus claim for loss of earnings did not inevitably mean that their evidence in respect of the claimant's care needs should be rejected. Nonetheless, if they were prepared to lie about one matter it was 'at least probable that they would similarly be willing to disregard the truth in relation to' another. [13] (2000) CA, unreported.

What, then, is taken into account in weighing the credibility of evidence? There is no single test. There are a number of factors which the courts and tribunals may treat as indicative of truth: (a) the weight of the evidence; (b) the objectivity of the evidence; (c) the inherent probability of the truth of the evidence; and (d) the manner in which the evidence is presented.

Weight of the evidence

How much evidence points to a particular conclusion and how persuasive is that evidence in terms of other factors (objectivity, inherent probability of the truth, manner of presentation)? Corroborative evidence of the disability, for example, evidence that the claimant has undergone significant medical intervention (perhaps involving repeated surgery) for the condition, suggests that, at the very least, the claimant is not *consciously* fabricating symptoms (although there might be an unconscious element of exaggeration). The inference is that someone who is malingering would not be likely to put themselves through a lot of treatment just to maintain a pretence.

Objectivity of the evidence

The objectivity of the evidence depends on two factors: (a) Who is giving the evidence? Evidence from a claimant or defendant is less likely to be objective, because there is an understandable risk that the evidence will be 'self-serving'. On the other hand, the evidence of an independent witness of fact will tend to carry more weight, as will evidence from expert witnesses, on the assumption that they have no particular axe to grind.[14] (b) What type of evidence? Documentary evidence, including video evidence, may be regarded as more 'objective'. A common refrain in the cases is that 'the videotape evidence is not consistent with the level of disability being claimed', and the natural inclination is to believe the evidence of one's eyes rather than the oral evidence of a claimant. Other conflicting evidence may undermine the claimant's credibility. For example, evidence that the claimant works as a golf caddy suggests that he is not 'virtually unable to walk'.[15] A video of him carrying a golf bag on a golf course would go to proof of this, but so would oral evidence from a reliable independent witness who saw him carrying the bag on the golf course.

Inherent probability of the truth of the evidence

Lawyers' common sense has a role to play here. A statement that the claimant is so disabled as to be unable to make a cup of tea where the claimant is capable of and does actually drive a motor car strains credibility. Similarly, a statement that the claimant can only walk two yards in five minutes strains credibility.[16] Paradoxically, the more extreme the claim in terms of improbability, the less likely it is that the court or tribunal will conclude that the claimant is malingering (in the sense of consciously trying to deceive) on the basis that a skilled liar is unlikely to make so exaggerated a claim unless he held an extremely low opinion of the intelligence of the judge of

---

[14] Sometimes, however, expert witnesses become highly partisan. In these circumstances the value of their evidence is likely to be undermined: *Joyce* v. *Yeomans* [1981] 1 WLR 549, 556. For example, in *Cooper* v. *P & O Stena Line Ltd* [1999] 1 Lloyd's Rep 734, 742, the judge described an expert witness for the defendant in the following terms: 'Mr. Wadsworth was not a satisfactory witness. His approach to pain was that if there was no orthopaedic basis for it, it was not genuine. He took that extreme view because he was convinced, without having any expertise in the field of rheumatology to justify his opinion, that pain syndromes such as fibromyalgia do not exist. This did not, in my judgment, demonstrate the open and fair mind required of an expert witness ... Mr. Wadsworth expressed his opinion in the witness box in discourteous and intemperate language saying, inter alia, that if the World Health Organization recognized the syndrome that was because the organization had had the wool pulled over its eyes and that the decision to recognize the syndrome must have been taken by a committee consisting of a bunch of rheumatologists.'

[15] This example comes from the author's personal experience as a deputy district chairman of appeal tribunals for social security benefits.

[16] Both of these assertions have been made to tribunals chaired by the author on more than one occasion. Of course, the claimant may simply be very bad at estimating distance, or it may be exaggeration, or it may be a lie. What a lawyer would not do is try to rationalize the statement as part of the individual's psychiatric condition.

the tribunal members. Exaggeration, whether unconscious or of the gilding of the lily variety, is the more likely conclusion.

Manner in which the evidence is presented

The manner in which the evidence is presented is usually relied upon quite heavily by judges, in terms of observing the witness in the witness box. This is also a significant factor in the reluctance of the Court of Appeal to overturn a judge's finding of fact. Appellate courts, who do not see witnesses but merely transcripts of evidence, are very conscious that the impression given by a witness, through non-verbal cues, often does not come across well from simply reading the words of the transcript. The manner in which the evidence is presented is used by judges to assess the credibility of all witnesses, including expert witnesses. Thus, apparently partisan or exaggerated evidence by an expert witness will reduce its credibility. In many respects, this can be the most the unreliable indicator of veracity. Different observers may well place different interpretations on similar behaviour. Thus, if the claimant appears to be in pain in the witness box, constantly shifting his position, groaning occasionally, etc. the court/tribunal may interpret this as: (a) evidence that he is genuinely in pain; or (b) evidence that he is exaggerating, or putting on a 'show' in order to persuade the court. Conversely, if he sits still in the witness box for a lengthy period of time this may be treated as: (a) evidence that he is not in pain and that therefore his assertions of constant pain are false or exaggerated; or (b) evidence that he is stoical, and not prone to exaggeration, which thereby improves his credibility as a witness when he asserts that he is actually in pain.

Malingering in the courts

In order to see how malingering has been dealt with in the courts a search for the term was undertaken on the two standard electronic legal databases ('Lexis' and 'Westlaw'). Combined, these databases provide a reasonably comprehensive database of reported cases since 1945, with some cases going beyond that.[17] There are approximately 250 reported and unreported cases (most concerned with personal injury claims) where 'malingering' is mentioned in the judgment, but in many of these (128 cases) it is only a passing reference to malingering as an aside (as where the judge says, e.g. 'there is no suggestion that the plaintiff was malingering'). There are a number of features of the cases that are worth highlighting:

1. A remarkably large proportion of the cases in which malingering or conscious exaggeration feature concern back injury or whiplash injuries.[18] Of the cases from the databases in which malingering was mentioned as a possibility about 50 per cent involved back injuries and/or whiplash injuries.[19] It may well be that the difficulty of demonstrating a direct organic cause of the pain that such injuries produced is a significant factor in the allegations of malingering.

2. A typical case involves a dispute between medical experts.[20] Impressionistically, it would appear that orthopaedic surgeons tend to take a more robust view of the capabilities of claimants than psychiatrists or those experts who specialize in pain management. The view, which probably reflects most lay people's attitude, that if there is no organic cause there can be no pain and therefore the claimant must be exaggerating or malingering, is not uncommon within the medical profession.

---

[17] It will also include unreported cases that reach the Court of Appeal or House of Lords. However, there are thousands of first instance cases that never get into the databases because they are unreported.

[18] David Mason, 'Whiplash' (1999) 149 NLJ 749: 'In 1995, 18 per cent of injury accidents involved rear end collisions. (Department of the Environment, Transport and the Regions, Road and Traffic Directorate Transport Statistics—Road Safety).'

[19] It is difficult to be more precise. Not all of the cases report the precise injuries sustained by the claimant.

[20] See, e.g. *Burke* v. *Royal Infirmary of Edinburgh NHS Trust* 1999 SLT 539 where there was a stark conflict between those medical experts who considered that the claimant's problems were genuine and those who considered him to be a malingerer.

3. In the cases where the allegation of malingering is made and persisted in (and in many the initial allegation may well be tempered or withdrawn), it is only a small number in which the court concludes that the claimant is actually a malingerer, in the sense of *deliberately and consciously feigning symptoms*. There are, however, far more numerous occasions where the court concludes that the claimant was exaggerating his symptoms—sometimes consciously, and sometimes unconsciously.

4. It is apparent that the *total* number of cases in which malingering is even mentioned is a tiny fraction of the total number of personal injury cases. There are a number of possible explanations for this:
    -   true malingering is not a very common phenomenon; or
    -   being a 'question of fact' rather than a question law, the cases tend not to get reported very often; or
    -   due to the seriousness of the allegation the issue is dealt with by the lawyers and the courts in different ways.

    There may be an element of truth in all of these explanations.

Malingering is not a common phenomenon

There is no empirical evidence as to the true extent of malingering in personal injury claims brought in the courts. In the context of claims for social security benefits the DSS has found very little evidence of malingering,[21] though the Department is careful to distinguish malingering from a claimant's overstatement of the degree of disability and needs, which 'should not be classed as malingering without there first having been established that apparent exaggeration of care needs and mobility requirements is not due to a misunderstanding of the questions listed in the claim packs or, indeed, the eligibility requirements for an award'.[22] In a study to measure the level of fraud and error in relation to incapacity benefit (which is payable where an employee is incapacitated for work) the Department for Work and Pensions carried out reviews on a random sample of 1401 individuals claiming this benefit and found only three cases of confirmed fraud.[23] It was estimated that the percentage of all incapacity benefit cases that are fraudulent is less than 0.5 per cent, whereas 1.9 per cent of cases had incorrect benefit in payment due to claimant error, and 2.1 per cent of cases had an official error.

Malingering is a question of fact

Strictly speaking, only cases that raise important issues of law should get reported, since it is only the principle of law involved in a case that can have any value as a precedent. In practice, with a proliferation of specialized series of law reports over the last 20 years or so, many cases get reported today, involving only questions of fact, that would never have seen the light of day in the past. Nonetheless, the question of whether a particular claimant was or was not malingering, being a 'question of fact', is not of particular interest to the law reporters. Thus, a search of the databases for 'malingering' will only pick up those cases which incidentally involve malingering.

---

[21] *Stress Related Illness—A Report for DSS Policy Group: Part II*, 1998, DSS, 19.11.1: 'Malingering is not common.'

[22] *Stress Related Illness—A Report for DSS Policy Group: Part II*, 1998, DSS, 19.11.2.

[23] *Fraud and Error in Claims to Incapacity Benefit: The Results of the Benefit Review of Incapacity Benefit*, Department for Work and Pensions, 2001. Cases were only classed as fraud on admission by the claimant or when third party corroborative evidence was obtained. Note that fraud does not necessarily take the form of malingering in the sense of feigning symptoms.

The seriousness of the allegation

The seriousness of the allegation of malingering, which is an allegation of fraud, is such that there should be very clear evidence before it is found as a fact.[24] This may lead to the issue being dealt with by the lawyers and the courts in different ways. Sometimes this can be simply a matter of using language carefully. A judge may phrase a judgment in perhaps gentler terms than the bare facts might warrant. An example of this can be seen in *Bridges* v. *P & NE Murray Ltd*[25] where on any reasonable, objective interpretation of the evidence the plaintiff was being 'economical with the truth'. There was damning video evidence of the plaintiff's ability to carry out many tasks that she claimed to be unable to perform. The judge declined to describe the plaintiff as a malingerer, though he did not accept her evidence. In the Court of Appeal Otton LJ commented that:

> I have little doubt that the judge was conscious from the outset that the plaintiff was in a delicate psychiatric state. . . . he adopted a format which while firm and unequivocal in many of its conclusions, nevertheless tempered the wind to the shorn lamb and spared the plaintiff a good deal of pain and humiliation.

Sometimes the court will conclude that the claimant is exaggerating symptoms, but that this is not conscious. In *Napier* v. *Chief Constable of Cambridgeshire Constabulary*,[26] following observation of video evidence of the claimant walking his dog and taking his child to and from school, the judge said:

> the claimant is [not] consciously exaggerating his symptoms when seen by the doctors, or when sitting stiff necked in court as he has, but [the video] does lead me to the conclusion that the pain and stiffness that he suffers in his neck is not as disabling as he has come to believe and that when he is not thinking about it, he can manage a fairly normal life-style.[27]

Unconscious exaggeration, though clearly not dishonest or even blameworthy, is nonetheless *exaggeration*, whether or not we conclude that the claimant was a truthful or honest witness. The claimant's symptoms remain objectively less severe than he claims to perceive them, and there is no good reason why a defendant should pay compensation for exaggerated symptoms. An award of damages should reflect 'objective' evidence about the degree of symptoms/suffering.[28]

Even conscious exaggeration may not be treated as malingering, but as merely a forgivable attempt to gild the lily so that observers do not underestimate the 'true' extent of the claimant's injuries, as he perceives them. For example, in *Rogers* v. *Little Haven Day Nursery Ltd*[29] Bell J concluded that although the claimant was exaggerating he was not malingering because: 'the exaggeration which I have described falls within the bounds of familiar and understandable attempts to make sure that doctors and lawyers do not underestimate a genuine condition, rather than indicating an outright attempt to mislead in order to increase the value of her claim beyond its true worth.' Sometimes it is a case of the claimant's tale having 'improved with the telling' over time.[30]

---

[24] This was acknowledged by the Department of Social Security. *Stress Related Illness—A Report for DSS Policy Group: Part II*, 1998, DSS, para. 19.11.4: 'The seriousness of an allegation of malingering is such that it must not be accepted without documented authoritative confirmation, since the procedures which may be followed upon the confirmation of malingering may well have grave consequences for the malingerer.' [25] *The Times*, 25 May 1999, CA.

[26] (2001) unreported, QBD.

[27] Of course, it is impossible to know from the judgment whether the judge actually believed that the claimant was not consciously exaggerating his symptoms. This may simply be an example of avoiding the *public* conclusion that the claimant was a liar, when the judge entertained serious doubts about his honesty.

[28] Exaggerated symptoms should be distinguished from a genuine but more extreme reaction to the event than would normally be expected. The so-called 'thin-skull rule' ('the defendant must take his victim as he finds him') applies to psychiatric conditions: *Malcolm* v. *Broadhurst* [1970] 3 All ER 508; *Page* v. *Smith* [1995] 2 All ER 736. [29] (1999) unreported, QBD.

[30] *Ludlow* v. *National Power plc* (2000) unreported, CA. In some cases, the judge may be so outraged that he directs that the papers in the case be referred to the Director of Public Prosecutions to consider whether a criminal prosecution for fraud is appropriate. See, e.g. *Cottrell* v. *Redbridge NHS Trust* (2001) 61 BMLR 72 where the claimant had sustained a genuine injury to his leg as a result of clinical

Avoiding the issue of malingering

The serious nature of an allegation of malingering, its potential consequences for the claimant, and the difficulty of proving fraud, make the courts and tribunals reluctant to reach a conclusion of outright malingering. Moreover, in most instances it is simply not necessary for the court to draw the inference of dishonesty since a case involving a suspicion of malingering can be dealt with in other ways, particularly through findings on causation or in some cases the threshold assessment of the degree of disability.

The causation question

In the context of certain legal issues, causation is central. For others it is irrelevant. All claims for compensation for personal injuries from an allegedly negligent defendant involve a causation question—the claimant must prove that the damage for which he seeks compensation was caused by the defendant's negligence (which, of course, must also be proved). Similarly, claims for industrial injuries benefit (disablement benefit) under the industrial injuries scheme involve a causation issue. The question is: is the claimant's disability *attributable* to a relevant industrial accident or a prescribed occupational disease? Where proof of causation is required the court or tribunal can side-step an allegation of malingering by concluding that the symptoms are due, for example, to: (a) a pre-existing condition (e.g. degenerative disease of the spine); or (b) the subsequent development of a condition unrelated to the accident (e.g. cervical spondylosis) which would have occurred irrespective of the accident. This bitter pill can be lightly coated in sugar by the conclusion that the relevant accident probably accelerated the onset of symptoms by a given period (provided, of course, that there is some medical evidence which supports such a conclusion, on the balance of probabilities). The claimant is then entitled to compensation, limited to that period. Effectively, the court or tribunal can say: 'We accept that you are suffering from the symptoms of which you complain, but the evidence indicates that they are not attributable to (or caused by) the relevant event [the defendant's negligence or the industrial accident].' This is just as true for psychiatric symptoms as for physical symptoms. Of course, if the claimant's psychiatric condition is causally linked to the defendant's negligence then he is entitled to be compensated for that psychiatric condition, but the burden of proof is the claimant's and exaggerated symptoms, whether conscious or unconscious, can be discounted as not *caused* by the accident (but rather by the claimant's reaction or personality). 'Compensation neurosis' or 'litigation neurosis' is usually taken to be causally linked, but the normal implication of this diagnosis is that the claimant will recover quickly once the litigation is resolved, and this has obvious implications for the size of an award of damages, since future psychiatric symptoms are being excluded from the assessment.[31]

Threshold tests of disability

In certain types of claim, entitlement to compensation or benefit is based simply on the proof of a particular condition or *degree* of disability or incapacity. It does not have to be proved *how* the disability or incapacity came about. For example, entitlement to the social security benefits of Disability Living Allowance and Incapacity Benefit depend upon proof of a particular type and degree of disability. The manner in which this was caused is irrelevant. Similarly, entitlement to compensation under a permanent health insurance policy may depend upon the degree of incapacity, rather than the manner in which it was caused. Causation is then irrelevant—since

---

negligence, but fabricated a totally fraudulent claim in respect of loss of earnings, entering into a conspiracy to deceive with his wife, his parents, and his daughter. Such references are comparatively rare: see Sprince, Chapter 18.

[31] See Mendelson, Chapter 17.

entitlement does not depend upon how the disability arose, but on the fact of disability. In this situation, one can avoid the conclusion that the claimant is malingering by a finding that, though the claimant has some degree of disability, it is not sufficient to meet the criteria for an award of benefit. Effectively, the court or tribunal can say: 'We accept that you are suffering from the symptoms of which you complain, but the evidence indicates that they are not sufficiently severe to meet the qualifying conditions.'

An example of this can be seen in section 72 of the Social Security Contributions and Benefits Act 1992 which governs an individual's entitlement to the 'care component' of disability living allowance. A person qualifies for the lowest rate of the care component if he is so severely disabled physically or mentally that 'he requires in connection with his bodily functions attention from another person for a significant portion of the day.'[32] This requires an assessment of whether the claimant has a physical or mental disability and: (a) requires attention from another person; (b) in connection with bodily functions; and (c) for a significant portion of the day. Although causation is irrelevant, a tribunal can say that: 'We accept that you have some needs for attention, but this does not amount to a need for attention *for a significant portion of the day.*' In other words, the necessary degree of disability is not present. Or the tribunal could say that: 'although in fact you do receive attention in connection with your bodily functions from other members of your family, this attention is not reasonably required.' There may be an implicit judgment, here, that the claimant is exaggerating symptoms, whether consciously or unconsciously, but it does not necessarily have to be made express. Although when giving reasons for a decision a tribunal may state that they do not accept the claimant's evidence because there was exaggeration, it is rarely possible, let alone necessary, to conclude that the claimant is malingering, since there is rarely direct evidence available to a tribunal that the claimant has a fraudulent intention.

'Genuine lies'

The problem of how to respond to an apparently lying claimant is illustrated by the case of *Bridges* v. *P & NE Murray Ltd*.[33] The plaintiff suffered whiplash in a relatively minor road traffic accident, causing vehicle repair costs of £346. By the time of trial the continuing organic disability (if any) was minimal. The plaintiff complained of grossly disabling symptoms. She claimed that as a result of the accident she suffered from total body pain or somatization disorder rendering her totally disabled. This diagnosis was generally accepted by the doctors, but the nature, extent and severity of the psychiatric condition depended upon the plaintiff's honesty and accuracy in her description of her alleged disabilities to the doctors and to the court. There was video evidence which showed the plaintiff functioning normally, without any apparent pain or discomfort. There was later video evidence, by which time the plaintiff had become aware that she was being observed, in which she had adopted a peculiar way of walking for which there was no organic explanation. The judge refused to address the question of the claimant's honesty, saying: 'Whether she can be described as honest or dishonest is perhaps merely a matter of labelling.'[34] The Court of Appeal dealt with the resulting problem by reference to the plaintiff's credibility as a witness. She was 'a patently unreliable witness, and her inability to tell the truth contaminated her evidence both as to her pre-accident and post-accident state.' One expert witness attempted to ascribe her pathological inability to tell the truth as unconscious and merely a symptom of her behavioural disorder. But as the judge said: 'The consequence of that approach would simply be

---

[32] Social Security Contributions and Benefits Act 1992, s. 72(1)(a)(i). Note that this is neither the only means of qualifying nor the only qualifying condition. There are additional qualifying criteria.   [33] *The Times*, 25 May 1999, CA.
[34] This is a remarkable statement from a judge. The 'label' honest or dishonest will separate many a convicted prisoner from citizens free to walk the streets.

that everything she says must be taken at face value.' Agreeing, the Court of Appeal commented, 'the judge was entitled to take a different view'. This is simply a polite way for the court to say: 'What nonsense!' And, indeed, it is nonsense. A claimant who is confronted with video evidence of, for example, her ability to lift heavy objects, walk long distances, or undertake heavy gardening activities, who persists in asserting that she is unable to perform these tasks either has some distortion of her visual perception or is lying. Of course, she may explain that these activities took place on her 'good days' and she is much worse on her 'bad days'. But to persist in the claim that she is *never* able to do them is just plain silly. The crucial point, however, is that whether the plaintiff in *Bridges* subjectively believed her own story, and therefore might be described as 'honest', was irrelevant to the outcome. As the judge said, and again the Court of Appeal agreed, 'there must be some room for common-sense and the evidence of one's own eyes.'

A willingness to treat even extreme examples of apparent dishonesty as merely symptoms of illness or disorder is the point at which most lawyers would part company with the medical diagnosis. It leads down the path of moral nihilism, where no-one can be held *responsible* for their actions. The reaction of the courts is predictable. A divergence between a medical approach and the lawyer's mindset becomes apparent. The doctor dealing with a patient in a clinical setting has a natural tendency to explain symptoms in terms of disease or disorder—after all, diagnosis and treatment is what doctors are trained in. Hence, exaggeration, dissimulation, minor lies about apparently trivial matters, and even obvious lies about central issues, can be interpreted as 'symptoms' of a psychiatric disorder. A lawyer is far more likely to interpret them as evidence of an attempt to deceive.

Conclusions

For a lawyer, malingering is a question of fact, not law, and therefore it does not involve complex conceptual issues, but is merely part and parcel of an everyday forensic exercise in establishing facts, based on credible evidence. It does, however, have a connotation of dishonesty which is potentially serious for the claimant, and which therefore requires very cogent evidence of the claimant's intention to deceive. Even apparently strong evidence, such as a video of the claimant performing tasks that he claims to be unable to perform, is not necessarily conclusive. The court may be reluctant to draw the inference of dishonesty, for a variety of reasons. But this does not mean that the claim is bound to succeed. A court is entitled to reject evidence as part of the fact-finding process, including evidence from the claimant, without condemning the witness as dishonest. The burden of proof lies with the claimant, and the exaggeration of symptoms, whether of the gilding of the lily variety or more extreme, and whether conscious or unconscious, remains an exaggeration of symptoms which it will be difficult to link causally to the conduct of a negligent defendant. Thus, although evidence that the claimant has lied, or even exaggerated, helps a defendant's case in that it undermines the credibility of the claimant's evidence, it is rarely essential for a defendant (and even less so for his expert medical witnesses) to establish outright malingering.

17 Outcome-related compensation: in search of a new paradigm

George Mendelson

A compensation neurosis is a state of mind, born out of fear, kept alive by avarice, stimulated by lawyers, and cured by a verdict.

Kennedy (1946)

Abstract

Terms such as 'compensation neurosis' and 'accident neurosis' have been used in medical and psychiatric literature to refer to the concatenation of physical and emotional symptoms experienced by those who had been involved in accidents giving rise to entitlement for compensation. In some instances, the person concerned may have sustained a physical injury at the time of the accident; in other instances no objectively demonstrable organic injury resulting from the accident had been documented. Implicit in the use of such terms has been the expectation that once litigation had been finalized the symptoms will resolve, and the individual will return to his or her pre-injury state, both with respect to health and employment. Follow-up studies of most personal injury litigants, however, have shown that this does not occur. The concept of there being a specific 'neurosis' that develops following personal injury, in the setting of entitlement to compensation or litigation, is not supported by a critical examination of this view using the customary validation criteria. Similarly, there is no support for the view that personal injury litigants or compensation recipients malinger so as to maximize their entitlements. Personal injury litigants and compensation recipients thus cannot be categorized as either 'mad' or 'bad'—either suffering from a specific psychiatric disturbance that will be 'cured' by the finalization of the claim or engaging in deception or fraud.

To understand the reactions of those who have suffered an injury in compensable circumstances it is necessary to consider a variety of factors—interpersonal, demographic, economic, occupational, cultural, societal, as well as developmental. It is only by constructing a new paradigm that takes into consideration these various factors that an understanding of such reactions can be achieved and, more importantly, that appropriate interventions can be undertaken to minimize the personal and social impact of accidental injury.

Introduction

Kennedy's definition of 'compensation neurosis' encapsulates the conventional view of personal injury litigants and applicants for compensation and other benefits as being essentially motivated by the prospect of financial gain.

This view can be traced to the development of the railways in Great Britain during the first half of the nineteenth century, when terms such as 'railway brain' and 'railway spine' came into use to describe persons who complained of physical and emotional symptoms that could not be explained by the presence of objectively demonstrable organic injuries. After Erichsen coined the phrase 'nervous shock' to indicate what he considered to be a 'molecular derangement' consequent upon railway accidents (Erichsen 1875), contrary views were expressed, for example, by Page, which held that the symptoms were due to the emotional rather than the physical impact of the accident (Page 1885).

Following the introduction of workers' compensation insurance in Germany during the 1880s (see Wessely, chapter 2), and the subsequent enactment of similar legislation in Great Britain, the United States, Australia, and other European countries, many writers held that the prospect of financial benefits motivated workers to feign injuries or to malinger (Collie 1913; Jones and Llewellyn 1917). A wide variety of terms were used to describe this putative phenomenon—terms that, to a large extent, expressed the prejudice of those who used them as 'diagnoses'. A selection of these terms is set out in Table 17.1.

It was following the publication of Henry Miller's Milroy lectures in 1961 that the concept of 'accident neurosis' gained in popularity. Miller put forward five propositions, which he developed from a follow-up of 50 highly selected accident litigants who had been referred to him on behalf of insurance companies. The five features of 'accident neurosis', according to Miller, were:

1. 'an absolute failure to respond to therapy until the compensation issue was settled';
2. 'the accident . . . must have occurred in circumstances where the payment of financial compensation is potentially involved';
3. 'it is comparatively uncommon where injury has been severe . . . the inverse relationship to the severity of injury . . . is crucial to its understanding';
4. 'after (the compensation issue was settled) nearly all the cases described recovered completely without treatment';
5. 'such a development is favoured by a low social and occupational status'.

Subsequent research did not support Miller's assertions about 'accident neurosis'; indeed, another British neurologist, Reginald Kelly, showed that each of the five propositions put forward by Miller was false and referred to these as 'myths' (Kelly and Smith 1981).

Table 17.1 Terms used to describe the sequelae of compensable accidents

Accident neurosis	Mediterranean disease
Aftermath neurosis	Profit neurosis
Attitudinal pathosis	Railway brain
Catastrophic neurosis	Railway spine
Compensation hysteria	Secondary gain neurosis
Compensationitis	Traumatic hysteria
Compensation neurosis	Traumatic neurasthenia
Entitlement neurosis	Traumatic neurosis
Erichsen's disease	Unconscious malingering
Functional overlay	Vertebral neurosis
Greenback neurosis	Wharfie's back
Litigation neurosis	Whiplash neurosis

Follow-up studies of litigants and claimants for compensation after personal injuries has been one of the ways in which the influence of compensation on outcome has been examined. Another method of studying this interaction has been through examining the response to treatment of compensation recipients and litigants. Some studies have also examined the influence of the system of compensation on the rate and duration of compensation claims, or have considered the nature of the symptoms described by claimants when compared with symptoms described by persons not involved in litigation or compensation.

This chapter will briefly review studies related to the influence of compensation and litigation on 'outcome'—both treatment outcome following compensable injuries and outcome on follow-up after the finalization of litigation and compensation payments. The influence of compensation status on symptoms such as chronic pain, as well as the prevalence of chronic pain complaints following compensable injuries under different systems of compensation have been discussed elsewhere (Mendelson 1994). I shall also discuss the various factors that influence the outcome of compensable injuries. Finally, the role of the health care professional in the assessment of the personal injury claimant or applicant for illness-contingent benefits will be considered.

The effect of compensation on treatment outcome

One of the propositions put forward by Henry Miller, in his influential 1961 Milroy lectures, was the assertion of 'an absolute failure to respond to therapy until the compensation issue was settled'. Other authors suggested that recipients of compensation benefits have more marked disability and show reduced motivation for effective treatment when compared with non-compensable patients with similar symptoms. For example, Fowler and Mayfield (1969), in a study comparing 327 patients receiving disability benefits with 613 patients not on compensation commented that the compensation beneficiaries, despite having fewer symptoms, had a significantly poorer occupational adjustment than the non-compensation group.

In general, studies of the effect of compensation and litigation on treatment outcome are in agreement that these have an adverse effect on treatment outcome and prognosis. For example, Hammonds et al. (1978) found that among 26 patients with chronic pain who were not receiving compensation, 18 (69 per cent) showed significant benefit from a rehabilitation programme, whereas only 15 out of 35 patients (43 per cent) of a group receiving pain-contingent financial benefits showed comparable improvement.

Sander and Meyers (1986) compared the period of work disability following a low back sprain/strain injury among two groups of patients, drawn from railway employees who were covered by a federal disability scheme in the United States. One group consisted of those injured at work; the other comprised those who had been injured off duty. The two groups were matched for type of injury and for gender. The 35 work-injured patients were away from work for a mean of 14.2 months, compared with a mean of 4.9 months for the 30 subjects injured off duty. The authors concluded that 'the financial rewards of compensation' were responsible for the prolonged recovery time of those injured at work.

In a similar study of the duration of time off work due to low back pain, Leavitt (1990) found that among a group of 1373 patients with work-related pain, 23.7 per cent were disabled for longer than 12 months, whereas among 417 patients with similar pain, but not receiving compensation, 13.2 per cent were off work for longer than 12 months. The difference was statistically significant.

Studies of the effects of conservative treatment of conditions such as rotator cuff tears (Hawkins and Dunlop 1995) and of thoracic outlet syndrome (Novak et al. 1995a) have also shown that compensation and litigation are associated with a worse prognosis.

The surgical literature also is replete with studies that have shown elective orthopaedic procedures to be less successful when the patient is in receipt of compensation or involved in litigation. This has been shown following shoulder surgery (Frieman and Fenlin 1995; Misamore *et al.* 1995) resection of neuromas (Novak *et al.* 1995*b*) carpal tunnel surgery (Higgs *et al.* 1995; Elmaraghy and Hurst 1996; Filan 1996) and spinal surgery (Schnee *et al.* 1997).

Although the studies noted above have indicated that the receipt of compensation, or involvement in litigation, have an adverse influence on treatment outcome and tend to prolong work disability, it has been shown that specific treatment programmes can significantly reduce the likelihood of progression to pain chronicity after a work injury. (Wiesel *et al.* 1984; Schofferman and Wasserman 1994; Ryan *et al.* 1995).

Similarly, Fordyce *et al.* (1986) have shown that a treatment programme for acute low back pain, which incorporates behavioural methods, is more effective than traditional management and prevents chronicity. Thus, the adverse effect of compensation and/or litigation on the outcome of some injuries sustained in compensable circumstances can be modified by specific interventions and treatment programmes that stress early mobilization and return to the work-place, appropriate activity and exercises, and avoidance of other factors that may promote learned pain behaviour.

Follow-up studies after conclusion of litigation

An early comment on the prognosis of personal injury claimants following the finalization of litigation was made by Bailey and Kennedy, who wrote in 1923 that

> It was at one time believed by physicians, and is still the very general opinion of laymen, that traumatic neurasthenia or hysteria begins to improve as soon as litigation is at an end, and that of all remedies, financial compensation is the most speedy and the most certain in action. Larger experience has shown that this view is not entirely correct. It is true that in the traumatic neuroses, as in diseases of any character, annoying and exciting agents exercise an unfavorable influence, and that improvement in symptoms ordinarily follows when such circumstances cease to exist. Nevertheless, there are many rebellious cases of accident neurasthenia in which there is no question of damages, but in which there may be inherent weakness or faulty suggestions other than those contained in litigation, and in a few of those which do become the subject of litigation the patients improve but little or not at all even when the suits are decided in their favor.

The 'larger experience' referred to by Bailey and Kennedy (1923) had been lost by the time that Henry Miller published his follow-up study of 50 personal injury litigants in 1961. Miller's views on the outcome of what he had termed 'accident neurosis' became the accepted wisdom for the next two decades, although other follow-up studies—and particularly those of Kelly—did not support Miller's assertions. (For a review of the early studies, see Mendelson 1983.)

Further studies published subsequent to the 1983 review have also demonstrated that there was no 'cure by a verdict' as had been proposed by both Kennedy and Miller.

Sprehe (1984) reported on a follow-up of 108 litigants, out of a total of 503 whom he examined and who 'had psychiatric disability as part of their overall disability rating in connection with their workers' compensation claim'. The patients had been seen during the decade 1971–1981, and follow-up was undertaken during 1981. Of the total group, 266 could not be traced, and out of the remaining 237 patients follow-up questionnaires were completed by 108; in most cases the questionnaire was forwarded to the patient and then returned by mail, but in several cases follow-up was by telephone.

Out of the 108 returned questionnaires, 79 cases had been finalized, including those of six subjects who had died. Of the 73 patients whose claims had been finalized and who were living, 56 (77 per cent) described themselves as either 'worse' or 'no change', and 17 (23 per cent) indicated that they were 'better'. Forty out of the 73 patients whose cases had been finalized were not working. Nine of these 40 patients had made 'a conscious election to retire' whereas the other 31 out of 73 patients (43 per cent) remained disabled following finalization of their claims and had not been able to return to work. There were another 14 patients who had returned to work but continued to experience significant symptoms and rated themselves to be 'in a worse job' than they had prior to the accident and injury.

Another follow-up study of 'accident neurosis' was reported by Tarsh and Royston (1985). These authors reviewed 35 claimants who had presented with 'gross perplexing somatic symptoms without demonstrable organic pathology', possibly due to conversion reactions. All the patients had been psychiatrically assessed by the first-named author prior to finalization of the compensation claim; all had been referred by solicitors acting on the claimant's behalf. The 35 patients described in this report were derived from a group of 50 who had shown particularly 'gross somatization' and 'their cases had given rise to medical perplexity and argument'. Five patients out of the group of 50 had died by the time of follow-up, and 10 could not be traced. The average age of the patients at the time of follow-up was 42 years, and there were nearly equal numbers of men and women. There was one patient who had been injured in an assault, and 75 per cent had been injured in work accidents.

The average duration of litigation in this group was more than 5 years, but the authors did not state the time elapsed between finalization of claim and follow-up. Among the 35 patients one had never worked, and two did not leave work at any time during the course of litigation. Of the remaining 32 patients, two resumed work prior to the finalization of the claim, and four returned to the same work after settlement. A further four patients returned to easier and less well paid work. The authors noted that of those who returned to work after settlement, one did so after a year, five after 2 years, one after 3 years, and the remaining patient after 5 years. Thus, out of the 30 patients who had not returned to work at the time of settlement 22 (73 per cent) failed to return to work during the follow-up period. The authors of this study commented that 'in the whole series, therefore, return to work was the exception rather than the rule'.

Binder *et al.* (1991) described a follow-up study of only 18 subjects, who had been involved in civil litigation following industrial or motor vehicle accidents. All the litigants had been referred for psychiatric assessment because of psychological symptoms. Eight litigants stated that their symptoms decreased in severity after the finalization of the claim. Ten subjects returned to work following their accidents, but the authors did not state whether this had been prior to, or after, the claims had been finalized.

In a follow-up study of 50 subjects with post-traumatic headache, who were reviewed after the finalization of litigation, Packard (1992) found that all the patients continued to experience persistent headaches one or more years after their claims had concluded. Only four patients reported an improvement in the headache pattern following finalization of their legal actions.

A follow-up of 760 personal injury litigants following, predominantly, work and automobile accidents, found that 396 subjects (52 per cent) had resumed work prior to the finalization of their claims (Mendelson 1995). Of the 363 litigants who were not employed at the time of settlement of their claims, 99 were lost to follow-up. Out of the 264 persons who were contacted, 198 were unemployed. Assuming that all those lost to follow-up were working, the study found that 198 out of 363 subjects (55 per cent) of those not working at the time their claims were finalized were not employed when reviewed, on average, 23 months after their cases were settled. The only significant predictive factor was age, with those working at follow-up being younger than those not employed.

The nosological status of 'compensation neurosis'

The concept of 'compensation neurosis' or 'accident neurosis' has been invoked for many decades in discussing the sequelae of compensable injuries, especially when symptoms and disability are disproportionate to the extent of the initial physical injury or objectively demonstrable organic abnormalities. These terms carry with them certain assumptions about the aetiology and prognosis of the patient's condition, and tend to be used as if they were specific diagnoses.

These terms, however, have no diagnostic validity. Using standard criteria of diagnostic validity, 'compensation neurosis' has been shown to be an invalid diagnosis (Mendelson 1985). 'Compensation neurosis' did not meet any of the four different criteria on which diagnostic validity rests (Kendell 1975).

The four ways of establishing diagnostic validity may be briefly summarized as follows:

1. *Content validity.* The demonstration that the defining characteristics of a given disorder were enquired into and elicited before that diagnosis was made.
2. *Construct validity.* The demonstration that aspects of psychopathology that can be measured objectively occur in disorders that assume their presence and not in those that assume their absence.
3. *Concurrent validity.* The demonstration that two independent techniques for arriving at a diagnosis both gave the same diagnosis.
4. *Predictive validity.* The demonstration that predictions derived from a diagnosis are subsequently borne out by events.

In particular, as shown in the above section, the concept of 'compensation neurosis' has no prognostic validity: it thus fails the test of predictive validity, which Kendell considered the most important of the 'implications' embodied by diagnostic concepts.

It well might be that a psychiatric classification such as *Diagnostic and Statistical Manual of Mental Disorders* (DSM-IV-TR) contains some mental disorders that do not meet Kendell's criteria; since the publications of DSM-III in 1980 there has been a continuing process of reviewing and modifying both the diagnostic criteria and the clinical entities included in DSM so as to enhance the validity of the disorders it contains. Some earlier entries have been omitted from the most recent version, while others have been modified or introduced.

While it could be argued that the concept of 'compensation neurosis' has survived (see Chapter 18), under one name or another, since the second half of the nineteenth century because it has fulfilled a clinical need, it is nevertheless the case that its basic postulate—that litigating patients improve when the case is finalized—is incorrect.

The status of malingering

Malingering has been defined as 'the willful, deliberate, and fraudulent feigning or exaggeration of the symptoms of illness or injury, done for the purpose of a consciously desired end' (*Dorland's Illustrated Medical Dictionary* 1974). The term 'malingerer' is of French origin, and was introduced in 1785 in the *Dictionary of the Vulgar Tongue*. It was originally used in a military setting, to describe persons who pretended to be sick so as to evade military duty.

Although 'malingering' is noted both in the DSM-IV-TR (American Psychiatric Association 2000) and in the *International Classification of Diseases* (World Health Organization 1992, ICD-10), both these systems of classification refer to malingering *not* as a diagnosis but as an act or a behaviour. In DSM-IV-TR, malingering (V65.2) is listed among 'Additional Conditions That May Be a Focus of Clinical Attention'. It is described as the intentional production of false or grossly exaggerated physical or psychological symptoms motivated by external incentives.

In ICD-10, malingering (conscious simulation) (Z76.5), also described as 'persons feigning illness with obvious motivation', is similarly not included within chapters dealing with specific psychiatric diagnoses, and is listed alongside 'issue of repeat prescriptions'. Thus, malingering does not fall within the lexicon of the diagnostician but is a form of behaviour to be assessed or evaluated on the basis of facts.

It is therefore incorrect for expert witnesses to offer the putative 'diagnosis' of malingering in written reports or in depositions, or when giving evidence in court. To do so is to usurp the role and function of the trier of fact—be it a jury, a tribunal, or a judge. Similarly, questionnaires and other methods touted as being 'measures' of malingering have no validity. The only means of determining whether or not a person is malingering is through the legal process, where all the relevant information is placed before the trier of fact and a legal decision is given as to the veracity of the person before the court.

Kay and Morris-Jones (1998) have discussed the assessment and management of litigants with complaints of pain, and noted that 'The assessment of exaggeration . . . is a personal assessment'. It is interesting to read in this article that 'the senior author thought that most of the patients attending pain clinics with musculo-skeletal litigation claims were exaggerating their disability (42 out of 43)'. According to the authors in 20 per cent of cases covert video evidence was obtained and 'in *all* of these cases the patient was found to be malingering or grossly exaggerating their symptomatology' (emphasis in original). There is no comment about the apparent discrepancy between the senior author's clinical assessment and the fact that video evidence was not produced in court for more than 20 per cent of the patients. There is also no comment about the degree of congruency between the clinical assessment and video evidence.

Writing in 1823, before the inauguration of the first railway link in 1830 between Liverpool and Manchester, Beck stated that:

> diseases are generally feigned from one of three causes—fear, shame, or the hope of gain. Thus the individual ordered on service, will pretend being afflicted with various maladies to escape the performance of military duty—the mendicant, to avoid labour, and to impose on public or private beneficence—and the criminal, to prevent the infliction of punishment. The spirit of revenge, and the hope of receiving exorbitant damages, have also induced some to magnify slight ailments into serious and alarming illness.

Beck (1823) urged that 'against such impositions, the police of every well regulated country should direct its energies'. He thus recognized that feigned diseases are a legal rather than a medical issue, and one that should be determined in courts of law.

Pilowsky (1985) has drawn attention to health practitioners who have taken upon themselves the role of detecting whether or not symptoms complained of by those seeking compensation or statutory benefits, as well as litigants, are 'genuine' or otherwise, and has described them as manifesting 'malingerophobia'. Regrettably, some members of the legal profession find it easier to seek the opinion of such 'experts' and abdicate their proper function as triers of fact, instead adopting the views about malingering and illness deception based on invalid clinical or psychometric tests.

The role of the health care professional in the assessment of claimants

As I have argued above, malingering is a legal concept and is the term used to denote fraud in a health context. There is no such diagnosis as malingering, and it is not a valid task of health care professionals to label individuals as malingerers. At the same time, clinicians do have a legitimate role in the assessment of personal injury litigants, and compensation and disability claimants.

The questions that clinicians can validly address in such circumstances are:

- Is there a diagnosable disorder/disease?
- What is the aetiology of the condition?
- What is the extent of impairment?—Is it temporary or permanent?
- Is the history consistent?—Is it plausible?
- Are findings on physical examination/mental state examination consistent/plausible?
- Has there been compliance with treatment and treatment recommendations?
- Has there been cooperation and motivation during rehabilitation?

While it is appropriate, and in some cases even necessary, for a clinician to offer an opinion about such issues to assist the trier of fact, to extrapolate from such clinical data and express the view that a person is lying and committing fraud is to step beyond the limits of clinical expertise.

Factors that influence outcome of compensable injuries

The literature that has been reviewed above has shown that there is no support for the assertion that there is any specific diagnosable 'disorder' resulting from accidental injury suffered under circumstances that give rise to an entitlement to compensation—that is, there is no such diagnosis as 'accident neurosis' or 'compensation neurosis'. I have also argued that there is no such diagnosis in medicine or psychiatry as 'malingering'.

It is therefore necessary to examine the various influences on the outcome of compensable injuries by looking beyond the conventional dichotomy of 'compensation neurosis' and malingering—is the person 'mad' or 'bad'—and to examine other factors that help to determine both response to treatment and the eventual outcome after the claim is finalized. There is a large literature dealing with such factors, and it is too extensive to summarise here. Table 17.2 sets out the most important of these factors, which are also of relevance in relation to disability and pension applicants (see Aylward, chapter 22).

The prospect of financial gain is only one of a number of factors that need to be taken into account; the concept of 'compensation neurosis' gives it an unwarranted primacy. While there are studies that have demonstrated the adverse influence of litigation/compensation on treatment outcome, there are also studies that have shown that actively pursuing litigation does not prevent recovery with appropriate treatment (Sapir and Gorup 2001).

Personality factors related to emotional deprivation in early life have been implicated among those that influence disability following injury (Fann and Sussex 1976), as well as dependency and immaturity. Enelow (1968) has stated that 'dependent, immature persons are very likely to surrender to disability as soon as they are injured.'

Societal factors, such as preferential treatment, also influence disability and such effects persist after litigation has been finalized (Hyman 1971). Attitudes towards certain types of accidents

Table 17.2 Factors that influence outcome of compensable injuries

Personality
  Childhood emotional deprivation
  Hypochondriacal traits
  Unmet dependency needs

Demographic factors
  Age
  Education level

Cultural factors
  Illness behaviour
  Folk belief concerning illness

Interpersonal dynamics
  Within the family
  Social milieu

Occupational factors
  Job dissatisfaction
  Work stress
  Type of work performed
  Employer/supervisor attitude

Psychological reaction
  Alteration in self-concept and body image
  Personality disorganization
  Regression
  Development of a mental disorder

Physical factors
  Presence and nature of physical injury or disease
  Extent of residual organic impairment

Economic factors
  Compensation payments
  Job security/level of unemployment
  Litigation
  Level of wages

Societal factors
  Acceptance of complaint as work related
  Expectations concerning prognosis
  Availability of rehabilitation

and injuries similarly influence illness behaviour, as demonstrated by studies of chronic neck pain following motor vehicle accidents (Schrader *et al.* 1996; Cassidy *et al.* 2000). While these studies have been criticized on methodological grounds, they nevertheless make the important point that illness behaviour is influenced by context, and that societal attitudes modify and shape such behaviour.

It is the contribution of these factors that ultimately determines the individual outcome following compensable injury and influences the presence and extent of any residual disability. The availability of compensation and the potential of a financial award are among a range of factors that need to be evaluated, and in the assessment of each individual it is necessary to develop a formulation and a new paradigm that takes into consideration all the factors of relevance to that person.

Conclusions

Following the development of the railways, commencing in 1830, which gave rise to accidents and injuries of a type that had been hitherto unknown, persons who had been involved in such accidents presented with symptoms and complaints that gave rise to 'new' diagnoses such as railway spine and railway brain, as well as 'nervous shock'. These terms were used to explain conditions that otherwise could not be understood using the medical knowledge at the time.

After the introduction of workers' compensation legislation at the end of the nineteenth century and during the early years of the twentieth century many authors postulated that it was the prospect of compensation and financial gain that motivated claimants and led to prolongation of disability.

This ultimately led to the concepts of 'compensation neurosis' and 'accident neurosis', with the implication that such symptoms will resolve once there was no further prospect of pecuniary gain. Another explanation offered for the presence of what were otherwise considered to be inexplicable symptoms was malingering.

Such 'explanations' are both inaccurate and simplistic. There are may factors that influence outcome following compensable injury and also influence the behaviour of disability claimants, and a new paradigm is needed that takes into consideration these variables and provides a comprehensive explanatory model that, ultimately, may lead to effective interventions which will reduce the adverse effects on both individuals and society of abnormal illness behaviour, unnecessary invalidism, and disproportionate disability.

Beck (1823) noted that the those who undertake assessments in situations where illness might be feigned have a 'double duty . . . to guard the interests of the public . . . and also those of the individual, so that he be not unjustly condemned'. This principle is also expressed in the aphorism that 'it is better to trust and be deceived, than to suspect and be mistaken'.

References

American Psychiatric Association (2000). *Diagnostic and statistical manual of mental disorders*, 4th edn, Text Revision. American Psychiatric Association, Washington, DC.

Bailey, P. and Kennedy, F. (1923). Injuries and disorders of the nervous system following railway and allied accidents. In *Legal medicine and toxicology* (eds F. Peterson, W. S. Haines, and R. W. Webster), 2nd edn, Vol. 1, pp. 397–440. WB Saunders Co., Philadelphia, PA.

Beck, T. R. (1823). *Elements of medical jurisprudence* (in two volumes). Websters and Skinners, Albany, NY. (Reprinted by The Lawbook Exchange, Ltd, Union, NJ, 1997.)

Binder, R. L., Trimble, M. R., and McNiel, D. E. (1991). Is money a cure? Follow-up of litigants in England. *Bulletin of the American Academy of Psychiatry and the Law*, **19**, 151–60.

Cassidy, J. D., *et al.* (2000). Effect of eliminating compensation for pain and suffering o the outcome of insurance claims for whiplash injury. *New England Journal of Medicine*, **342**, 1179–86.

Collie, J. (1913). *Malingering and feigned sickness*. Edward Arnold, London.

Dorland's Illustrated Medical Dictionary (1974). WB Saunders, Philadelphia, PA.

Elmaraghy, M. W. and Hurst, L. N. (1996). Single-portal endoscopic carpal tunnel release: agee carpal tunnel release system. *Annals of Plastic Surgery*, **36**, 286–91.

Enelow, A. J. (1968). Industrial injuries: prediction and prevention of psychological complications. *Journal of Occupational Medicine*, **10**, 683–7.

Erichsen, J. E. (1875). *On concussion of the spine, nervous shock and other obscure injuries of the nervous system in their clinical and medico-legal aspects*. William Wood & Company, New York, NY.

Fann, W. E. and Sussex, J. N. (1976). Late effects of early dependency need deprivation: meal ticket syndrome. *British Journal of Psychiatry*, **128**, 262–8.

Filan, S. L. (1996). The effect of workers' or third-party compensation on return to work after hand surgery. *Medical Journal of Australia*, **165**, 80–2.

Fordyce, W. E., Brockway, J. A., Bergman, J. A., and Spengler, D. (1986). Acute back pain: a control group comparison of behavioral vs. traditional management methods. *Journal of Behavioral Medicine*, **9**, 127–40.

Fowler, D. R. and Mayfield, D. G. (1969). Effect of disability compensation: disability symptoms and motivation for treatment. *Archive of Environmental Health*, **19**, 719–25.

Frieman B. G. and Fenlin, J. M. (1995). Anterior acromioplasty: effect of litigation and workers' compensation. *Journal of Shoulder and Elbow Surgery*, **4**, 175–81.

Hammonds, W., Brena, S. F., and Unikel, I. P. (1978). Compensation for work-related injuries and rehabilitation of patients with chronic pain. *Southern Medical Journal*, **71**, 664–6.

Hawkins, R. H. and Dunlop, R. (1995). Nonoperative treatment of rotator cuff tears. *Clinical Orthopedics*, **321**, 178–88.

Higgs, P. E., Edwards, D., Martin, D. S., and Weeks, P. M. (1995). Carpal tunnel surgery outcomes in workers: effect of workers' compensation status. *Journal of Hand Surgery [Am]*, **20**, 354–60.

Hyman, M. D. (1971). Disability and patients' perceptions of preferential treatment: some preliminary findings. *Journal of Chronic Diseases*, **24**, 329–42.

Jones, A. B. and Llewellyn, L. J. (1917). *Malingering or the simulation of disease*. William Heinemann, London.

Kay, N. R. M. and Morris-Jones, H. (1998). Pain clinical management of medico-legal litigants. *Injury*, **29**, 305–8.

Kelly, R. and Smith, B. N. (1981). Post-traumatic syndrome: another myth discredited. *Journal of the Royal Society of Medicine*, **74**, 275–7.

Kendell, R. E. (1975). *The role of diagnosis in psychiatry*. Blackwell, Oxford.

Kennedy, F. (1946). The mind of the injured worker: its effects on disability periods. *Compensation Medicine* **1**, 19–21.

Leavitt, F. (1990). The role of psychological disturbance in extending disability time among compensable back injured industrial workers. *Journal of Psychosomatic Research*, **34**, 447–53.

Mendelson, G. (1983). The effects of compensation and litigation on disability following compensable injuries. *American Journal of Forensic Psychiatry*, **4**, 97–112.

Mendelson, G. (1985). 'Compensation neurosis'—an invalid diagnosis. *Medical Journal of Australia*, **142**, 561–4.

Mendelson, G. (1994). Chronic pain and compensation issues. In *Textbook of Pain* (eds P. D. Wall and R. Melzack), 3rd edn, pp. 1387–400. Churchill Livingstone, Edinburgh.

Mendelson, G. (1995). 'Compensation neurosis' revisited: outcome studies of the effects of litigation. *Journal of Psychosomatic Research*, **39**, 695–706.

Miller, H. (1961). Accident neurosis. *British Medical Journal*, **i**, 919–25; 992–8.

Misamore, G. W., Ziegler, D. W., and Rushton, J. L. (1995). Repair of the rotator cuff. A comparison of results in two populations of patients. *Journal of Bone and Joint Surgery [Am]*, **77**, 1335–9.

Novak, C. B., Collins, E. D., and Mackinnon, S. E. (1995a). Outcome following conservative management of thoracic outlet syndrome. *Journal of Hand Surgery [Am]*, **20**, 542–8.

Novak, C. B., van Vliet, D., and Mackinnon, S. E. (1995b). Subjective outcome following surgical management of upper extremity neuromas. *Journal of Hand Surgery [Am]*, **20**, 221–6.

Packard, R. C. (1992). Posttraumatic headache: permanency and relationship to legal settlement. *Headache*, **32**, 496–500.

Page, H. W. (1885). *Injuries of the spine and spinal cord without apparent mechanical lesion, and nervous shock, in their surgical and medico-legal aspects*. J & A Churchill, London.

Pilowsky, I. (1985) Malingerophobia. *Medical Journal of Australia*, **143**, 571–2.

Ryan, W. E., Krishna, M. K., and Swanson, C. E. (1995). A prospective study evaluating early rehabilitation in preventing back pain chronicity in mine workers. *Spine*, **20**, 489–91.

Sander, R. A. and Meyers, J. E. (1986). The relationship of disability to compensation status in railroad workers. *Spine*, **11**, 141–3.

Sapir, D. A. and Gorup, J. M. (2001). Radiofrequency medical branch neurotomy in litigant and nonlitigant patients with cervical whiplash: a prospective study. *Spine*, **26**, 268–73.

Schnee, C. L., Freese, A., and Ansell, L. V. (1997). Outcome analysis for adults with spondylolisthesis treated with posterolateral fusion and transpedicular screw fixation. *Journal of Neurosurgery*, **86**, 56–63.

Schofferman, J. and Wasserman, S. (1994). Successful treatment of low back pain and neck pain after a motor vehicle accident despite litigation. *Spine*, **19**, 1007–10.

Schrader, H. *et al.* (1996). Natural evolution of late whiplash syndrome outside the medicolegal context. *Lancet*, **347**, 1207–11.

Sprehe, D. J. (1984). Workers' compensation: a psychiatric follow-up study. *International Journal of Law and Psychiatry*, **7**, 165–78.

Tarsh, M. J. and Royston, C. (1985). A follow-up study of accident neurosis. *British Journal of Psychiatry*, **146**, 18–25.

Wiesel, S. W., Feffer, H. L., and Rothman, R. H. (1984). Industrial low back pain: a prospective evaluation of a standardized diagnostic and treatment protocol. *Spine*, **9**, 199–203.

World Health Organization (1992). *The ICD-10 classification of mental and behavioural disorders: clinical descriptions and diagnostic guidelines*. WHO, Geneva.

18 Malingering and the law: a third way?

Alan Sprince

Abstract

This chapter examines the phenomenon of malingering in the context of contemporary English law. It does so in three interlinking sections. In the first section, the various references to malingering in the modern legal context are identified and categorized. The second section examines the way in which the law actually addresses those malingering issues. Such an examination exposes something of a disparity between the noticeable number and nature of references to malingering in the modern cases and their ultimate insignificance in direct substantive terms. In the final section, the same material is subjected to critical analysis in order to offer an explanation for that discrepancy and, with it, perhaps the basis for an indirect legal contribution to the wider discourse.

References to malingering in the modern legal setting

References to malingering in contemporary English law can be found in two main sources: (a) legal theory; and (b) legal practice.

Legal theory: legal academic attempts to describe and define malingering

So far as the legal theory is concerned, it is instructive in this context to consider the occasional attempts by academic lawyers to describe, and even in a rudimentary way to conceptualize, malingering. For instance, while such references do not purport to provide an authoritative definition of malingering for general legal purposes, they seem, in passing, to have touched briefly on some relevant definitive features. Within the legal system, the term 'malingering' is meant to be given its appropriate meaning of the deliberate, conscious feigning of symptoms for an ulterior purpose.

For example, in Napier and Wheat's (1995) book on the recovery of damages for psychiatric injury, the authors refer to malingering, characterizing a malingerer as '... someone who deliberately pretends to be suffering from an illness or disability ... for gain' (Napier and Wheat 1995, p. 100). The Law Commission (1998, para 3.30) describes malingering in exactly the same terms, again mentioning the phenomenon in passing in its report on the same 'nervous shock' subject-matter that Napier and Wheat cover.

Notably, these descriptions of malingering include additional material seemingly geared to ensuring that lawyers employ the concept with appropriate precision. Napier and Wheat (1995, p. 101), for example, offer lawyers guidance on how, in any given case, they might identify malingering. There is, moreover, a degree of attempted sophistication about their approach. While careful not to detract from their central concern that lawyers should adopt a methodical approach to the identification process, the authors are suitably circumspect about the practical utility of the DSM-IV criteria for that purpose. They refer to the general concerns expressed by medical commentators and suggest how each criterion might be recast in the specific legal context (Scrignar 1988).

Most significantly, perhaps, both sets of authors' attempts to secure some degree of precision do not stop at positive guidance on how lawyers might accurately conceptualize and identify malingering. Both supplement these efforts by identifying that which they fear could militate against precise usage. More particularly, both identify and seek to eliminate the potential for lawyers to confuse malingering with other unrelated concepts. The rudimentary general legal conceptualization of malingering offered in these sources, therefore, contains *exclusion*, as well as inclusion criteria.

Predictably, factitious disorder (American Psychiatric Association 1994) is singled out as the most potentially confusing concept. While alerting lawyers to the essential similarity between malingering and factitious disorder, both Napier and Wheat (1995, p. 100) and the Law Commission (1988, paras 3.30–3.32) also succinctly identify the subtle, but critical, point of distinction. They explain that conscious deception characterizes both, but that only malingering also requires there to be a particular motivational factor.

In the same vein, both Napier and Wheat (1995, p. 49) and the Law Commission (1988, para 3.31, fns. 90, 91) urge lawyers not to confuse malingering with 'compensation neurosis'. While careful to acknowledge that this phenomenon has gradually been re-evaluated and its practical significance minimized, both sources isolate the theoretical points at which it can be distinguished from malingering (see Chapter 17). They suggest that what they describe as malingering's 'rational expectation of gain' also features generally in compensation neurosis, but that it does not do so as part of a conscious feigning of symptoms (Napier and Wheat 1995, p. 118; The Law Commission 1998, paras 3.30–3.32).[1]

Legal practice: specific case references

A more prominent source of malingering reference emerges from an examination of the frequency and type of specific references to the term in the cases that make up modern legal practice.

Frequency

As for frequency, any responsible conclusion must be tentative. This is because of the relative qualities and limitations of two relevant indicators. One is statistical, probably reliable in its own right, but incomplete in the context of this enquiry; the other is anecdotal, ostensibly less reliable in statistical terms, but, intuitively, probably more dependable in this context.

As for statistics, a search of the reports of English cases brought for formal adjudication and recorded in paper-based 'law reports' and (increasingly nowadays) on electronic legal databases reveals approximately 250 references to 'malingering' and 'malingerer', with the majority

---

[1] On reflection, this reasoning can now be questioned. Generally, 'compensation neurosis' has become a somewhat discredited and, thus, less frequent diagnosis since Napier and Wheat's and The Law Commission referred to it in 1995 and 1998, respectively. More specifically: Is the expectation of the malingerer necessarily rational?; Could it not be said that compensation neurosis involves personal gain directed intention?; Is the difference between them one of not consciously feigning symptoms in compensation neurosis?; If so, it is noteworthy that neither Napier and Wheat nor The Law Commission provide any guidance as to how one can operationally (i.e. clinically) distinguish compensation neurosis and factitious disorder. (I am grateful for the anonymous referee for raising these potential problems with the reasoning employed by Napier and Wheat and The Law Commission.)

appearing in the modern era. In this context, however, the indicative limitations of this result are likely to be significant. As the vast number of cases are compromised before formal adjudication and, therefore, wholly unrecorded, it would be necessary to draw on other sources in order to form a more complete picture of the likely frequency of malingering references in modern legal practice. When, therefore, that statistical indicator is matched with the (admittedly anecdotal) evidence from legal practitioners in connection with those unrecorded cases, it seems that malingering, while by no means common, is at least reasonably noticeable to those involved in processing English legal cases (see Chapter 16).

Type

As for type, it is possible to identify several generic case categories in which references to malingering seem most typically to arise.

Military

For example, malingering references arise in the context of military law (see Palmer, Chapter 3). This is not surprising. As Mendelson (1995) points out, the phenomenon that modern lawyers would label 'malingering' actually acquires its legal provenance through long-established association with equivalent military regulation. She cites classical and medieval legal codes which, while not employing specific malingering nomenclature, were clearly devised to punish (often by death) those who simulated disease or self-mutilated in order to evade the call to battle. From the end of the eighteenth century, the specific term 'malingering' acquired its first formal legal usage when it was employed in that military context to describe and punish servicemen conducting themselves in that manner.

The modern military designation adopts essentially the same approach. There is separate legislation for each division of the military.[2] Together, the relevant statutes offer the only modern legal definition of malingering, each characterizing it as: (a) falsely pretending to be suffering from sickness or disability; (b) injuring oneself with intent to avoid service; and (c) doing or failing to do anything to produce, or prolong or aggravate, any sickness or disability, with intent to avoid service. A person convicted of the offence of malingering is liable to imprisonment for a term not exceeding 2 years. Case are heard before a special military tribunal, as a court-martial, with rights of appeal to a Court-Martial Appeal Court[3] (see Palmer, Chapter 3).

Social security

Malingering references can also arise in cases heard by tribunals with specific jurisdiction over the law regulating the administration of the state welfare system that, *inter alia*, provides benefits to those unable to find work or who have been incapacitated as a result of their work.

In relation to those receiving welfare benefits on the basis that they claim to be unable to find work, there is potential for an allegation of malingering to arise in two distinct types of case. First, a claim to benefit might be resisted if there is a suspicion that the claimant has feigned illness in order to avoid work that is available. Second, the claim might be similarly resisted even when the claimant is (secretly) working and, by feigning illness, has claimed to be unemployed.

By definition, malingering allegations are more likely to arise in connection with the operation of the state welfare system that provides benefits to those who can establish that they have a

---

[2] See section 42 of The Army Act 1955; s. 27 of the Naval Discipline Act 1957 s. 42 of The Air Force Act 1955.
[3] Armed Forces Act 1996, ss. 5, 15–17 and Schs. 1 and 5; the Armed Forces Discipline Act 2001, ss. 14–25; The Court-Martial (Appeals) Act 1968.

sufficient degree of work-related incapacity or disablement. Typical cases would tend to involve suspicion over the genuineness of the incapacity or disablement that the applicant claims entitles him or her to benefit. The Social Security Appeals Tribunal hears appeals from initial determinations as to entitlement to benefit under the legislation. Appeals from that tribunal lie, first, to a Social Security Commissioner and then to the Court of Appeal (in both cases, on a point of law).

Employment

It is also possible for malingering references to arise in cases heard by tribunals with specific jurisdiction over the law that regulates employees' rights. Initially, such cases are processed by the Employment Tribunal. Appeals lie, first, to the Employment Appeals Tribunal, and then to the Court of Appeal (in both cases on a point of law).

Relevant references arise where dismissal follows an allegation of malingering and/or a dispute about the genuineness of the symptoms of a supposedly sick employee. The potential for such claims to be resisted on these bases corresponds with the findings in recent research into the roles played by non-medical factors and outright deception as determinants of sickness absence and early retirement due to ill health (Johns 1997; Poole 1997).

Civil compensation claims

Research also indicates that references to malingering can arise in cases that are determined under the mainstream civil and criminal court system. Allegations of malingering have been raised in civil cases since the second half of the nineteenth century, coinciding with the increase in the relevant medical literature during that period (Mendelson 1995, p. 426). The absence of demonstrable physical injury meant that early civil claims for 'nervous shock' were especially prone to being resisted by way of an allegation that the plaintiff was wholly simulating his symptoms and, thereby, malingering (Mendelson 1998, Chapters 2 and 3). Dismissing such a claim in *Victorian Railway Commissioners* v. *Coultas*,[4] Sir Richard Couch famously voiced a fear that to do otherwise might result in' . . . a wide field opened to *imaginary* claims'.[5] At the same time, defendants sued for conventional physical injury began to aver that the plaintiff was similarly feigning or exaggerating injury.

While nervous shock cases now tend to be dominated by restrictive rules designed to meet the fear of a flood of *genuine* claims (Jones 2000), the same references to malingering still arise in standard compensation actions brought for physical injury following an accident. Occasionally, defendants use video and other forms of surveillance with a view to catching the claimant suspected in this way.

A related grouping of civil cases in which references to malingering arise include those in which claims brought under contracts of insurance or a pension scheme to sickness benefit or a pension are resisted on a similar basis and heard by the same courts. Civil cases will be heard by the County Court or High Court (depending mainly on the value of the action). Appeals then lie to the Court of Appeal (Civil Division) and, thereafter, to the House of Lords.

Criminal law potential

There is also potential for malingering references to arise in the context of the criminal law. Criminal liability is determined initially either by Magistrates in the Magistrates Court or judges

---

[4] (1888) 13 App Cas 222.   [5] (1888) 13 App Cas 222–225, emphasis added.

and juries in the Crown Court (depending on type of offence) and then, on appeal, first to the Court of Appeal (Criminal Division) and then to the House of Lords. The distinctiveness of both criminal law as a branch of English law and of the criminal courts that determine liability in relevant cases makes it natural to distinguish potential references to malingering along civil and criminal lines.

That said, any categorization built on such a theoretical distinction should not ignore the practical interrelationship between the case types, especially in the malingering context. In practice, malingering's criminal context mostly arises out of other actions initially processed by non-criminal courts.

Indeed, other than in the military context, there is no independent criminal offence of malingering. In any given non-criminal action where malingering is in issue, however, the deception component might be sufficiently prominent and proven for the malingerer *both* to lose his claim (in whole or in part) *and* to end up on the receiving end of a separate criminal prosecution for one of the more general, deception-based offences under criminal law (Jones 2002).

There are three such types of offence that could, in theory, be triggered in that way.

(1) a claim to benefit under social security law could be rejected in circumstances in which allegations of malingering are so clearly established as to amount to one of the fraud-based criminal offences specific to the social security legislation.

(2) the alleged malingering in any of the above-mentioned non-criminal contexts might be so clearly established that the deception amounts to an offence under the Theft Acts. The most likely offence would be that of obtaining (or attempting to obtain) 'property' by deception under section 15 of the Theft Act 1968, on the basis that 'property' for these purposes would include any wages that the malingerer deceitfully secured or attempted to secure.[6]

(3) the alleged deception in the originating non-criminal action could subsequently acquire its criminal context simply because it was practised through court proceedings. The most relevant such 'offence against the administration of justice' would be perjury. English law first criminalized perjury in 1563, the essence of the offence then, as now, being that the accused was guilty of providing false sworn testimony in court. Also, as now, the gravity of such an offence was reflected in the nature of the punishment that it could attract. Sixteenth century English criminal law required that perjurers lucky enough to avoid imprisonment, but unlucky enough to be too poor to pay hefty fines, be 'pilloried' in the public square and have their ears nailed. The modern offence is contained in Section 1 of the Perjury Act 1911, under which it is an offence punishable by up to 7 years imprisonment for a person lawfully sworn as a witness in judicial proceedings to make a statement about something which is 'material' which he knows is false or does not believe to be true.

Perjury has achieved some prominence recently, with successful prosecutions having been brought against former UK Cabinet minister, Jonathan Aitken, and former Conservative Party chairman, Jeffrey Archer. Both Aitken and Archer became criminal defendants after it became clear that they had fabricated evidence in earlier civil claims for libel that they had brought as claimants. Aitken's libel case had actually collapsed on that basis; infamously, Archer had won and more than 10 years elapsed before it emerged that he had misled the court.

The nature of the legal response

This section examines the way in which English law actually addresses the malingering component in modern legal practice identified in the previous section.

---

[6] Theft Act 1968, s. 4(1).

In doing so, it also seeks to evaluate the nature of the ultimate contribution that that legal response might offer to the wider malingering discourse. After all, just because malingering references can be identified in the legal setting, it does not follow that, when processed, they would translate into an identifiable and meaningful legal position on the subject.

The expectation: a meaningful legal contribution

Reflecting on the relevant material, however, it would at first sight seem reasonable to expect that the law makes a substantive legal contribution to the malingering debate, both in qualitative and quantitative terms. As for the former, the general, discursive material from the likes of Napier and Wheat and the Law Commission seems geared to safeguarding and developing the quality of the law's position on malingering. Though brief, it is explicitly educative in approach, guiding lawyers beyond basic descriptors and towards a more sophisticated appreciation of relevant identification criteria and distinguishing characteristics.

While important, a sophisticated legal appreciation of the nature of malingering would, however, be virtually worthless in this context without the stock of relevant material through which that legal position might achieve some prominence. It is, therefore, convenient that other aspects of the material discussed in the first section would, at first sight, also seem to provide the corresponding quantitative indicators. For instance, though by no means abundant, malingering references seem to punctuate modern legal practice with sufficient frequency for lawyers themselves to be at least reasonably familiar with the notion of malingering.

Moreover, the relevant references to malingering would also seem to be of a type suited to delivering a meaningful legal contribution to the wider material. For example, those references arise in cases processed under the so-called 'Common Law' system operated under English law. The main characteristic of such a system is the importance it attaches to the law that comes from the courts and that will bind future courts. If, therefore, malingering features in cases before them, the decisions of the presiding judges might be expected to generate a relevant stock of 'malingering law'.

In cases heard by the civil courts and the tribunals of specialist jurisdiction, the alleged malingerers are (save in the case of the military tribunal) pursuers of claims that they could lose (either totally, on liability, or in part, as to quantum) as well as win. If the claimant's status as an alleged malingerer arose by reference to the way in which the claim has been resisted, then it might be assumed that defeat on the malingering-related quantum or liability issue would brand the unsuccessful claimant with the mark of the proven malingerer.

At the same time, the prospect of the pursuer of a claim before a legal system to become pursued under it appears at first sight to be especially relevant in the malingering context. It may be that, as a general proposition, the potential for there to be interplay between the civil and criminal law in this way has rarely been realized.[7] It has been one thing to acknowledge that a claim's failure might often give rise to the very real suspicion that the party pursuing it was attempting to perpetrate a deception. It has, however, been quite another for it to be similarly clear both that deception was sufficiently material to the pursuit of the claim and that it was sufficiently established through the whole or partial failure of those proceedings. Indeed, the crime of perjury has, for these reasons, become notorious as one of the least prosecuted offences under the law, despite obvious concern that numerous cases, both civil and criminal, are likely to have provided examples of it having been committed (Slapper 2001).

---

[7] Aitken and Archer provide two well-publicized modern exceptions.

Yet there would seem good reason to assume that the initial failure (in whole or in part) of a claim that had been resisted by way of an allegation of malingering might provide the exceptional conditions for generating subsequent prosecutions for perjury in particular. Strictly, because malingering also requires that the deception be specifically motivated by rational gain[8] and that it be practised through the simulation of symptoms, where perjury requires neither, it is (as Aitken and Archer illustrate) possible to have perjury without malingering. It is virtually impossible, however, to have malingering in the legal contexts so far identified without there also being perjury. The common deception component sees to that. The deception inherent in malingering would, it is assumed, be the very reason the malingerer lost (in whole or in part) the initial action he mounted as claimant, so enabling it to become both the very reason why he ended up as defendant before the criminal court and the evidence of deceit that would go quite some way to convicting him.

Experience: highly limited legal contribution

In the event, that suggested legal position has not materialized, however reasonable it might be to have expected otherwise. Indeed, far from providing anything of substance to add to the wider discourse, the actual legal position on malingering has, on examination, provided almost as little of direct worth as it did in the conversion hysteria context, in spite of the relative imbalance in available material (Jones and Sprince 2001).

There is, for instance, no evidence that the conceptual sophistication that some legal commentators have achieved at a theoretical level has yet trickled down into legal practice. If anything, practical legal usage of the term 'malingering' remains loose and barely conceptualized. Where such lack of sophistication serves to limit the quality of any wider legal contribution to the malingering discourse, it is the limited quantity of useful case law that most restricts the law's capacity to make a substantive contribution to the wider debate. An important stock of 'malingering law' has not emerged from the identifiable stock of cases in which references to malingering arise.

Where claims made have been resisted in whole or in part by reference to malingering, the relevant court or tribunal in them has rarely reached a positive finding that an individual is or is not malingering. Moreover, where any such cases have gone on appeal to the Court of Appeal and the House of Lords, the malingering element rarely even arises. Equally, where the pursuer of such a claim has gone on to lose in whole or in part, defeat has rarely triggered a prosecution under the criminal law for one of the deception-based offences apparently so naturally associated with the malingerer's *modus operandi*. At the same time, while the relevant jurisdiction has by no means become redundant, relatively few suspected cases of malingering are actually determined by formal courts martial.

An explanation for the disparity

The previous section exposed a disparity between, on the one hand, the number and nature of references to malingering in the modern cases and, on the other, their ultimate insignificance in direct substantive terms. This section offers an explanation for that disparity and, with it, an indirect legal contribution to the wider discourse.

---

[8] Arguably, it may not matter if the deception was motivated by irrational gain, provided that this was not considered psychiatric. (I am grateful for the anonymous referee for raising this issue.)

An over-familiarity?

Given that the disparity results from the combined effect of each of its contributing elements, it is valid to speculate that the relative frequency of malingering references in modern English legal practice might be as inordinately excessive as the insignificant amount of substantive case law seems exceedingly limited.

Indeed, when noting that relative imbalance in the legal references to conversion hysteria and malingering, it was submitted that a dearth of the former might in part be due to an excess of the latter, given the tendency for lawyers in practice to take a somewhat robust, often cynical, attitude to apparently 'unexplained' symptoms (Jones and Sprince 2001). Malingering's capacity to function in that way as the 'dustbin' into which lawyers discard (rather than explain) that which they cannot explain with the naked eye would, in this context, account for both unsophisticated legal usage and a resultant *over*-employment. On reflection, the lengths that Napier and Wheat and the Law Commission go to ensure that lawyers appreciate both what characterizes malingering and what distinguishes it from other phenomena can be taken to signify these very concerns. In short, their exhortations also draw attention to the problem they seek to remedy, serving as implicit recognition that, without such further elaboration, lawyers might be prone to confuse malingering with those other conditions. Indeed, elsewhere in the same material, both leave little room for doubt that they suspect that any such confusion might itself be part of a *conscious* legal motivation to eschew the more sophisticated approaches that are available and simply to label as malingering much that does not present as 'physical' (Napier and Wheat 1995, p. 100, 118; The Law Commission 1998, para 3.31). In other words, the lawyer's lingering scepticism over the validity of psychiatric harm generally still tempts him to attribute symptoms that cannot be readily explained as physical to conscious gain-motivated simulation on the part of the claimant/patient.

A limited stock of malingering law: the distinct legal process

As for the other contributor to the discrepancy under review, the absence of an identifiable source of malingering law itself can be explained by reference to the same contrast between the legal and medical forensic processes that was drawn on to explain similar apparent legal inactivity in the context of conversion hysteria (Jones and Sprince 2001, p. 160).

Law and fact

Central to this is the distinction courts draw between law and fact. Any given dispute calls for the court to resolve disputes on the latter, by hearing evidence, and then to apply either an undisputed legal principle or a disputed one that it has resolved to the facts it determined.

The role of the medical expert in any given case is to provide evidence to assist the court in resolving a dispute over the factual basis of the action. By definition, the medical expert is not a legal expert and so has no direct involvement in any application of legal principle to the facts. Those legal principles fall to be determined and applied by the courts, especially the senior courts such as the Court of Appeal and the House of Lords. The system of binding precedent confers the highest authority on the decisions of these senior courts.

This basic law/fact division, coupled with the way in which the dispute context influences the legal processes for determining questions on both sides of it, can, in turn, serve as the means of explaining the relative imbalance between the ultimate quality and utility of any legal and medical pronouncements on malingering.

Higher courts: appeals on points of *law*

While the medical professional has no direct involvement in the determination of relevant legal principle, the court clearly does. Yet there are virtually no Court of Appeal or House of Lords decisions encompassing a malingering question even though one might have been raised when the case was heard at first instance. As a general rule, however, appeals to the Court of Appeal and the House of Lords are confined to questions of legal principle. Any malingering question will not, therefore, readily qualify as an issue of legal principle fit for determination by the Court of Appeal and the Law Lords.

Malingering as fact: materiality, burden, and standard of proof

As a corollary, the malingering issue would be treated as raising a question of fact for determination by the relevant non-senior court with the help of expert and other evidence. The relative frequency with which such questions appear to be raised before such courts would, in theory, provide the potential for the absence of authoritative legal pronouncements on malingering to at least be mitigated by a number of relevant findings of fact. That even this has not materialized can be attributed to the distinct fact-finding process employed by those courts.

The legal fact-finding process differs from the medical professional's diagnostic determinations because it takes place in a dispute-centred context. While both the court and the doctor will treat their respective determinations as 'facts', the legal finding of fact is the product of a very narrow enquiry, delineated by the requirements of dispute resolution. In short, many facts sought and found by the medical professional might not even come for determination by the court should the dictates of that responsibility agenda (in turn set by the questions of materiality and burden/standard of proof discussed below) not require there to be such a positive finding.

The actual mechanism through which the legal fact-finding process is conducted requires, first, that any given factual issue is in some way material to the case, and then, most importantly, that the court is actually formally required to make a finding on it. That this may open up the possibility that an issue might be material but might not require formal determination may seem odd to the medical professional. Where malingering is put in issue, the modern clinician may pursue the question to the point of its diagnostic resolution one way or the other. For the court, the same malingering issue might meet the test of materiality (being, by definition, an important element in the parties' dispute), but not, in the event, require formal resolution as a fact (for reasons discussed in the next paragraph). In other words it might be useful to resolve such an issue but it might not be legally necessary.

In turn, the criteria that determine whether the court is required to make a formal finding of fact on any given issue is itself the product of the dispute context that drives the legal decision-making process. While numerous facts may be material to the dispute between the parties, the court restricts itself to establishing only those facts necessary for it to determine responsibility. In an adversarial system the court treats that determination not as the sort of independent fact-finding exercise that characterizes inquisitorial systems of law, but rather as a response to one party's assertions as to the alleged responsibility of the other. This is formalized in the so-called burden of proof whereby one party has the onus of convincing the court to accept the case it puts. In civil cases, the burden is on the claimant; in criminal cases, it is on the prosecution. Such burdens of proof are discharged according to varying standards of proof: the balance of probabilities in civil cases; and beyond a reasonable doubt in criminal prosecutions.

In general, therefore, the burden of proof doctrine restricts the scope of the facts that a court must find. It limits them to those material factual issues advanced by the party carrying the relevant burden of proof. While the other party might also advance a factual basis to resist the case put against them, the burden on them is merely to do sufficient to ensure that the case against them is not proved. In general, they are not obliged to prove the case they put in response. So, therefore, in the civil context, a defendant seeking to resist a claimant's claim that a coin landed 'heads' may lead evidence that the opposite was true, but he is not formally required to prove that it landed 'tails'.

In claims pursued before the legal system and resisted by reference to malingering, the malingering question falls naturally outside of the scope of the factual and legal material that falls to the claimant to prove. It will, by definition, be a defendant assertion. As a result, the court in such a case will not be required to make a factual finding on the question as part of its formal response to the claimant's allegations as to defendant responsibility. If, therefore, the court finds that the claimant in such a case has not discharged the burden of proving his case on the malingering-related liability or quantum issue, that does not mean that it has made a concomitant finding that the defendant was correct to assert malingering. In effect, the court can declare that it does not accept the claimant's version of the facts without declaring the claimant a liar as the defendant might have alleged. It can find that the claimant has not proved his claim that a coin landed 'heads' without thereby confirming that it landed 'tails'.

The burden of proof doctrine, therefore, limits the stock of decisions in which the court finds it necessary not merely to reject an alleged malingerer's claim but also to find as a fact that he malingered in the process. As a corollary, without a formal finding of malingering in such cases, there is no clear deception component to trigger a prosecution for one or more of the deception-based offences under the criminal law, in spite of the ready theoretical association between those offences and malingering.

Conclusions

In examining malingering in the legal context, this chapter has been careful not to pretend that malingering is, ever has been, or ever will be, a *legal* phenomenon (Mendelson 1995). Nor has it suggested that a legal perspective on malingering might provide the 'missing link' for those in the medical profession who have taken on responsibility for developing its phenomenology. If anything, the law's position on malingering is characterized by the absence of substantive and definitive features and by an indifference to any imperative to acquire them.

As such, this chapter's contribution is to submit that legal position as a counterpoint to a medical approach that is seemingly driven towards achieving the 'holy grail' of reliable diagnostic determination or elimination. The contrasting legal standpoint, with its occasional readiness to accommodate 'not proven' as a finding of equal validity to the standard positive and negative alternatives, might at first sight look like a 'cop out' to a medical community striving for conclusiveness. Yet, while such conclusiveness remains no more than a chimera, the legal approach might offer a temporary 'third way' model for medical thinking that might otherwise consider anything short of a definitive position as failure.

Acknowledgements

The author is grateful to his colleagues, Stephen Hall-Jones, Mitchell Davies, and Debra Morris, for their kind and patient assistance with earlier drafts of this chapter.

References

American Psychiatric Association (2000). *Diagnostic and statistical manual of mental disorders*, 4th edn, text revision. American Psychiatric Association, Washington, DC.

Johns, G. (1997). Contemporary research on absence from work: correlates, causes and consequences. In *International review of industrial and organizational psychology* (eds C. Cooper and I. Robertson). Wiley and Sons, Chichester.

Jones, M. A. (2002). *Textbook on torts*, 8th edn, pp. 147–69. Oxford University Press, Oxford.

Jones, M. A. and Sprince, A. (2001). Conversion hysteria: a legal diagnosis. In *Contemporary approaches to the study of hysteria* (eds Halligan, Bass, and Marshall), pp. 155–70. Oxford University Press, Oxford.

Mendelson, D. (1995). The expert deposes, but the Court disposes: the concept of malingering and the function of a medical expert witness in the forensic process. *International Journal of Law and Psychiatry*, **18**(4), 425–36.

Mendelson, G. (1998). *The interfaces between law and medicine, the history of liability for negligently occasioned psychiatric injury (nervous shock)*, Chapters 2 and 3. Dartmouth.

Napier, M. and Wheat, K. (1995). *Recovering damages for psychiatric injury*. Blackstone Press, London.

Poole, C. J. M. (1997). Retirement on grounds of ill health: cross-sectional survey of six organizations in United Kingdom. *British Medical Journal*, **314**(7085), 929–32.

Scrignar, C. B. (1988). *Post-traumatic stress disorder: diagnosis, treatment, and legal issues*, 2nd edn, pp. 89–90. Bruno Press, New Orleans, LA.

Slapper G. (2001). The peculiar crime of perjury. *New Law Journal*, August, **1206**.

The Law Commission (1998). *Liability for psychiatric illness*, Law Com No. 249.

19 How can organizations prevent illness deception among employees?

Charles Baron and Jon Poole

Abstract

There is increasing evidence to show that in certain circumstances employees will deceive their employers about their health so as to avoid work or for financial gain by way of sick pay, early pensions, injury awards or litigation. In the process, doctors may also be deceived and inadvertently collude with the patient. Examples are provided of policies and procedures which should help to prevent or reduce the likelihood of illness deception by employees.

Introduction

Sickness absence and early retirement due to ill health have traditionally been used as indices of the health of employees. Each has a direct and quantifiable negative effect on costs and productivity of the organisation. This review presents evidence from published studies, national statistical data, and professional experience, which indicates that non-medical factors, to include illness deception, play an important role as determinants of these occupational health indices. Although most employees are honest about their health under most circumstances, there is evidence that points to intentional manipulation of a desired outcome either by withdrawal from work or by claims for financial benefit through exaggeration and occasional fabrication of medical history, symptoms and signs. There is also some evidence that doctors may collude with their patients to help them fulfil these ends (see Chapter 15). Furthermore, the actions of organisations may condone and encourage this process through their policies, poor working conditions, reluctance to rehabilitate ill employees, and ambiguity about applying rules.

Doctors are often faced with conflicting roles in managing the health–work interface. The general practitioner (GP) will put the interests of the patient first and is particularly sensitive about maintaining a good long-term relationship with the patient. The consideration of illness deception in patients is avoided by many doctors as it raises difficult personal and ethical issues which may compromise the doctor–patient relationship. We believe that open and objective debate about this taboo subject will help to facilitate the management of patients who deceive or mislead doctors to obtain a desired outcome. In addition, by understanding the complex interactions around employees within an organisation, it may be possible to minimise illness deception behaviour and mitigate its effects on sickness absence and early retirement. This should be a constructive and positive process, which should be to the benefit of employees, the employing organisation and society as a whole.

Sickness absence

Studies of absence from work attributed to sickness have been mainly of a cross-sectional design linking absence records with demographic details. It is affected by a variety of factors which include illness, factors at home and at work, and the employee themselves such as their ability to cope in adversity. Some evidence for non-medical factors affecting sickness absence is described below.

Variation within organizations

In a survey of 212 Local Authorities in England, the median absence rate was 4.3 per cent, equivalent to 9.8 days per employee per year (LGEO 2000). For non-manual employees the median rate was 4.0 per cent (9.1 days) and for manual employees, 5.7 per cent (13.0 days). Marked variation occurred between employees, the lower quartile rate was 3.4 per cent (7.8 days) and the upper quartile rate 5.1 per cent (11.6 days). A comparison of absence rates in 40 UK fire brigades showed similar variations in absence, with the average number of shifts lost per year in 1998–99 varying from five in the 'best performing' brigade to 16 in the 'worst performing' (HMFSI 2000). While there may be geographical differences in the experience of health problems among employees of the same organization, the magnitude of these differences suggests that there are other, non-medical factors affecting absence rates.

Do people lie about sickness?

In a qualitative study originally designed to identify gender differences in absenteeism, hospital workers who had just returned from a scheduled day off or an unscheduled day off that was classified by the employer as due to sickness absence were interviewed about their absence (Haccoun and Dupont 1987). In the latter group, 72 per cent admitted to not being sick on their (sick) day off. Whilst this percentage seems to be particularly high and may not be applicable to other organisations, it does suggest that some sickness absence is not for medical reasons.

Job satisfaction

In a study of factors affecting post-operative recovery rates, delayed return to work after elective laparoscopic cholecystectomy was shown to be much more likely in patients assessed as having low job satisfaction (OR 12.56, 95% CI 3.34–47.2) (Froom et al. 2001). In a case referent study in Denmark of employees with absences longer than 10 weeks, the odds ratio for the existence of low job satisfaction as compared with referents was 2.1 (CI 1.2–3.5) (Eshoj et al. 2001).

Other occupational psychosocial factors

Occupational psychosocial factors have been implicated as determinants of musculoskeletal disorders (Waddell 1998) and stress disorders (Cox et al. 2000). It seems likely therefore that a person's perception of a bad or unsupportive work environment will influence their desire to withdraw from work and the way that symptoms are presented to a doctor.

A prospective study of 12 555 French Electricity and Gas Board employees examined the results of annual self-administered questionnaires linked to company absence records between 1989 and 1995 (Niedhammer *et al.* 1998). This demonstrated that those with jobs with high decision latitude had 15–25 per cent fewer spells and days than those with lower levels of decision latitude after adjusting for confounders. In addition, those with a higher perceived level of social support at work had 15–20 per cent fewer spells and days absence than those with lower perceived social support after adjusting for confounders.

A study of Finnish hospital physicians demonstrated that those working in poorly functioning teams were 1.8 times more likely to take long spells of absence than those working in well-functioning teams (CI 1.3–3.0) (Kivimaki *et al.* 2001).

Attitudes and culture of the employer

In a two-phase longitudinal study, absence levels for individuals and work groups were measured before and 12 months after the qualitative phase (Gellatly and Luchak 1998). Researchers interviewed hospital workers to discover the bases of employees' beliefs about what is acceptable and expected in terms of absence behaviour. They found that perceptions about absence were influenced by prior personal absence, the average level of absence within the immediate work group, and the absence culture to which they belonged. Perceived absence norms were also shown to also predict future personal absence 1 year later.

Attitudes at home

In a study of 10 308 British civil servants (Whitehall II) high levels of confiding/emotional support at home was found to correlate with sickness absence suggesting that support of this nature encouraged illness behaviour (Rael *et al.* 1995).

Financial compensation affecting absence and recovery

Another non-medical factor affecting the presentation and management of medical conditions is the pursuit of financial compensation after injury. In a prospective study of the effects of removing compensation for pain and suffering from claims for whiplash injury after road traffic accidents, the incidence of claims decreased by 43 per cent for men and by 15 per cent for women between the tort period and the no-fault period (Cassidy *et al.* 2000). The median time from the date of injury to the closure of a claim decreased from 433 days (95% CI 409–457) in the last 6 months of the tort period to 194 days (95% CI 182–206) in the first 6 months of the no-fault period and 203 days (95% CI 193–213) in the second 6 months of no-fault. The intensity of neck pain, the level of physical functioning, and the presence or absence of depressive symptoms were strongly associated with the time to claim closure in both systems. The authors concluded that the elimination of compensation for pain and suffering is associated with a decreased incidence and improved prognosis for whiplash injury.

The impact of financial incentives on disability, symptoms, and objective findings was evaluated by a meta-analysis of 18 studies after closed-head injury (Binder and Rohling 1996). The authors concluded that there was evidence of more disability in patients with financial incentives despite less severe injuries. In another meta-analysis of 32 studies of patients receiving compensation for chronic pain, receipt of financial compensation was associated with a greater experience of pain and reduced treatment efficacy (Rohling *et al.* 1995).

Apparent increase in illness without medical explanation

Claimants for state sickness benefits have steadily increased in the United Kingdom from 1984 to 1995, mainly due to increases in the number of long term sick (Moncrieff and Pomerleau 2000). The non-employed made up a rising proportion of recipients and regional incapacity rates were strongly associated with socioeconomic factors, particularly social class. These observations have lead to the suggestion that sickness benefits increasingly represent disguised unemployment.

The number of person days of sickness for back pain has dramatically risen in the United Kingdom from around 25 million days in 1985 to around 125 million days in 1995, which cannot be explained by a change in the prevalence of back disorders (Waddell 1998). In a 1-year prospective intervention study in industry, researchers assessed the effects of distributing a psychosocial educational pamphlet about the benefits of a positive approach to back pain and reducing avoidance behaviours such as extended sickness absence (Symonds *et al.* 1995). Control subjects in other factories received either a non-specific pamphlet or no intervention. In the company whose employees received psychosocial pamphlets, a significant reduction occurred for the number of spells with extended absence and the number of days of absence (70 and 60 per cent, respectively) compared with extrapolated values. Erroneous beliefs (and therefore not deception) may explain some of these findings.

A dramatic rise in the numbers of cases presenting with so called repetition strain injury or RSI was seen in Australia in the 1980s. Many of the cases were the subject of compensation claims against employers. Gun (1990) described the numbers and incidence of such cases in South Australia between 1980–81 and 1985–86. His figures were derived from the Australian Bureau of Statistics who started to classify them as industrial accidents leading to lost time in 1980. He found that there was a high incidence among blue-collar manual workers 'engaged in work situations which engendered feelings of boredom, powerlessness and alienation'. Superimposed on this high base rate, was a peak in 1984–85 that later declined to below previous rates in 1986–87. In addition there was a 17-fold increase in cases in the female, clerical sector from 12 cases in 1980–81 to 204 in 1984–85 declining to 85 cases in 1986–87. While it may be argued that there was an increase in the use of computer keyboards at around this time, this was the case throughout the developed world and changes of this magnitude were not seen in other western countries at the same time. It seems unlikely therefore that this was the sole cause of such an increase in the incidence of these conditions.

Whilst it may be too simplistic to suggest that these examples indicate illness deception on a large scale, the possibility that illness deception provides an explanation for some of these trends must be given consideration.

Early retirement due to ill health

Most occupational pension scheme rules provide for members who become disabled from working by reason of ill health or injury to be granted an early release of enhanced pension benefits. The criteria for this early release vary between schemes. Usually, there is a requirement for the claimant to demonstrate permanent incapacity (normally defined as incapacity to do their normal job or comparable work until the normal age of retirement). There is evidence however that non-medical factors affect the way in which early pensions due to ill health are granted.

In its report on retirement in the public sector, the Audit Commission demonstrated that nearly 40 per cent of all retirements in Local Authorities in England were due to ill health. However the percentage of early retirements due to ill health relative to all retirements between authorities varied from 5 to 70, suggesting that retirements were not all related solely to levels of medical incapacity (Audit Commission 1997).

In a survey of the UK fire service, wide variation in the proportions of ill health retirements were found between the 50 brigades in 1998–99 (HMFSI 2000). The 'worst performing' brigade, however, reported that approximately 3.3 per cent (330 per 10 000) of serving whole-time fire-fighters had retired through reasons of ill-health in that year. The 'best performing' brigade however reported this figure to be 0.69 per cent (69 per 10 000). The authors of the report drew the conclusion that there must be non-medical factors operating to explain these large differences.

A cross-sectional survey of ill health retirements in six UK organizations showed rates of ill-health retirement to vary from 20 to 250 per 10 000 contributing members, and in two of the organizations the rate varied geographically within the same organisation (Poole 1997). In four of the organizations studied, modes in rates of early retirement due to ill health concurred with enhancements in financial benefits (Fig. 19.1). There is no medical reason for this phenomenon, which is likely to be due to manipulation of the pension scheme regulations for financial advantage.

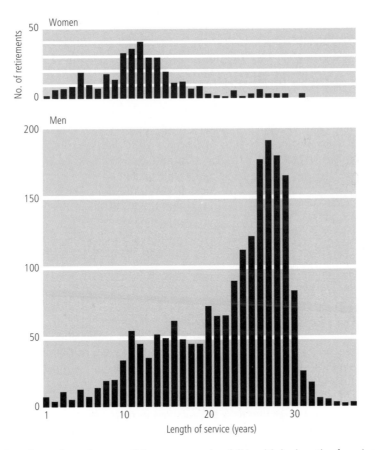

Figure 19.1 Numbers of employees retiring on grounds of ill health by length of service and sex during 1994–95 in organization C. Enhancements in benefits are payable after 10 and 27 years of service. From Poole, C. J. M. (1997). Retirement on grounds of ill health: Cross-sectional survey in six organisations in United Kingdom. *British Medical Journal* **314**, 929–32.

Clinical experience of occupational physicians

Malingering among employees is rare in our experience. Most patients present with an honest medical history, which is consistent with objective clinical findings and with the observations of third parties. Most of our experience of illness deception has been encountered during the task of assessing financial awards associated with disability, usually in connection with applications for early retirement due to ill health or occupational injury awards. Patients have been encountered who have given us information about their past medical history, functional ability or job, which on checking is found to be false or misleading. Some patients have been discovered working elsewhere whilst off sick or to be participating in activities that are incompatible with their claimed disabilities (e.g. running marathons or competitive rally driving in someone who 'cannot' carry out manual tasks because of pain and poor mobility).

Exaggeration of symptoms and behaviour which is not consistent with clinical expectations has also been observed. A patient told one of us that as a consequence of an accident at work he could not use one of his arms, but on court surveillance by his employers he was seen to use it normally. In extreme cases, colleagues have described being threatened, complained about to their employers' or reported to the General Medical Council by patients who were unhappy that their claim for financial benefit was not supported. We have also encountered patients who have asked for information to be removed from medical reports which did not support their claim for financial benefits.

Do doctors collude with patients?

Certified absence from work (FMed 3), financial awards for injuries, early retirement benefits for ill health, and state benefits for illness or disability all require support from a medical practitioner. It follows therefore that doctors who support claimants in circumstances of illness deception may be colluding with them (see Chapter 15). Doctors may, in some cases, be deceived by the patient, or perhaps more commonly, be suspicious but unable to demonstrate evidence of deceit.

In a qualitative study of the role of GPs in sickness certification, researchers showed that GPs will admit to signing certificates when the medical evidence does not justify it (Hiscock and Richie 2001). We have experience of receiving certificates of incapacity and letters from doctors, which make assertions (to their patient's advantage) that are not supported by objective medical evidence. There are a number of reasons why doctors may 'collude' in the signing of certificates (Hiscock and Richie 2001). Various factors influence the way in which the process of judging incapacity takes place. These include patient behaviour, number of patients to be seen in the surgery, and inadequacy of consultation times. As a result, some GPs believe that it is often easier to 'just sign' than to engage in a lengthy discussion or examination. Maintaining a good relationship with the patient is also an important consideration and will influence certification practice, as will how well the GP knows the patient as GPs may find it easier to negotiate an alternative to certification with patients they know well. GPs also admit to a lack of sufficient occupational information on which to base advice and employees may mislead their doctors with regard to aspects of their employment.

Doctors also want to be liked by their patients and to be perceived as good or caring. Some doctors may be professionally unconfident and feel vulnerable to challenge by the patient or his advisors. In cases where there have been threats or intimidation, it may be easier to 'go with the flow' than risk formal complaints with the potentially harmful effects that these may have on their careers. Given all of the above, it is not surprising that doctors occasionally will collude with their patients to help them to either avoid work or pursue financial advantage.

Discussion

Evidence is presented above for non-medical factors playing an important part in determining patterns of sickness absence, dramatic rises in the prevalence of certain illnesses, financial awards for injury or disabilities, and early retirement due to ill health. Clinical experience of the authors and others indicate that in some cases this is directly attributable to illness deception by patients. Illness deception and manipulation are involved to some extent with these non-medical phenomena. The doctors involved in advising on these issues may collude with some patients in certain circumstances. Proving and challenging illness deception is extremely difficult in the absence of video evidence or self-confession, particularly where psychological or pain symptoms are the main disabling features. The detection of illness deception runs contrary to the empathetic instincts of most doctors and would compromise a normal doctor–patient relationship.

The familiar quotation 'all men have their price' which is usually attributed to Sir Robert Walpole (1676–1745) is pertinent. The assumption is that everyone has a potential level of dishonesty that can be encouraged by the offer of higher rewards. Rewards need not always be monetary. This concept can be easily applied to illness deception. One might envisage a scale of 'health honesty' from 0 to 100. The patient who never lies or exaggerates about his health would score 100 and the one who is a frank malingerer would score 0. If the psychosocial work environment is made worse for our honest patient, then it is reasonable to postulate that he is likely to score less. Factors that may encourage him or her to take time off work 'dishonestly' include a job that is unsatisfying or boring and for which there is no control. Such a person may also feel less 'guilty' about dishonesty if he or she works for an organization, the management of which he does not trust, or where there is no perceived support, or the team is poorly functioning. If the culture of the organization is such that taking sick leave or leaving 'on ill health' is seen as reasonable, legitimate behaviour, he or she may have much less difficulty in displaying dishonest behaviour than if this behaviour was culturally unacceptable. Such a model can be used as a basis for preventative strategies for employers.

Prevention

We recommend that organizations introduce the following policies and procedures to reduce the risk of illness deception. Even where this form of behaviour is rare, these actions should provide a demonstrably fairer and better working environment.

1. Organizations in which it is custom and practice to receive ill health and injury awards after an optimum number of years should review their policies and procedures.
2. Negative psychosocial risks should be addressed. These may involve the job (e.g. a lack of decision latitude), the work team (e.g. dysfunctional working due to interpersonal problems within the team) or the organization as a whole (e.g. inconsistent application of the rules).
3. Other occupational risks (physical, chemical, and biological) which make the environment less attractive or more frightening to work in, should be assessed and controlled in compliance with health and safety legislation.
4. Erroneous belief systems that lead to dysfunctional behaviour (including unjustified, extended withdrawal from work) should be addressed by general and individual education programmes at work.
5. Employees should be aware of their attendance record in comparison with their peers and the organization as a whole. There should be a clear understanding by employees that sickness absence should be solely for reasons of ill health. Absence should be monitored and managed equitably across the whole organization.

6. Decisions about financial benefits or early retirement due to ill health should be taken by doctors in whom there is no potential for conflicts of interest. A two-doctor system where the second doctor is solely an advisor to the benefit provider or the pension scheme should achieve this.

7. Occupational physicians taking ill-health pension decisions should be given appropriate training and work to explicit evidence-based guidelines. They should audit their recommendations on an annual basis and compare them with benchmarks from comparable organizations.

8. If alternative (non-medical) routes to early retirement do not exist then they should be made available.

9. Systems which provide a pecuniary disincentive to recovery or return to normal functioning for complaints which are solely subjective should be reformed.

10. Employers should provide more options for rehabilitation to help GPs negotiate earlier return to work and avoidance of early retirement. These might include modified and phased return to work programmes, provision of early treatment such as occupational physiotherapy and counselling, or the provision of other early interventions such as education programmes about mechanical back pain. This policy will also help to address employee perceptions about a lack of support by the organization.

11. There should be more timely advice and support for GPs in making certification decisions such as from departments of occupational health in local NHS Trusts.

12. Organizations should foster better relations between their occupational physicians and local GPs. This may result in a better understanding for GPs of the workplace through good early communications. More information about jobs and the options available in the workplace will aid the GP in negotiating with the patient.

Future research

The use of these interventions should be evaluated more formally. While measures of illness deception are not available, it may be necessary to use outcomes that are thought to be proxies for these, such as sickness absence, early retirement due to ill health, and compensation for injury to evaluate the effectiveness of these recommendations.

References

Audit Commission (1997). *Retiring nature—early retirement in local government.* Audit Commission.

Binder, L. M. and Rohling, M. L. (1996). Money matters: a meta-analytic review of the effects of financial incentives on recovery after closed-head injury. *American Journal of Psychiatry*, **153**, 7–10.

Cassidy, J. D., Carroll, L. J., Cote, P., Lemstra, M., Berglund, A., and Nygren, A. (2000). Effect of eliminating compensation for pain and suffering on the outcome of insurance claims for whiplash injury. *New England Journal of Medicine* **342**, 1179–86.

Cox, T., Griffiths, A., Barlow, C., Randall, R., Thomson, L., and Rial-Gonzalez, E. (2000). *Organisational interventions for work stress: a risk management approach*, HSE Books, Sudbury.

Eshoj, P., Jepsen, J. R., and Nielsen, C. V. (2001). Long-term sickness absence—risk indicators among occupationally active residents of a Danish county. *Occupational Medicine—Oxford*, **51**, 347–53.

Froom, P., Melamed, S., Nativ, T., Gofer, D., and Froom, J. (2001). Low job satisfaction predicts delayed return to work after laparoscopic cholecystectomy. *Journal of Occupational and Environmental Medicine*, **43**, 657–62.

Gellatly, I. R. and Luchak, A. A. (1998). Personal and organizational determinants of perceived absence norms. *Human Relations*, **51**, 1085–102.

Gun, R. T. (1990). The incidence and distribution of RSI in South Australia 1980–81 to 1986–87. *Medical Journal of Australia*, **153**, 376–80.

Haccoun, R. and Dupont, S. (1987). Absence research: a critique of previous approaches and an example for a new direction. *Canadian Journal of Administrative Sciences*, **4**, 143–56.

Hiscock, J. and Richie, J. (2001). The role of GPs in sickness certification. National Centre for Social Research on behalf of Department for Work and Pensions, Leeds.

HMFSI (2000). Fit for duty—a thematic review of sickness absence and ill-health retirements in the fire service in England, Wales and Northern Ireland. Home Office—HM Fire Service Inspectorate, London.

Kivimaki, M., Sutinen, R., Elovainio, M., Vahtera, J., Rasanen, K., Toyry, S., Ferric, J. E., and Firth-Cozens, J. (2001). Sickness absence in hospital physicians: 2 year follow up study on determinants. *Occupational and Environmental Medicine*, **58**, 361–6.

LGEO (2000). Local Government Sickness Absence Levels 1999/2000. Local Government Employers Organisation (Employment Surveys and Research Unit), London.

Moncrieff, J. and Pomerleau, J. (2000). Trends in sickness benefits in Great Britain and the contribution of mental disorders. *Journal of Public Health Medicine*, **22**, 59–67.

Niedhammer, I., Bugel, I., Goldberg, M., Leclerc, A., and Gueguen, A. (1998). Psychosocial factors at work and sickness absence in the Gazel cohort: a prospective study. *Occupational and Environmental Medicine*, **55**, 735–41.

Poole, C. J. M. (1997). Retirement on grounds of ill health: cross sectional survey in six organisations in United Kingdom. *British Medical Journal*, **314**, 929–32.

Rael, E. G., Stansfeld, S. A., Shipley, M., Head, J., Feeney, A., and Marmot, M. (1995). Sickness absence in the Whitehall II study, London: the role of social support and material problems. *Journal of Epidemiology and Community Health*, **49**, 474–81.

Rohling, M. L., Binder, L. M., and Langhinrichsen-Rohling, J. (1995). Money matters: a meta-analytic review of the association between financial compensation and the experience and treatment of chronic pain. *Health Psychology*, **14**, 537–47.

Symonds, T. L., Burton, A. K., Tillotson, K. M., and Main, C. J. (1995). Absence resulting from low back trouble can be reduced by psychosocial intervention at the work place. *Spine*, **20**, 2738–45.

Waddell, G. (1998). *The back pain revolution*. Churchill Livingstone, London.

Section 6

Contributions from cognitive neuroscience

20 Lying as an executive function

Sean Spence, Tom Farrow, David Leung, Samir Shah, Becky Reilly, Anna Rahman, and Amy Herford

Abstract

A number of lines of evidence suggest that lying represents a 'higher', executive function supported by relatively recently evolved brain systems. However, brain activity during lying is only beginning to be elucidated. We developed an objective approach to its investigation, utilizing a computer-based 'interrogation' and fMRI. Interrogatory questions probed recent episodic memory in three cohorts of healthy volunteers ($n = 30, 31$, and 48, respectively) studied outside, and 10 volunteers studied inside the MR scanner. In a counter-balanced design subjects answered 36 questions both truthfully and with 'lies'. Lying was associated with longer response times ($P < 0.001$) and greater activity in bilateral ventrolateral prefrontal cortices ($P < 0.05$, corrected). Less significant foci were observed in other, dorsal and medial prefrontal regions (including anterior cingulate cortex). These findings were consistent, irrespective of whether questions were presented in a visual or auditory modality. Ventrolateral prefrontal cortex may be engaged in generating lies or 'withholding' the truth. Other studies, emerging from other laboratories, have subsequently supported the hypothesis that experimental deception is an executive task, associated with prefrontal activation. Anterior cingulate cortex has been activated in two of the three studies reported to date. The anatomy of deception is likely to be further elucidated through novel brain imaging techniques.

Introduction

lie ... an intentionally false statement

(The Concise Oxford Dictionary)

deception ... a successful or unsuccessful deliberate attempt, without forewarning, to create in another a belief which the communicator considers to be untrue.

(Vrij 2001, p. 6)

Judging by the writings of antiquity, lying and deceit have been among human concerns for millennia. The instruction of Ptahhotep, originating more than five thousand years ago in Pharaonic Egypt, enjoins the reader to:

'Control your mouth ...', 'keep to the truth, don't exceed it', 'do not repeat calumny'.

(Chinweizu 2001)

Similarly, the Hebrew Bible refers to verbal lies:

> Thou shalt not bear false witness against thy neighbour.
>
> (Exodus 20:16, King James Version)

> They deceive their friends
> and never speak the truth;
> they have trained their tongues to lying . . .
>
> (Jeremiah 9:5, Revised English Bible)

Speech ethics may have been of particular importance in the ancient Mediterranean world because of a reliance upon the oral transmission of culture (Bauckham 1999). Nevertheless, despite this apparent emphasis upon honesty in human discourse there are emerging evolutionary, developmental, and neurodevelopmental–psychopathological literatures which suggest that deception (in animals and humans) and lying (specifically in humans, utilizing language) are consistently increased among organisms with more sophisticated nervous systems (Giannetti 2000). Such behaviours follow a predictable, 'normal', developmental trajectory in human infants (O'Connell 1998) and are 'impaired' among human beings with specific neurodevelopmental disorders (such as autism; Happe 1994). Hence, there would appear to be an interesting tension between that which is socially undesirable (cf. Vrij 2001) but 'normal' and that which is perhaps socially commendable but pathological. Higher organisms have evolved the ability to deceive each other (consciously or otherwise), while humans, in a social context, are (overtly, consciously) encouraged to refrain from doing so. Of course, it may be hypothesized that it is precisely *because* the human organism has such an ability (to deceive another) that it is called upon to exercise control over this behaviour.

What is the use of lying?

Given the 'normal' appearance of lying and deception in childhood, a number of authors have speculated upon the 'purposes' served by these behaviours. Here, purpose is essentially teleonomic, an after-the-fact application of an ability that may have arisen spontaneously (persisting through natural selection). One view has been that deceit establishes a boundary between 'self' and 'other', specifically between the child and her mother (Ford *et al.* 1988). Knowing something that her mother does not know allows the child to constrain the omniscience of the former while allowing her (the child) a certain degree of control. Indeed, the desire for control (over information) may contribute to pathological lying in dysfunctional adolescents and adults (Ford *et al.* 1988).

Lying also eases social interaction, by way of compliments and information management. Strictly truthful communication at all times would be difficult and perhaps rather brutal (Vrij 2001). Hence, it is unsurprising that 'normal' subjects (when studied) admit to telling lies on most days. Studies, often of college students, suggest that lying and dissimulation facilitate impression management, especially at the beginning of a romantic relationship; though mothers continue to be lied to frequently (Vrij 2001, pp. 8–9)!

Deception may be a vital skill in the context of conflict, especially that between social groups, countries, or intelligence agencies. When practiced in this context it might also be perceived as 'good'. However, when one is branded 'a liar', any advantage formerly gained may be lost. Though fluent liars may make good companions (at times), being known as a liar is unlikely to be advantageous (Vrij 2001).

In an extensive review of the psychology of deception, Vrij (2001) has demonstrated that whereas humans often lie, they are generally poor at detecting deception by others. Indeed, statistically, they exhibit a 'truth bias': both 'lay' and professional 'lie-detectors' over-estimate the truthfulness of their interlocutors. Nevertheless, professional lie-detectors report more confidence in their judgement.

Principles of executive control

Controlling behaviour in everyday life is crucial though highly likely to be constrained by cognitive neurobiological resources (Spence *et al.* 2002). Executive function is not necessarily 'conscious', although it may be (Badgaiyan 2000; Jack and Shallice 2001). Higher centres, such as prefrontal cortex, become involved when behaviour is non-routine, difficult or spontaneous (Spence *et al.* 2002). Otherwise, 'lower' centres such as motor regions and basal ganglia may subserve much that is automated or routine. A recurring theme in the psychology of deception is the difficulty of deceiving in high-stake situations: information previously divulged must be remembered, emotions and behaviours 'controlled', information managed (Vrij 2001). These are inherently executive procedures. Hence, much of the behaviour of the liar may be seen from a cognitive neurobiological perspective as falling on a continuum with other situations in which behavioural control is exerted, albeit using limited (attentional) resources. Some examples may illustrate the principles underlying such behavioural control.

The emergence of movement

One of the clinical means by which a psychiatrist may assess whether a patient with schizophrenia receiving neuroleptic medication exhibits involuntary movements is through the use of distraction, for example, when the patient is standing and performing (requested) alternating hand movements. While distracted by the manual task, the patient may begin to 'tramp' on the spot (with his feet), his tongue perhaps exhibiting dyskinesia (Barnes and Spence 2000, p. 188). While his central executive is engaged by the complex manual tasks 'it' may not be inhibiting these other, involuntary, movements (pseudo-akathisia and dyskinesia). Similarly, a patient with hysterical conversion symptoms such as motor paralysis may move the affected limb when she is distracted or sedated, suggesting that her executive processes were engaged in maintaining the 'functional' symptom when it was present (Spence 1999). In certain situations, liars may also betray deception by their bodily movements. While telling complex lies they may make fewer expressive hand and arm movements (Vrij 2001). The implication here is that similar executive resources are utilized for expressive gesture and the inhibition of 'truthful' responding. The slower, more rigid behaviour exhibited by liars (while inhibiting truthful responding) has been termed the 'motivational impairment effect' and police officers have been advised to observe witnesses from 'head to toe' rather than focusing on their eyes (Vrij 2001).

The suppression of speech

Finally, we might posit that the liar is attempting to avoid making a 'slip of the tongue', by which he might be discovered. Although Freud's writings in this area are explicitly concerned with unconscious processes, there is a tacit understanding that such 'slips' implicate executive dysfunction. In *The Psychopathology of Everyday Life*, Freud states:

> What happens is that, with the relaxation of the inhibiting attention—in still plainer terms, *as a result of* this relaxation—the uninhibited stream of associations comes into action.
>
> (Original italics, Freud 1991, p. 103)

Subsequently, he seems to re-emphasize the executive:

> I really do not think that anyone would make a slip of the tongue in an audience with his Sovereign, in a serious declaration of love or in defending his honour and name before a jury—in short, on all those occasions in which a person is heart and soul engaged.

(Freud 1991, p. 147)

Hence, we might equate the 'heart and soul engaged' with the conscious executive system. Indeed, there is recent empirical evidence for the Freudian concept of 'repression' being modelled as an executive function ('suppression'). Anderson and Green (2001) demonstrated that normal subjects could be made to suppress certain word associations, that subsequently the suppressed words would be recalled less frequently, and that access would remain reduced even after changes of stimulus probe.

Thus, it is perhaps unsurprising that accomplished liars are more likely to evince executive skills, for example, verbal fluency, cognitive flexibility, and a good memory. A literature review of 'pathological lying' reflected that despite high levels of central nervous system pathology such 'liars' demonstrated preserved or even enhanced verbal skills (King and Ford 1988).

Executive tasks necessitate longer response times

A final point worth raising is that response times (RTs) are generally increased when subjects perform executive tasks, relative to baseline conditions. Executive function is constrained by resource limitations and more processing time is required on more difficult tasks (Spence *et al.* 2002). Hence, RTs may be increased when subjects give dishonest answers (cf. the 'truth') as demonstrated by recent behavioural studies (e.g. Seymour *et al.* 2000). Also, despite RT being a variable that is potentially open to conscious manipulation, these studies have demonstrated that constraining RT variability (i.e. by stipulating that responses be made in under 800 ms) prevents healthy subjects from influencing their RTs in order to elude discovery (Seymour *et al.* 2000).

Lying as a cognitive process

Deceiving another human subject is likely to involve multiple cognitive processes, including social cognitions concerning the victim's thoughts (their current beliefs) and the monitoring of responses made by both the liar and the victim in the context of their interaction. In an unconstrained natural environment, motor control processes are likely to contribute to the generation of some novel motor responses ('lies') and the inhibition of pre-potent responses ('truths'). In such a model, the basic assumption is that the truth equates to a 'pre-potent' response (assuming that the subject actually knows the answer). Hence, it may be hypothesized that the generation of truly novel responses (lies) in contrast to pre-potent, known, responses (truths) will be associated with greater prefrontal cortex activation (see Spence and Frith 1999, for a review of *dorsal* brain regions activated during willed actions). The active inhibition of such pre-potent responses (truths) may also be hypothesized to implicate *ventral* prefrontal regions (e.g. Starkstein and Robinson 1997).

In a constrained situation, lying may be limited to merely saying the 'opposite' of that which is believed (by the liar) to be true. For instance, answering 'yes' instead of 'no'. It is of note that both the popular forms of the polygraph test (the Control Question Test and the Guilty Knowledge Test) restrict subjects' possible answers to 'yes' or 'no' (Vrij 2001). We posited that if the social elements of lying to another human subject could be minimized in the experimental setting, then the cognitive processes supporting such a mode of responding (with opposites) might be preferentially revealed. By using a highly constrained protocol, in which subjects were required to withhold truthful responses and answered with their opposites (i.e. 'yes' for 'no'), we examined the behavioural and functional anatomical correlates of this form of lying.

In order to enhance the face validity of our method, we focused on subjects' accounts of their recent behaviours (engaging autobiographical, episodic memory).

Experimental method

One hundred and nine healthy subjects (43 males, 66 females) participated in three behavioural studies, conducted outside the scanning environment (Spence *et al.* 2001; Farrow *et al.* submitted for publication). Ten healthy males undertook a functional MRI (fMRI) experiment (reported in Spence *et al.* 2001). The demographic and psychometric profiles of all subjects are shown (Table 20.1).

On the day of the study, each subject completed a 36-item questionnaire, specifically designed to record (truthfully) whether they had performed certain specified acts on that day. The questionnaire began with the stem: 'In the course of today, have you done any of the following?' This was followed by 36 exemplars (e.g. 'Made your bed', 'Taken a tablet', etc.). Subjects answered 'yes' or 'no' to each item. These responses provided templates for the rating of their subsequent performance on the experimental tasks.

The 36 questions were then re-administered (in counter-balanced sequences) in two computer-administered 'interrogations' (one utilizing a visual mode of question presentation, the other an auditory mode) where the response was governed by designated colour-based rules (below).

In the *visually* presented interrogation, each question appeared on a laptop computer screen for 5 s. Subjects replied 'yes' or 'no' using designated keypads. The words 'yes' and 'no' appeared beneath each question, both in green or red (colours alternating at 30-s intervals). Subjects' answers were determined by a 'colour rule' relating to the colour of these prompts. Each subject had been told by one investigator to 'lie' in response to green or red. Over two experimental runs, each subject answered every question once with the 'truth' and once with a 'lie'. Response

Table 20.1 Demographic and response data from subjects performing lying tasks outside and inside scanner

	Outside scanner 1	Outside 2	Outside 3	Inside scanner
Number of subjects	30	31	48	10
Males	12/30	16/31	15/48	10/10
Right-handed (EHI)	26/30	27/31	0/48	10/10
Mean age (range) years	24 (19–29)	23 (19–31)	38 (21–76)	24 (23–25)
Mean predicted verbal IQ (NART) (range)	118 (110–123)	123 (117–126)	116 (95–129)	120 (111–127)
Response times (ms)				
Visual protocol				
Truth: mean ± s.d.	1607 ± 710	1467 ± 717	1529 ± 651	1600 ± 592
Lie: mean ± s.d.	1820 ± 795*	1628 ± 753*	1744 ± 703*	1793 ± 636*
Auditory protocol				
Truth: mean ± s.d.	2485 ± 579	2503 ± 591	2293 ± 426	2438 ± 448
Lie: mean ± s.d.	2689 ± 611*	2670 ± 536*	2472 ± 513*	2632 ± 498*

*In each case, lie versus truth, 2-tailed, paired T test, $P < 0.001$.

times and accuracy were recorded and verified (each subject's initial questionnaire serving as their template).

In the *auditory* mode, each subject heard the questions in the computer-sampled voice of one of the investigators (the same male voice across all studies). Subjects replied 'yes' or 'no' using the same designated keypads (as above). The words 'yes' and 'no' appeared on the computer screen, in green or red (alternating at 30-s intervals) and the same colour rule applied for each subject. The experiment again comprised two runs, so that by the end, each subject had answered every question once with the 'truth' and once with a 'lie'. Response times and accuracy were again recorded and verified. This methodology was applied to three cohorts of volunteers, the third comprising specifically left-handed subjects.

Similar procedures were also applied to ten subjects in the scanning experiment. Auditory stimuli were presented via MR-compatible headphones. Visual stimuli were presented on a projector screen at the foot of the MR scanner bore and viewed by the subject via a headcoil-mounted mirror. Again, subjects made overt motor responses, using a button-box held in the right hand. Only one of the investigators knew the colour rule pertaining to each subject. Subjects were informed that two other investigators (in the MR observation room) would attempt to detect the colour rule on the basis of their motor responses. Four functional scans were acquired (two each for the visual and auditory interrogatory protocols).

FMRI imaging

All imaging was performed on a 1.5-T MR system. For each of the four functional scans, 64, 20-slice brain volumes were acquired using an echo planar imaging (EPI) sequence. Each functional scanning 'run' comprised the introductory stem (in either the auditory or visual modality), followed by six 30-s epochs, during which 'truth' and 'lie' responses alternated in a standard counterbalanced, between-sessions 'box car' design (Spence *et al.* 2001).

Data were analysed using Statistical Parametric Mapping (SPM99, Wellcome Department of Cognitive Neurology, London, UK) implemented in MATLAB (Mathworks Inc., Sherborn, MA, USA) on a PC. A fixed-effect analysis was performed on the data from the ten subjects. With respect to each selected contrast, a statistical parametric map was generated with an extent threshold of five voxels and a significance threshold of $P < 0.05$, corrected for multiple comparisons. We adopted this conservative threshold to reduce the possibility of 'false positive' results (Type 1 errors).

Results

In all four groups of subjects studied, both inside and outside the scanner, RTs were significantly longer when lying ($P < 0.001$, Table 20.1). There was an absolute difference between lying and truthful responses of approximately 200 ms. This level of statistical significance and absolute time difference applied to both the visual and auditory versions of the protocol (inside and outside the scanner). Mean accuracy across all trials was in excess of 95 per cent 'correct' (i.e. 'truth' or 'lie' responses, consistent with original questionnaire data).

Analysis of the fMRI data from both modalities of the protocol (visual and auditory) revealed very similar activation results (Table 20.2). Performing the visual protocol, subjects exhibited greater activity in the following areas when lying (relative to telling the truth): bilateral ventro-lateral prefrontal and medial premotor cortices. Other regions (particularly in left prefrontal and inferior parietal cortices) exhibited weaker effects that failed to survive statistical correction.

Table 20.2 Brain regions showing increased activation during lying responses (relative to 'truthful' responses), $P < 0.05$, corrected at voxel- and cluster-levels

Protocol	Cortical region (Brodmann area)	Coordinates	Z value
Visual task	Right ventrolateral prefrontal (BA 47)	56, 16, −8	5.29
	Left ventrolateral prefrontal (BA 47)	−52, 18, −8	5.30
	Medial premotor (BA 6)	0, 18, 54	5.52
		4, 26, 44	4.68
		−2, 38, 36	4.51
Auditory task	Right ventrolateral prefrontal (BA 47)	56, 18, −6	5.66
	Left ventrolateral prefrontal (BA 47)	−52, 18, −6	5.00
Both tasks	Right ventrolateral prefrontal (BA 47)	56, 18, −6	7.70
	Left ventrolateral prefrontal (BA 47)	−52, 18, −6	7.23
	Medial prefrontal (BA 32/8)	4, 26, 42	6.34
	Medial premotor (BA 6)	0, 18, 54	6.18
	Left lateral premotor (BA 6)	−38, 8, 56	5.00
	Left inferior parietal (BA 40)	−48, −52, 54	5.05

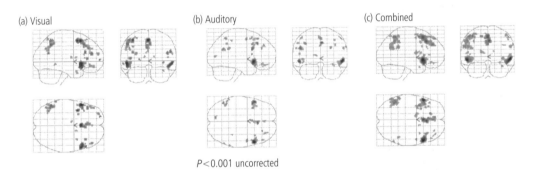

(a) Visual   (b) Auditory   (c) Combined

$P < 0.001$ uncorrected

Figure 20.1 Brain regions showing significantly greater neuronal response to lying on the visual protocol (a), auditory protocol (b), and combined analyses of both protocols (c). These figures show statistical parametric maps thresholded for display purposes at $P < 0.001$ (uncorrected). In each group, the upper left figure is a sagittal view (from the right side), the upper right figure is a coronal view (from behind), and the lower left is a transverse view (from above the brain).

On the auditory protocol, lying (relative to truth) was associated with greater activity in: bilateral ventrolateral prefrontal cortices and less significant foci in medial premotor regions.

When data from each of the fMRI lying protocols were combined, lying (relative to truthful responding—in a conjunction analysis) was associated with greater activity in: bilateral ventrolateral prefrontal cortices (VLPFCs), medial prefrontal (anterior cingulate) and premotor cortices, and left inferior parietal and lateral premotor cortices (Table 20.2 and Fig. 20.1).

Discussion of our findings

Our data show that on two (modality-specific) versions of a simple lying task, normal subjects exhibited consistent behavioural and functional anatomical responses. When lying, their RTs were significantly increased and there was reliable activation within specific regions of prefrontal cortex.

The brain region maximally implicated in both versions of our lying task was bilateral Brodmann area 47. In the monkey, Walker (1940) outlined a topographically similar region, calling it area 12. This region receives local projections from dorsolateral, anterior and medial prefrontal cortices (including anterior cingulate; Passingham 1993; Pandya and Yeterian 1996). It receives distant projections from temporal association cortices and amygdala (Passingham 1993). These projections carry visual, auditory, and tactile information although the role of area 47 seems to be independent of stimulus modality; connected instead with conditional learning and response inhibition (Passingham 1993). Hence, lesions of this region in non-human primates produce deficits on conditional response tasks (including certain forms of the 'go, no-go' paradigm), which may elicit response perseveration (Iversen and Mishkin 1970; Butters *et al.* 1973; Passingham 1993). In humans, lesions may also be associated with perseveration and a failure to inhibit prepotent responses (Starkstein and Robinson 1997). Functional imaging studies of healthy subjects have previously described ventrolateral prefrontal activation during response inhibition (Casey *et al.* 1997; Garavan *et al.* 1999).

Given the role of VLPFC in conditional learning and motor response inhibition there are two possible explanations for our current findings, which we are unable to differentiate using the current data. Activations of these homologous regions may be due to response reversal (alternation learning), which is inherent in the protocol described. Alternatively, our findings may relate specifically to an inhibitory function, the 'withholding of the truth' that is central to our current experimental design. However (in contrast to a 'go, no-go' protocol), our protocol always requires the subject to respond to each stimulus, so that any withholding of the truth (in response to specific stimuli) is always accompanied by the production of a 'lie' response. Hence, further investigation is required to differentiate response inhibition from response alternation.

A deficit in such an inhibitory mechanism has been previously hypothesized to explain the 'failure' of autistic subjects to deceive others (Hughes and Russell 1993). This theory holds that these subjects cannot lie because they are unable to suppress 'action towards the object' (an object that they are attempting to conceal in order to deceive another).

Our finding of increased response time during lying, in all groups of subjects, on both versions of our protocol, inside and outside the scanner, is congruent with a recent report of a convicted murderer, studied while lying and telling the truth (Vrij and Mann 2001; and see Vrij and Mann, Chapter 27). Although recounting similar material on both occasions, this subject exhibited slower speech with longer pauses and more speech disturbance when lying (Vrij and Mann 2001). He also exhibited less 'illustrators'—less bodily movement (Chapter 2 of Vrij 2001). Previous meta-analyses of behavioural lying studies have also pointed to speech disturbance, increased response latency and a decrease in other motor behaviours in the context of attempted deception (see Vrij and Mann 2001). Although responses on our tasks were non-verbal, the behavioural and functional anatomical profile revealed (above) may indicate a common process underlying these findings and others; namely, an inhibitory mechanism being utilized by those attempting to withhold the truth (a process associated with increased response latencies).

It is noteworthy that the difference between lying and truth RTs for all groups on both presentation modalities was around 200 ms. This is consistent with behavioural data from a 'guilty knowledge' task using an 'oddball paradigm', performed both with and without ERP recording (in Farwell and Donkin 1991, and Seymour *et al.* 2000, respectively). Such increases in RT during the 'lie' conditions in our studies are consistent with our hypothesis that lying is an executive task.

There are limitations to our current protocol, two of which are notable. The first is the relatively constrained option for motor response when lying (i.e. the subjects had only one possible 'lie' response to make, which they did not devise themselves). This means that subjects were not required to devise new 'lies' in our experiment. Hence, we have probably identified only a subset of those brain regions engaged in deception: those specifically activated by suppressing a pre-potent response (the truth) and producing its opposite (the lie). It may be countered that those regions activated are merely activated by this response reversal (responding 'yes' where 'no' would be truthful) but this is also inherent in a lying scenario *in vivo* in which there are only two responses allowed; and may be informative for this reason. Such limited responding also forms the basis of the polygraphic methods referred to above. A second problem is that there was an intentional lack of emotionally laden material in our questionnaire. This enabled us to reduce possible confounding variables but was clearly at variance with the 'real-life' ecology of lying (see Vrij and Mann, Chapter 27). Subjects in our study were fully compliant with the task (as evidenced by their response accuracy) and were not asked emotive questions. They were not attempting to lie in 'high-stake' (e.g. forensic) situations (Vrij and Mann 2001). These design limitations are being addressed in ongoing work.

Finally (and related to the first limitation above), we were surprised not to find more significant activation of left dorsolateral prefrontal cortex (DLPFC) in this study; it emerged as only a weak effect on the visual form of the task. Left DLPFC is implicated in response generation (Frith *et al.* 1991; Spence *et al.* 1998) and it is likely that our task did not place sufficient demand upon subjects generating their own (chosen) responses (there being only a single alternative to the 'truth' for each response elicited).

When data from both imaging studies were combined, in a conjunction analysis, to examine the difference in brain activity between lying and truthful responding, irrespective of stimulus modality, the statistical significance of a number of regional activations increased (Table 20.2). Of particular interest is the activation of medial prefrontal cortex, a region thought to be engaged by 'theory of mind' cognition, which has also been implicated in recent reports of lying studies emerging from other laboratories (and has been implicated in the cognitive neurobiology of autism).

Subsequent fMRI studies

Since publication of our own imaging methodology (Spence *et al.* 2001), two further studies have appeared in the peer-reviewed literature, each of which uses fMRI to investigate deception (Langleben *et al.* 2002; Lee *et al.* 2002). In the first, Langleben and colleagues used a variation of the Guilty Knowledge Test (as utilized in polygraphy). In this study, 18 subjects withheld knowledge of a playing card, which they held in their hands. Subjects made motor responses, pressing 'no' (instead of 'yes'). Compared with baseline conditions (in which they made truthful responses) such a 'lie' response elicited greater activation in medial prefrontal cortex (anterior cingulate cortex, ACC) and left premotor, motor, and parietal cortices. The authors did not elicit activation of VLPFC. The method used differed from that of our study but certain similarities are of interest. Both studies involved a motor (cf. verbal) response modality, in which subjects indicated the opposite of truth (i.e. 'no' for 'yes'). The material and modalities of presentation differed, as did certain technical scanning parameters (e.g. scanner field strengths). Yet both studies elicited activation of ACC (at coordinates 3, 28, 43 in our study, when data were combined on conjunction analysis (Table 20.2), and 4, 26, 42 in the Langleben study). The foci maximally activated in ACC were very similar and lie within its cognitive division (Bush *et al.* 2000). Also, neither study found any areas where activity was greater during the 'truth' condition (a finding consistent with both groups' contention that truthful responding represents the baseline condition).

A third study, by Lee *et al.* (2002), is perhaps closer to ours in that it probes autobiographical memory (as well as digit recall). These authors studied five subjects under four conditions: accurate recall, random responding, 'incorrect' responding, and active feigning (in which subjects tried to be bad without being *too* bad—in other words, by avoiding performance at levels below chance; a potential clue to feigning in the clinical setting). These authors did not report findings derived from the 'random' and 'incorrect' conditions, but their findings comparing feigned impairment and accurate recall implicate large regions of bilateral frontal, parietal, and temporal cortices, together with subcortical foci. There are apparently no foci of activation shared by this and the preceding two studies (by Langleben *et al.* and ourselves), although, perhaps the closest parallel with both the latter would have been with the 'incorrect' responding protocol used by Lee *et al.* (2002) but not reported. However, once again it appears that prefrontal cortex is implicated when subjects deliberately provide false information. Lee *et al.* (2002) reported no areas where accurate responding was associated with greater activity than feigned inaccuracy (again suggesting that accurate/truthful responding is a baseline state).

Conclusions

Our data and those of other groups suggest that by using highly constrained behavioural protocols investigators may begin to delineate the cognitive components of experimental deception in human subjects. Functional MRI provides a feasible method for investigating their neural correlates. Though these protocols require refinement, the published data clearly implicate specific regions of frontal cortex in the functional anatomy of deception. None of these studies reported areas of greater activation during truthful responding (consistent with truthful responding being relatively pre-potent). In our four cohorts (Table 20.1), response times were longer during attempted deception (again, indicative of executive function), a finding consistent with pre-existing behavioural studies and more recent, ecologically relevant studies conducted in the forensic setting (Vrij and Mann 2001).

Acknowledgements

We thank the subjects who participated in these studies, which were supported by the University of Sheffield. TFDF was supported by the John Templeton Foundation.

References

Anderson, M. C. and Green, C. (2001). Suppressing unwanted memories by executive control. *Nature*, **410**, 366–9.

Badgaiyan, R. D. (2000). Executive control, willed actions, and non-conscious processing. *Human Brain Mapping*, **9**, 38–41.

Barnes, T. R. E. and Spence, S. A. (2000). Movement disorders associated with antipsychotic drugs: clinical and biological implications. In *The psychopharmacology of schizophrenia* (eds M. A. Reveley and J. F. W. Deakin), pp. 178–210. Arnold, London.

Bauckham, R. (1999). *James*. Routledge, London.

Bush, G., Luu, P., and Posner, M. I. (2000). Cognitive and emotional influences in anterior cingulate cortex. *Trends in Cognitive Sciences*, **4**, 215–22.

Butters, N., Butter, C., Rosen, J., and Stein, D. (1973). Behavioural effects of sequential and one-stage ablations of orbital prefrontal cortex in the monkey. *Experimental Neurology*, **39**, 204–14.

Casey, B. J., Castellanos, F. X., Giedd, J. N., Marsh, W. L., Hamburger, S. D., Schubert, A. B., Vauss, Y. C., Vaituzis, A. C., Dickstein, D. P., Sarfatti, S. E., and Rapoport, J. L. (1997). Implication of right frontostriatal circuitry in response inhibition and attention-deficit/hyperactivity disorder. *Journal of the American Academy of Child and Adolescent Psychiatry*, **36**, 374–83.

Chinweizu. (2001). From Ptahhotep to postcolonialism. *Times Literary Supplement* 17 August, p. 6.

Farrow, T. F. D., Reilly, R., Rahman, T. A., Herford, A. E., Woodruff, P. W. R., and Spence, S. A. (submitted). Sex, lies and personality: The relevance of gender and EPQR-S scores to lying time.

Farwell, L. A. and Donchin, E. (1991). The truth will out: interrogative polygraphy ('lie detection') with event-related brain potentials. *Psychophysiology*, **28**, 531–47.

Ford, C. V., King, B. H., and Hollender, M. H. (1988). Lies and liars: psychiatric aspects of prevarication. *American Journal of Psychiatry*, **145**, 554–62.

Freud, S. (1991). *The psychopathology of everyday life*, pp. 94–152. Penguin, London (first published 1901) (Translated by A. Tyson).

Frith, C. D., Friston, K., Liddle, P. F., and Frackowiak, R. S. J. (1991). Willed action and the pre-frontal cortex in man: a study with PET. *Proceedings of the Royal Society of London [B]*, **244**, 241–6.

Garavan, H., Ross, T. J., and Stein E. A. (1999). Right hemisphere dominance of inhibitory control: an event-related functional MRI study. *Proceedings of the National Academy of Sciences USA*, **96**, 8301–6.

Giannetti, E. (2000). *Lies we live by: the art of self-deception*. Bloomsbury, London. (Translated by J. Gledson.)

Happe, F. (1994). *Autism: an introduction to psychological theory*. Psychology Press, Hove.

Hughes, C. H. and Russell, J. (1993). Autistic children's difficulty with mental disengagement from an object: its implications for theories of autism. *Developmental Psychology*, **29**, 498–510.

Iversen, S. D. and Mishkin, M. (1970). Perseverative interference in monkeys following selective lesions of the inferior prefrontal convexity. *Experimental Brain Research*, **11**, 376–86.

Jack, A. I. and Shallice, T. (2001). Introspective physicalism as an approach to the science of consciousness. *Cognition*, **79**, 161–96.

King, B. H. and Ford, C. V. (1988). Pseudologia fantastica. *Acta Psychiatrica Scandinavia*, **77**, 1–6.

Langleben, D. D., Schroeder, L., Maldjian, J. A., Gur, R. C., McDonald, S., Ragland, J. D., O'Brien, C. P., and Childress, A. R. (2002). Brain activity during simulated deception: an event-related functional magnetic resonance study. *NeuroImage*, **15**, 727–32.

Lee, T. M. C., Liu, H.-L., Tan, L.-H., Chan, C. C. H., Mahankali, S., Feng, C.-M., Hou, J., Fox, P. T., and Gao, J. H. (2002). Lie detection by functional magnetic resonance imaging. *Human Brain Mapping*, **15**, 157–64.

O'Connell, S. (1998). *Mindreading: an investigation into how we learn to love and lie*. Arrow Books, London.

Pandya, D. N. and Yeterian, E. H. (1996). Comparison of prefrontal architecture and connections. *Philosophical Transactions of the Royal Society of London [B]*, **351**, 1423–32.

Passingham, R. (1993). *The frontal lobes and voluntary action*. Oxford University Press, Oxford.

Seymour, T. L., Seifert, C. M., Shafto, M. G., and Mosmann, A. L. (2000). Using response time measures to assess "guilty knowledge". *Journal of Applied Psychology*, **85**, 30–7.

Spence, S. A. (1999). Hysterical paralyses as disorders of action. *Cognitive Neuropsychiatry*, **4**, 203–26.

Spence, S. A., Farrow, T. F. D., Herford, A. E., Wilkinson, I. D., Zheng, Y., and Woodruff, P. W. R. (2001). Behavioural and functional anatomical correlates of deception in humans. *NeuroReport*, **12**, 2849–53.

Spence, S. A. and Frith, C. D. (1999). Towards a functional anatomy of volition. *Journal of Consciousness Studies*, **6**, 11–29.

Spence, S. A., Hirsch, S. R., Brooks, D. J. and Grasby, P. M. (1998). Prefrontal cortex activity in people with schizophrenia and control subjects. Evidence from positron emission tomography for remission of 'hypofrontality' with recovery from acute schizophrenia. *British Journal of Psychiatry*, **172**, 316–23.

Spence, S. A., Hunter, M. D., and Harpin, G. (2002). Neuroscience and the will. *Current Opinion in Psychiatry*, **15**, 519–26.

Starkstein, S. E. and Robinson, R. G. (1997). Mechanism of disinhibition after brain lesions. *Journal of Nervous and Mental Diseases*, **185**, 108–14.

Vrij, A. (2001). *Detecting lies and deceit: the psychology of lying and the implications for professional practice*. Wiley, Chichester.

Vrij, A. and Mann, S. (2001). Telling and detecting lies in a high-stake situation: the case of a convicted murderer. *Applied Cognitive Psychology*, **15**, 187–203.

Walker, A. E. (1940). A cytoarchitectural study of the prefrontal area of the macaque monkey. *Journal of Comparative Neurology*, **73**, 59–86.

21 Differential brain activations for malingered and subjectively 'real' paralysis

David A. Oakley, Nicholas S. Ward, Peter W. Halligan, and Richard S. J. Frackowiak

Abstract

Differential diagnosis of conversion disorder and malingering presents a significant challenge to clinicians as it is ultimately based on a judgement of the patient's subjective experience of their symptoms and the intention to deceive for personal gain. Functional neuroimaging provides a possible basis for making that distinction. We review the relevant literature and report a neuroimaging study in which hypnosis was used to create in one condition a subjectively 'real' limb paralysis and another condition in which the same participants feigned the same symptom to deceive a naïve clinician. As anticipated, the two conditions could not be reliably distinguished by clinical observation or by electrophysiological measurement. There were, however, between- and within-hemisphere differences in brain activations in the two conditions, both when actively tested and during rest. This suggests that different brain processes are involved when a symptom is subjectively experienced as real compared to when it is intentionally feigned. An interpretation is offered for the functional significance of the different patterns of brain activation seen. This result is relevant to the differential diagnosis of conversion disorder and malingering and gives some clues as to the possible neuropsychological mechanisms involved. It also underlines the usefulness of hypnosis as an experimental tool in neuropsychology.

Introduction

When encountering medical symptoms such as motor paralysis, clinicians typically have to distinguish between (at least) two types of potential diagnosis. The first, more traditionally biomedical is that the paralysis originates from some demonstrable pathology of the peripheral or central nervous system; the second does not fulfil this criterion and the paralysis can be broadly considered as an 'unexplained medical symptom' or, more specifically, as an 'unexplained neurological symptom' (Brown and Ron 2002). Inclusion within this second group, however, could occur for a number of different reasons—none of which is mutually exclusive. It may be that an underlying pathological agent does in fact exist but has yet to be identified. In this case, it may just be a matter of time, test sensitivity and technical breakthrough before a proven physiological abnormality and a relevant causal link will be established. On the other hand, no underlying structural pathology may be involved—or, even if one exists, is not sufficient alone to account for the extent of the symptoms presenting. If this line of explanation is taken then there are at least three distinct interpretations that can be offered. First, the symptoms mighty be regarded as intentionally fabricated to satisfy an unconscious psychological need to adopt the 'sick-role'. Modern psychiatry (see DSM-IV 1994) deems this a legitimate mental disorder and describes it as a 'factitious disorder'. A second possibility, is that the symptoms are psychologically mediated but are genuinely experienced by the patient who has no awareness of involvement in generating the symptom. This has also long been considered a formal psychiatric diagnosis currently located within the general category classification of 'somatoform disorders' (DSM-IV 1994). Where the symptoms are of an acute sensory, motor, or cognitive nature suggestive of a neurological condition, the diagnosis of 'conversion disorder' can be made (see Halligan *et al.* 2001). In keeping with its psychoanalytic roots, no conscious intention to mislead the clinician or to generate the symptoms is assumed. The psychopathology is thought to be unconscious and to involve intra-psychic attempts to resolve underlying psychological conflict or need (Bass 2001).

Finally, a person may pretend to have an illness as a way of deriving personal benefit such as a financial reward, or to avoid an unwanted role, obligation, or social sanction. This is malingering, and so far has not been claimed by psychiatry to be a mental disorder. As such, malingering is not a condition but rather describes an act or set of behaviours that could be seen as adaptive when considered in terms of the financial and social circumstances of the individual assumed to be engaged in the deceit. While the definition of malingering is clear, it is far from easy to distinguish between a factitious disorder, malingering, and hysterical conversion, particularly since the first two by definition involve intentional wilful deception, and the differential diagnosis has to be made on the basis of the 'presumed goals' of the subject as determined by the doctor in the clinic (Bass 2001).

Given the rise in medically unexplained symptoms (Nimnuan *et al.* 2000, 2001), there is a growing practical need to distinguish between these competing explanations and in particular between malingering and conversion disorder (often referred to as 'conversion hysteria' or simply as 'hysteria'). In these cases, identical behavioural signs and symptoms do not provide a compelling platform of evidence from which to distinguish the origins of a patient's subjective experience and volitional intention or otherwise to deceive another. It is virtually impossible in practice for any clinician to separate conscious feigning for extrinsic gain (i.e. the patient is malingering) from those instances where the symptoms are genuinely experienced as subjectively 'real' (i.e. the patient is suffering from conversion disorder). In both situations, the verbal testimony is the same—for example, 'My left leg is paralysed, I cannot move it'—and the behavioural evidence equally unhelpful given its congruence with the claimed symptoms. Nevertheless, making the clinical distinction between malingering and conversion disorder is clearly important, not least in view of the numbers of patients involved and the clinical, financial, social, and legal implications that follow from one diagnosis rather than another. Despite the absence of reliable base-rates for malingering, there is considerable circumstantial evidence to suggest that where a compensation or welfare infrastructure exists (whether governmental or insurance-based) malingering is more than a possibility (see Chapter 1). The evidence for conversion disorder is also surprising. Current estimates indicate that it is as common as multiple sclerosis and schizophrenia (Akagi and House 2001). In the United Kingdom, estimates of prevalence for conversion disorder in the general population are between 33 and 53 per 100 000; in neurological clinics the estimated prevalence is 0.29–3.8 per cent and in liaison psychiatry settings 4.9–18.8 per cent (Akagi and House 2001).

Over the past decade, functional neuroimaging has provided researchers with potential neural indicators for distinguishing symptoms that are considered subjectively 'real' and behaviourally indistinguishable and those thought to be or know to be intentionally fabricated for an extrinsic reward. Recently, Lee *et al.* (2002) using functional magnetic resonance imaging (fMRI) demonstrated the involvement of a prefrontal–parietal circuit in six healthy male volunteers subject requested to feign memory impairment, although no pre-experimental predictions were put forward to constrain the potential brain activations that might be expected for this type of feigning.

In this chapter, we review some of the previous attempts to understand conversion disorder using neuroimaging and provide new evidence that show that the brain correlates for hysterical and malingered symptoms may be different. We then provide a description of a prospective experimental paradigm that recently investigated the brain areas involved in subjectively real and feigned paralysis within the same subjects. Finally, we offer a tentative account of the activations found that, together with related neuroscience findings, makes it possible to meaningfully distinguish these qualitatively different and socially important conditions.

Developing an experimental paradigm

Notwithstanding social, legal, and ethical sanctions, our starting point has to be that while most of us are not, or have not been, motivated to do so, we are all nevertheless capable of malingering. Hence when we wanted to compare feigned and subjectively real symptoms experimentally, we chose the specific but not uncommon neurological symptom of unilateral lower limb paralysis and adopted hypnosis as the method of choice by which to generate the subjectively real symptoms in volunteers. Thus, for the purpose of this two-way comparison we used a hypnotically induced leg paralysis as an easily manipulated and controllable experimental analogue for the clinically well-known conversion symptom of the same impairment. Drawing parallels between hypnosis and hysteria has a long history and the behavioural and phenomenological similarities between hypnotically induced phenomena, such as paralysis, anaesthesia, blindness, deafness, etc., and their conversion disorder counterparts remain as compelling today as they were to Charcot and his contemporaries (Charcot 1886–90; Oakley 1999, 2001; McConkey 2001; Brown 2002a,b). In particular, both hypnotic phenomena and conversion disorder symptoms are experienced as involuntary and as being subjectively 'real' experiences.

Direct evidence that both conversion hysteria paralysis and hypnotic paralysis share common mechanisms comes from two neuroimaging (positron emission tomography, PET) studies. The first one investigated brain activations when a patient with conversion disorder attempted to move her paralysed left leg compared to activations occurring during similar attempted movements of her normally functioning right leg (Marshall *et al.* 1997; Athwal *et al.* 2001). Both legs were restrained to prevent actual leg movements from occurring—since the focus of the investigation was not the recruitment or non-recruitment of motor execution areas but rather the earlier mental states of intentionality that are necessary before making, or not making, a voluntary limb movement. Preparing to move either leg produced normal activations of motor and premotor areas, however attempts to execute the movement of the 'paralysed' left leg failed to activate primary motor areas. The attempted movement instead produced activations of right orbitofrontal and right anterior cingulate cortex. These areas were not activated during attempts to move the non-paralysed leg where the expected activations of contralateral motor cortex occurred as normal. The findings were interpreted as inhibition of a 'willed (intended) movement' by contralateral orbitofrontal and anterior cingulate cortices. A subsequent case study using the same experimental paradigm, PET scanner and procedures, but this time with a volunteer subject with a hypnotically suggested paralysis of the left leg, produced a similar pattern of brain activations during attempted movements of the two legs (Halligan *et al.* 2000). Collectively, this was taken as evidence to support the view that hypnotically induced paralysis is based on brain processes similar to those found operating during conversion disorder. Employing hypnotic paralysis as an experimental analogue for conversion paralysis allowed us to test for the first time the controversial hypothesis that malingered and subjectively experienced paralysis involve different neural systems.

Predicting neural activations in motor hysteria

Tiihonen *et al.* (1995) described one of the first functional imaging studies (single positron emission computerized tomography, SPECT) of hysteria in the case of a 32-year-old female with left-sided hysterical paralysis and sensory disturbance. The hysterical episode lasted several days and ^{99m}HMPAO SPECT brain imaging was employed 2 days after the onset, when symptoms were present, and again 6 weeks later, following symptom resolution. The scans were taken during electrical stimulation of the median nerve of the left arm with the aim of investigating brain activity that, in normals, predicted an increase in blood flow in contralateral parietal areas corresponding to primary sensory cortex. During the period of left-sided weakness and sensory disturbance there was activation in the right frontal region and an unexpected decrease in blood flow in the right parietal region. Following symptom resolution, blood flow in the frontal regions equalized and blood flow in the right parietal region increased to the level expected during this type of median nerve stimulation.

The authors interpreted their patient's symptoms of parasthesia and paralysis in terms of activation of inhibitory areas involving the frontal lobes and a simultaneous deactivation of the sensory cortex of the parietal lobes. As only two scans were taken, both during sensory stimulation, it was not possible to determine whether frontal activity was increased throughout the illness. An important aspect of this study was the fact that it showed the presence of a physiological abnormality associated with hysteria that subsequently normalized upon symptom resolution.

Another SPECT imaging study by Vuilleumier *et al.* (2001) investigated seven patients with unilateral conversion symptoms comprising sensorimotor loss in the upper and/or lower limb. Again this study employed peripheral stimulation. In four of these patients, they found that responses to bilateral vibratory stimulation of the limbs were associated with reduced levels of activity in thalamus and basal ganglia (caudate and putamen) contralateral to the affected side of the body when compared to levels of activation in these areas produced by the same stimulation 2–4 months later when their symptoms had recovered. Critically this study did not request patients to perform or attempt to initiate a voluntary motor movement and the analysis was complicated by the fact that both sides of the body (affected and non affected) were stimulated in the experimental condition. Vuilleumier *et al.* (2001), however, suggest that orbitofrontal and cingulate cortex activity may influence motor functions through their inputs to basal ganglia and thalamic circuits, rather than acting directly to inhibit primary motor cortex as Marshall *et al.* (1997) had previously suggested. The decreased activity in the basal ganglia thalamic circuits in turn they proposed may set the motor system in a functional state of impaired motor readiness and response initiation resulting in abnormal voluntary behaviour.

One previous imaging study attempted to discover the potential neural differences between conversion disorder and its consciously simulated counterpart (Spence *et al.* 2000; Spence 2001). Spence *et al.* (2000) used PET to compare brain activations in two patients with hysterical weakness of their left arm, (a third subject with right arm weakness was also included) with six normal subjects who performed the same simple motor decision task and finally with two control subjects who had been asked to 'feign difficulty moving their left upper limbs'. More specifically, they were 'required to pretend they had difficulty' and slow 'their responses to match those of patients' (Spence *et al.* 2000, p. 1244). It is not made clear from this description that malingering was achieved in these subjects, given that the instructions referred to imitating poor performance and the absence of an explicit intention to deceive rather than comply with the experimenter's instruction. Furthermore, unlike the previous studies on hysteria, movements of the affected limb were involved. Subjects were required to make freely selected movements of a joystick, a task known to activate dorsolateral prefrontal regions (Frith *et al.* 1991). Compared to normal subjects and patients with conversion disorder, subjects 'pretending to perform the task poorly' showed hypo-activation of right anterior prefrontal cortex when using their left arm. The patients with conversion disorder, however, showed hypo-activation of left prefrontal cortex compared to the feigners and normal subjects. This prefrontal hypoactivation had two peaks, one above and one just below inferior frontal sulcus, suggesting that their region involved both dorsolateral and ventrolateral prefrontal cortex. A relative hypo-activation of left dorsolateral prefrontal cortex when performing actions with the affected limb in the conversion disorder patients would be consistent with a large literature linking this cortical area with the generation of voluntary actions and would further implicate motor conversion disorder as a disorder of willed action (Spence 1999). Hypo-activation in the ventral part of prefrontal cortex however requires a different interpretation, in that this region has been found to be active (i.e. relatively hyperactive) in tasks requiring the suppression of movement (Konishi *et al.* 1999). The results by Spence are consequently difficult to interpret because 'relative hypoactivation' of area A compared to area B might be due to decreased activation (compared to baseline) in area A, or increased activation (compared to baseline) in area B. Nevertheless, these between-group differences in activation of frontal cortical areas were used to support the view that conversion disorder patients were not consciously feigning their symptoms.

Collectively, the imaging studies we have reviewed indicate: (a) that brain circuits involved with initiating and preparing to execute motor movements (including orbitofrontal cortex, prefrontal cortex, anterior cingulate cortex, thalamus, and basal ganglia) may be involved in suppressing the normal voluntary motor activity that occurs in conversion disorder; (b) that similar brain activations are activated when conversion disorder patients and hypnotic subjects report experiencing the effects of comparable changes in their voluntary motor performance; and (c) brain activations are different when comparing conversion disorder patients with limb weakness and normal subjects who have been asked to pretend to perform poorly on the same simple motor tasks.

Since similar neural mechanisms appear to be involved in both hypnosis and hysterical conversion disorder, and since the behavioural effects of both are indistinguishable, hypnotically produced phenomena serves as a valid, controllable experimental analogue for conversion disorder symptoms particularly as well-documented cases of individuals with pure motor conversion symptoms who are willing to engage in functional imaging studies are not common. On this assumption, it follows that, as in conversion disorder, there should be a difference in brain activation when a subjectively 'real' hypnotic phenomenon, such as a leg paralysis, is compared with its consciously feigned counterpart.

Furthermore, since our intention was to provide as close an analogue as possible to the conventional definition of malingering, the feigning condition in our study involved two critical features not used in previous studies namely: (a) a specific requirement for the subject to attempt to deceive a naïve clinician regarding their impairment; and (b) a financial reward for doing so successfully. A further advantage of our study was the fact that we were making these comparisons within the same subjects and not between different subjects.

The present study

Methods

Twelve, right-handed male participants (ages 18–21) scoring at least eight (out of 12) on the Harvard Group Scale of Hypnotic Susceptibility: Form A (HGSHS:A; Shor and Orne 1962) were identified from a hypnotic susceptibility database and had been screened for their ability to produce a subjectively 'real' (i.e. involuntary) hypnotic leg paralysis. They were hypnotized using an eyes-closed, relaxation induction followed by descent imagery for deepening and self-selected 'special place' imagery as the baseline hypnotic condition. Presence of this baseline condition was checked before each scan by means of voluntary finger signals from the subject and was reinstated by further suggestions where necessary. PET scanning used the standard oxygen-15 technique with a CTI ECAT HR plus scanner (CTI, Knoxville, TN, USA) operating in three-dimensional mode. A total of 12 measurements of brain activity (scans) were taken. Spatial pre-processing and statistical analysis of images were performed with SPM99 (Wellcome Department of Imaging Neuroscience, http://www.fil.ion.ucl.ac.uk/spm).

For half of each scanning session, participants were given a suggested flaccid paralysis of the left leg (paralysis condition) and for the other half, both legs were normal but the participant was instructed to feign flaccid paralysis of the left leg (malingering condition) so as to deceive an experimenter with experience in clinical neurology who was blind to the experimental condition. A small financial incentive was offered to those capable of successfully deceiving the uninformed experimenter as to the source of their paralysis. The order of these two conditions was counter-balanced across participants. Continuous surface electromyographic (EMG) recordings were taken from quadriceps femoris and biceps femoris muscles in both legs throughout scanning to monitor muscle activity.

Of the 12 scans performed for each participant, six were 'resting' scans and six were active scans in which the participant was asked by the uninformed experimenter to move his left leg in time with a metronome (0.5 Hz). The paralysis and feigning conditions were each performed as a block of six scans (rest–active–rest–active–rest–active), the order of which was randomized in a counter-balanced fashion across subjects. In the rest scans, subjects were simply asked to remain relaxed and were told that they would not be asked to move. The metronome sound was present during rest scans but the subject was instructed that a response was not required. The naive experimenter was able to observe the participants during all 12 scans and halfway through each of the experimental conditions, he carried out a neurological examination of both legs. The EMG records revealed no significant movement of the left leg during any of the scan conditions and the uninformed experimenter was not successful in distinguishing between paralysis and malingering conditions at above chance level. There were, however, differences in brain activations between the two conditions.

Findings

The main effects of attempting to move (active–rest) during each condition revealed distinct patterns of task related activity (Table 21.1, Figs 21.1a and b). We were then interested in exploring the similarities and the differences between these task-related activations. In order to look for similarities we performed conjunction analysis of the main effects (Price and Friston 1997), which demonstrated relatively increased activation in a number of regions bilaterally, although more strongly in the right hemisphere (Fig. 21.1c and Table 21.2). In particular, attempted movement related activations were seen in bilateral SMA, insula and inferior parietal cortex, as well as bilateral putamen, and cerebellar hemispheres during both hypnosis conditions. Lateralized increases were also noted in right thalamus, and left anterior cingulate gyrus.

We examined for differences in task-related (active–rest) brain activations in the two conditions by direct comparisons. During subjective paralysis compared to feigning (Table 21.3, Fig. 21.2a), increased activation was seen in right posterior medial orbitofrontal cortex (Fig. 21.3a), left putamen and thalamus, and right cerebellum. During feigning compared to subjective paralysis (Table 21.3, Fig. 21.2b), activation was seen in left ventrolateral prefrontal cortex (BA45) (Fig. 21.3b), and a number of right-sided regions, including medial parietal cortex, intraparietal sulcus, parietal operculum, and superior temporal sulcus.

Table 21.1 Main effects of attempted movement

Region	Talairach coordinates in MNI space			Z-value
	x	y	z	
(a) During perceived paralysis				
R putamen	28	−2	6	5.73
L putamen	−18	−6	8	5.33
L thalamus (mediodorsal)	−4	−20	8	4.85
R orbitofrontal cortex	18	12	−14	4.58
L cerebellum	−22	−48	−40	4.63
L SMA	−2	−12	−64	4.15*
(b) During feigning				
R parietal operculum (S II)	50	−28	24	5.71
L inferior frontal sulcus	−36	34	24	5.27
R SMA	6	−18	62	5.27
R ventral premotor cortex	52	6	8	5.17
L cerebellum	−32	−52	−36	5.06
R cerebellum	26	−44	−38	4.83
L inferior parietal cortex	−44	−54	46	4.77

All coordinates (in standard stereotactic space) refer to maximally activated foci as indicated by the highest Z-score within a cluster of activations: x, distance (mm) to right (+) or left (−) of midsagital line; y, distance anterior (+) or posterior (−) to vertical plane through the anterior commissure; z, distance above (+) or below (−) the intercommissural (AC–PC) line. The AC–PC line is the horizontal line between the anterior and posterior commissures. All voxels are significant at $p < 0.05$ (corrected for multiple comparisons across whole brain).
* Represents the peak voxel in a cluster significant at $p < 0.05$ (corrected for multiple comparisons across whole brain).
R = right, L = left, SMA = supplementary motor area, AC = anterior commissure, PC = posterior commissure.

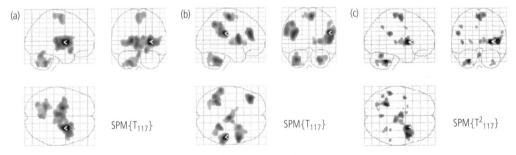

Figure 21.1 SPM{Z}s representing the categorical comparison of attempting to move the left leg compared to rest during (a) subjectively real paralysis, (b) feigned paralysis; and (c) the conjunction of the main effects (a and b). The SPM{Z}s are shown as maximum intensity projections. The brain is shown from the right, top, and back. Results for (a) and (b) are shown at cluster level significance (clusters are significant at $p < 0.05$, corrected for multiple comparisons across whole brain) for display purposes. All voxels in (c) are significant at $p < 0.05$, corrected for multiple comparisons across whole brain.

Our prefrontal region was almost identical to that indicated as less active in hysterics compared to feigners (i.e. relatively overactive in feigners compared to hysterics) by Spence *et al.* (2000), but was clearly situated below the inferior prefrontal sulcus, indicating that this activation is situated in ventrolateral not dorsolateral prefrontal cortex.

Looking at the two rest conditions—activations in paralysis/rest compared to feigning/rest were in right posterior cingulate sulcus, right transverse parietal sulcus and left intraparietal sulcus (Table 21.4, Figs 21.4a and 21.5). The converse comparison (feigning/rest–paralysis/rest)

Table 21.2 Conjunction of task-related main effects

Region	Talairach coordinates in MNI space			Z-value
	x	y	z	
L SMA	−2	−12	62	5.83
R SMA	10	−26	66	5.62
L inferior parietal	−52	−38	24	5.83
	−44	−56	40	5.27
R inferior parietal	56	−40	26	5.09
L insula	−40	−2	2	5.61
R insula	46	6	4	6.59
L cingulate gyrus	−8	2	38	5.08
L cerebellum	−26	−48	−40	6.37
R cerebellum	32	−50	−46	5.04
Cerebellar vermis	0	−58	−26	5.63
L putamen	−22	6	6	5.03
R putamen	28	6	4	6.53
R thalamus (ventromedial)	12	−14	6	5.09

Voxels for which the conjunction of main effects of attempting to move compared to rest for either subjectively real paralysis (B1–A1) or feigning (B2–A2) are significant. All voxels are significant at $p < 0.05$ (corrected for multiple comparisons across whole brain).
L = left, R = right, SMA = supplementary motor area.

Table 21.3 Task-related differential activations

Region	Talairach coordinates in MNI space			Z-value
	x	y	z	
(a) Paralysis compared to feigning				
R orbitofrontal cortex	18	12	−16	3.72
R cerebellum	12	−54	−50	3.56
L thalamus (mediodorsal)	−30	2	−4	3.35
L putamen	−4	−10	2	3.32
(b) Feigning compared to paralysis				
L VLPFC (BF 45)	−46	34	14	3.81*
R parietal operculum	48	−28	28	3.64
R posterior superior temporal sulcus	54	−54	6	3.47
R intraparietal sulcus	28	−50	38	3.46
R medial parietal cortex	2	−58	54	3.29

Peak voxels resulting from the comparison of (attempted) movement related increases in rCBF during (a) subjectively real paralysis compared to feigning ([B1–A1] − [B2–A2]), and (b) feigning compared to subjectively real paralysis ([B2–A2] − [B1–A1]). All voxels are significant at $p < 0.001$ (uncorrected for multiple comparisons across whole brain).
* The corrected p-value for the activation at left ventrolateral prefrontal cortex is $p = 0.025$, based on a small volume correction using a search volume of 20 mm radius centred at $x = −48$, $y = 36$, $z = 28$, based on previously published work (Spence *et al.* 2000).
L = left, R = right, VLPFC = ventrolateral prefrontal cortex.

showed higher activation in the feigning/rest condition on the left side in nucleus accumbens, orbitofrontal cortex, and thalamus (Table 21.4, Figs 21.4b and 21.6).

Meaning of the relative activations

Activations associated with preparing to move or imagining movement

The conjunction analysis demonstrated that during both subjectively real paralysis and feigning, attempts to move the left leg compared to rest activated a number of regions demonstrated

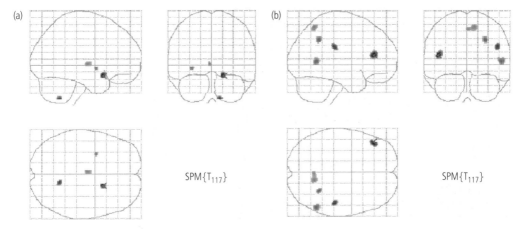

Figure 21.2 SPM{Z}s representing differential task related increases in rCBF during (a) subjectively real paralysis compared to feigning [paralysis (attempted movement–rest)] versus [feign (attempted movement–rest)] and (b) feigning compared to paralysis [feign (attempted movement–rest)] versus [paralysis (attempted movement–rest)]. The SPM{Z}s are shown as maximum intensity projections (as in Fig. 21.1). A1 = rest (paralysis), B1 = attempted movement (paralysis), A2 = rest (feign), B2 = attempted movement (feign). Voxels are significant at $p > 0.001$, uncorrected for multiple comparisons. The corrected p-value for the activation at left ventrolateral prefrontal cortex is $p = 0.025$, based on a small volume correction using a search volume of 20 mm radius centred at $x = -48, y = 36, z = 28$, based on previously published work (Spence et al. 2000).

by previous neuroimaging studies, to be involved when preparing to move (Dieber et al. 1996; Krams et al. 1998) and when imagining movement (Stephan et al. 1995). Thus, the absence of leg movement in both conditions appears to be due to a failure of movement initiation, not of movement preparation. In other words, the effects of the suggestion for paralysis acted further 'downstream' from motor preparation at the point where voluntary initiation of movement appeared to be important.

Activations associated with subjectively real symptoms (hypnotic paralysis)

Previous imaging studies of conversion paralysis for the left leg (Marshall et al. 1997) and its hypnotic analogue (Halligan et al. 2000) compared attempting to move the paralysed leg with attempting to move the normal leg against restraint and found increased activations in the paralysis condition in right anterior cingulate cortex and right orbitofrontal cortex (BA 10/11) (Marshall et al. 1997; Halligan et al. 2000). We did not make the same comparison in the present study, but if these two areas are actively involved in mediating the paralysis we would expect to see them differentially activated when the paralysis condition is compared to the no-paralysis condition (i.e. the malingering condition). Spence et al. (2000) found reduced activation of right anterior prefrontal cortex (BA 10) in their test condition in control participants with voluntary intentions to feign when compared with patients with conversion disorder. Given the relative comparisons involved, these findings would lead us to predict a relatively greater activation of right anterior prefrontal cortex in our subjectively real paralysis condition compared to malingering. Vuilleumier et al. (2001) found reduced activity to bilateral sensory stimulation in basal ganglia (caudate and putamen) and thalamus contralateral to the weak limb when the patients were diagnosed as suffering from conversion patients compared to levels subsequently found at recovery. This study, however, differs from ours in two important ways—first, the comparisons are based on brain activations during

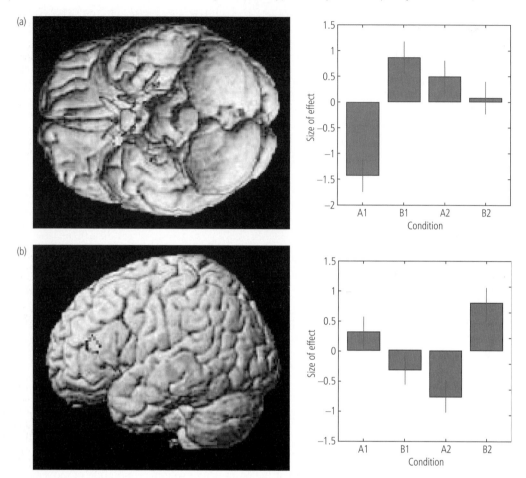

Figure 21.3 (a) Voxels in right posterior medial orbitofrontal cortex significant for the comparison paralysis (attempted move–rest) versus feigning (attempted move–rest), represented on a rendered brain seen from the inferior aspect. Voxels are significant at $p < 0.001$ (uncorrected for multiple comparisons across whole brain). (b) Voxels in left ventrolateral prefrontal cortex significant for the comparison feigning (attempted move–rest) versus paralysis (attempted move–rest), represented on a rendered brain seen from the left lateral aspect. After small volume correction (see Results section) these voxels are significant at $p < 0.05$ (corrected for multiple comparisons). The corresponding plots of effect size are displayed adjacent to the rendered brain. A1 = rest (paralysis), B1 = attempted movement (paralysis), A2 = rest (feign), B2 = attempted movement (feign).

vibratory stimulation of both the unaffected and the affected limbs and more importantly, attempted movements were not required of the patients in the Vuilleumier *et al.* study. Nevertheless, Vuilleumier *et al.* interpreted their finding as indicating that the basal ganglia and thalamus were part of a circuit along with orbitofrontal cortex and anterior cingulate cortex which underlie the inhibition of primary motor cortex during conversion paralysis and weakness. Consequently, we might expect to see some evidence of altered activity in the thalamus and basal ganglia in our paralysis condition during attempted movement by comparison with the malingering condition with relatively higher levels of activation being present ipsilaterally. In fact, our two rest conditions, which we will consider later, provide a more direct comparison to the Vuilleumier *et al.* study in

Table 21.4 Changes in rCBF related to rest

Region	Talairach coordinates in MNI space			Z-value
	x	*y*	*z*	
(a) *Paralysis (rest)–feigning (rest)*				
R posterior cingulate sulcus	14	−46	60	4.93*
R transverse parietal sulcus	16	−68	36	4.77*
L intraparietal sulcus	−34	−42	46	4.51‡
(b) *Feigning (rest)–paralysis (rest)*				
L nucleus accumbens	−4	−6	−10	4.19‡
L orbitofrontal cortex	−14	30	−26	4.15‡
L thalamus	−8	−14	−2	3.75‡

Peak voxels representing the comparisons of the rest conditions for (a) paralysis–feigning (A1–A2), and (b) feigning–paralysis (A2–A1).
* Peak voxels significant at $p < 0.05$, corrected for multiple comparisons across whole brain.
‡ Peak voxels within clusters significant at $p < 0.05$, corrected for multiple comparisons across whole brain.
L = left, R = right.

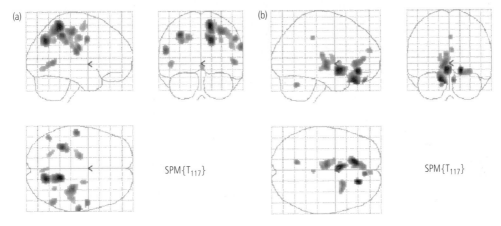

Figure 21.4 SPM{Z}s representing the categorical comparison of the resting conditions, (a) subjectively real paralysis versus feigning, and (b) feigning versus subjectively real paralysis. The SPM{Z}s are shown as maximum intensity projections (as in Fig. 21.1). All voxels are significant at $p < 0.001$, uncorrected for multiple comparisons across whole brain, for display purposes.

that they do not involve attempted movement, though again the difference in peripheral stimulation remains.

When the paralysis condition (active–resting) was directly compared with the malingering condition (active–resting) our results appear closely in line with the expectations of relatively increased activations unique to the paralysis condition seen in left thalamus, left basal ganglia (putamen), and right orbitofrontal cortex. However, contrary to expectations, no differential anterior cingulate cortex activation was observed. In contrast to predictions derived from Spence *et al.* (2000), we did not specifically find increased activations in right anterior prefrontal cortex (BA 10). Overall, though our findings confirm those of Halligan *et al.* (2000) and extend them to other brain areas implicated in motor conversion disorder. As such they support the view that hypnotically induced paralysis depends on similar mechanisms to those found in conversion

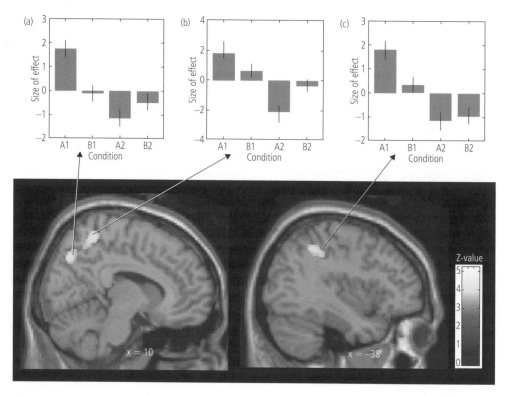

Figure 21.5 SPM{Z}s representing the categorical comparison of subjectively real paralysis (rest) versus feigning (rest), displayed on brain slices. Clusters are significant at $p < 0.05$ (corrected for multiple comparisons across whole brain). The corresponding plots of effect size are displayed for (a) right transverse parietal sulcus, (b) right posterior cingulate sulcus, and (c) left intraparietal sulcus. A1 = rest (paralysis), B1 = attempted movement (paralysis), A2 = rest (feign), B2 = attempted movement (feign).

motor disorder. This in turn further confirms the use of hypnotic paralysis as a valid experimental analogue for conversion paralysis.

Activations associated with malingering (feigned paralysis)

There is little by way of previous imaging evidence to make strong predictions for the likely patterns of activation specific to malingering (of proven leg paralysis) given that our study entailed the absence of motor movement in all subjects. Spence *et al.* (2000) reported reduced activation of left dorsolateral prefrontal cortex (BA9/46) in their conversion hysteria patients compared to the subjects who were simulating poor performance on the same task. Though they did not report it, the accompanying brain map also shows reduced activations in left ventrolateral prefrontal cortex (BA 45) in this same group. On this basis, we would expect to see relatively greater activations of left prefrontal cortex in our malingering condition compared to the paralysis condition. We found that the comparison of the feigned condition compared to the paralysis condition demonstrated relative increases in activation in left ventrolateral prefrontal cortex, right precuneus, right intraparietal sulcus, and right superior temporal sulcus. It can be seen from the plots of the relative changes in regional cerebral blood flow (rCBF) during each condition that these changes can be interpreted as relative increases in rCBF during feigning, or relative decreases of rCBF during paralysis.

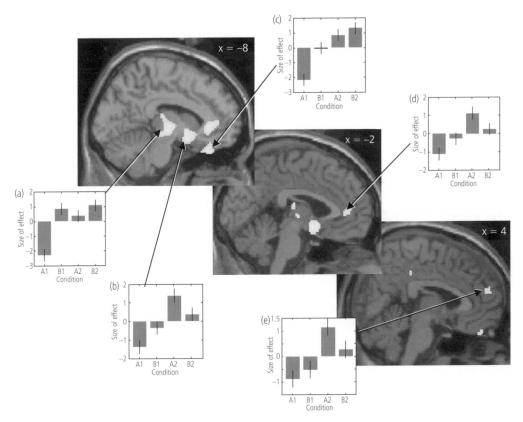

Figure 21.6 SPM{Z}s representing the categorical comparison of feigning (rest) versus subjectively real paralysis (rest), displayed on brain slices. Clusters (a), (b), and (c) are significant at $p < 0.05$ (corrected for multiple comparisons across whole brain); clusters (d) and (e) are significant only at $p > 0.001$, uncorrected. The corresponding plots of effect size are displayed for (a) left thalamus, (b) left nucleus accumbens, (c) left orbitofrontal cortex, (d) left anterior cingulate cortex, and (e) right paracingulate gyrus. A1 = rest (paralysis), B1 = attempted movement (paralysis), A2 = rest (feign), B2 = attempted movement (feign).

Increased activation in ventrolateral prefrontal cortex during feigning is consistent with the notion that subjects instructed to feign are consciously inhibiting a motor response. This is interesting in its own right since no specific guidance was offered to subjects as to how they should expedite the malingering phase. The indication from the activations appears to be that they were countermanding an original preparation to move which may have originated outside conscious awareness. Activation of the ventrolateral prefrontal cortex has been seen in other tasks involving inhibition of motor tasks such as go–no-go paradigms (Konishi *et al.* 1999), but is also thought to be involved in the learning of new associations between cues and motor responses (Passingham *et al.* 2000). We argue that the activation in ventrolateral prefrontal cortex seen in feigners is due not only to the inhibition of a motor act, but could also be related to the learning of a new association between the auditory cue and the inhibition of movement. We know that subjects are not merely ignoring the cue, as regions involved in motor preparation are significantly activated. We also hypothesize that sustained activation of this region (as opposed to diminishing activation once the new association has been learned) is due to concentration by subjects on the new association in order to increase the chances of them deceiving the observer. However, we cannot rule out the fact that there may indeed be a decrease in activation in this prefrontal region during the paralysis condition. Dorsolateral prefrontal cortex is activated in tasks involving the internal generation of choice of action (Frith *et al.* 1991), and underactivation of dorsolateral prefrontal cortex has been reported during motor-related conversion disorder (Spence *et al.* 2000) and in patients with schizophrenia experiencing passivity phenomena (Spence *et al.* 1997). We see no such changes in the more dorsal prefrontal region, but only in the ventral region.

Increased activation during feigning is also seen in a number of right-sided cortical regions that have known anatomical connections in the macaque monkey (Lewis and Van Essen 2000; Leichnetz 2001). Toni *et al.* (2002) recently demonstrated activation in a number of regions, including superior temporal gyrus, during motor preparation, and suggested that the interaction of this region and the frontoparietal network that was also activated in their study, enables integration of perceptual and executive processes, in the context of visuomotor associations. Intraparietal sulcus is a region involved in higher order sensory integration (Macaluso *et al.* 2002) and Rushworth *et al.* (2001) demonstrated that left intraparietal sulcus was involved in 'motor attention'. Since it is highly likely that subjects were attending to their left legs, particularly so in the case of the feigners, then it appears that right intraparietal sulcus may also have a role to play in attention during motor tasks.

The relative overactivation of the medial parietal association cortex (precuneus) in the feigning condition is also of interest. The precuneus is involved in higher order sensory integration and is known to have reciprocal connections with prefrontal areas (Goldman-Rakic 1988) as well as intraparietal sulcus and superior temporal sulcus (Leichnetz 2001). Interaction between precuneus and prefrontal areas is thought to be involved in states of self awareness (Kjaer *et al.* 2001) and has been implicated in situations involving task switching (Dove *et al.* 2000), or attentional switches between different object features (Nagahama *et al.* 1999). Feigning paralysis of the left leg in the face of continued movement-related cues requires monitoring of both self and the changed significance of the cue (i.e. to do the opposite of the instruction and not move), thus it is not surprising that activation of a network of regions involved in higher order processing, integration and monitoring is seen. We do not make the claim that this network is specific for deceit or feigning, but many of the cognitive processes required to perform such acts will involve the network we have described.

In a broader sense, our results suggest that the neural mechanisms involved in these two behaviours are qualitatively different and that subjects with hypnotically induced paralysis, like patients with hysteria, were not simply choosing not to move. This result provides one possible objective basis for distinguishing a subjectively 'real' symptom from a behaviourally indistinguishable symptom which is intentionally simulated under conditions of extrinsic motivation (malingering).

Activations associated with rest conditions

As the hypnotic paralysis suggestion and the instruction to malinger leg paralysis were continuously present throughout the respective experimental conditions, the resting scans are another potential source for distinguishing between subjectively 'real' paralysis and the malingered paralysis conditions. There are two possibilities here. One is that the hypnotic suggestion and instructions to deceive another person affect brain processes only at the time they are actively enacted—in which case the rest scans in the two conditions should be the same. Alternatively, one or both of the conditions could exert a continuous differential effect in which case the two sets of rest scans could produce different activation patterns. If this were to be the case, then there would be very little upon which to base a prediction as to the relative differential activations we might expect. The fact that the participants in this study were being observed constantly by the naive experimenter meant that they were continuously aware of the need to deceive him throughout the malingering condition irrespective of the type of scan (active or rest) being conducted. This might be expected to engage brain areas involved in Theory of Mind or 'mentalizing', in particular medial prefrontal regions such as paracingulate cortex (Frith and Frith 1999; Shallice 2001; Gallagher *et al.* 2002). As noted earlier, the fact that there is no movement requirement makes our rest condition similar in some respects to the group study of Vuilleumier *et al.* (2001). Specifically our 'paralysis rest' condition is similar to Vuilleumier *et al.*'s conversion disorder patients with the symptom present and our 'malingering rest' condition parallels their symptom recovery condition (though our participants were not subjected to vibratory stimulation of the limb). On this basis, we might expect to see some evidence of altered activity in the thalamus and basal ganglia in our paralysis rest condition compared to the malingering rest condition with relatively lower levels of activation being present contralaterally.

When we compared paralysis/rest with feigning/rest we found predominantly right-sided activations in parietal and posterior cingulate regions. Comparing feigning/rest with paralysis/rest showed higher activation on the left in orbitofrontal cortex, nucleus accumbens, and thalamus. In addition, the right paracingulate gyrus ($x = 4$, $y = 48$, $z = 20$, Z-score $= 3.38$) and left anterior cingulate cortex ($x = -6$, $y = 42$, $z = 10$, Z-score $= 3.56$) were more active at rest during feigning than for hypnotic paralysis, but at a reduced threshold ($p > 0.001$, uncorrected for multiple comparisons).

It is important to note that there are clear differences in the laterality and location of activations in the two rest conditions. Of the two predicted sets of activations, we did not find evidence of contralateral hypoactivation of thalamus and basal ganglia in the paralysis/rest condition though again it may be that this would appear only with concurrent sensory stimulation of the limbs. We did, however, find some evidence for the anticipated involvement of Theory of Mind areas in the feigning/rest condition in the increased activation of paracingulate gyrus, which may be involved when attempting to deceive another person (Gallagher *et al.* 2002). Overall, these observations suggest that there was a continuing effect of the hypnotic paralysis suggestion, the malingering instruction, or both in rest trials when the leg paralysis was not being actively tested.

Summary and suggestions for future work

The similarities observed in brain activations during hypnotic paralysis and malingered paralysis suggest that the normal ability to prepare for or imagine a movement remains intact in both conditions. The fact that the participants had received hypnosis instructions throughout all conditions (to control for any specific effects of hypnosis) also suggests that hypnosis per se does not disturb normal brain functions.

The brain activations seen only during the subjectively real symptoms (hypnotic paralysis) condition were consistent with those seen in previous studies of both hypnotic paralysis and motor conversion disorders. This is significant since our confirmatory observations involve the largest group size (12 participants) reported in this literature so far for this experimental condition. More importantly, there was confirmation of striking neural differences between the paralysis and malingering conditions—this is the first demonstration with substantial numbers of an objective neural and indeed hemispheric differentiation in the same participants between a subjectively real 'symptom' and its consciously feigned equivalent. It is also the first to do so using hypnosis to generate the target 'symptom' and the first to incorporate a true malingering condition (i.e. deception) rather than simple simulation or just pretending to perform the task poorly.

Hypnotic paralysis would appear to be a useful model with which to further explore the neurobiological basis of hysterical paralysis and volitional motor inhibition with the intention to deceive. In addition to replicating the current studies, future studies need to look at several related and hitherto difficult research and clinical questions such as the possibility of determining within a single subject whether there is evidence of malingering in a patient diagnosed as having conversion disorder. Finally, functional imaging studies are only the starting point for work in this area and are not its ultimate goal. The challenge for functional imaging remains whether it is capable of moving beyond the identification of isolated brain regions and to use these findings to develop wider cognitive accounts of the processes involved in volition, deception, and intentionality (see Spence *et al.*, Chapter 20 and Malle, Chapter 6).

Acknowledgements

N. S. W. and R. S. J. F. are supported by the Wellcome Trust, P. W. H. is supported by the Medical Research Council, and D. A. O. was supported by a Leverhulme Research Fellowship.

References

Akagi, H. and House, A. (2001). The epidemiology of hysterical conversion. In *Contemporary approaches to the study of hysteria: clinical and theoretical perspectives* (eds P. W. Halligan, C. Bass, and J. C. Marshall), pp. 73–87. Oxford University Press, Oxford.

Athwal, B. S., Halligan, P. W., Fink, G. R., Marshall, J. C., and Frackowiak, R. S. J. (2001). Imaging hysterical paralysis. In *Contemporary approaches to the study of hysteria: clinical and theoretical perspectives* (eds P. W. Halligan, C. Bass, and J. C. Marshall), pp. 216–34. Oxford University Press, Oxford.

Bass, C. (2001). Factitious disorders and malingering. In *Contemporary approaches to the study of hysteria: clinical and theoretical perspectives* (eds P. W. Halligan, C. Bass, and J. C. Marshall), pp. 126–42. Oxford University Press, Oxford.

Brown, R. J. (2002a). The cognitive psychology of dissociative states. *Cognitive Neuropsychiatry*, **7**, 221–35.

Brown, R. J. (2002b). Dissociation, epilepsy and non-epileptic seizures. In *The neuropsychiatry of epilepsy*, (eds M. R. Trimble and B. Schmitz), pp. 189–209. Cambridge University Press, Cambridge, UK.

Brown, R. J. and Ron, M. A. (2002). Conversion disorders and somatoform disorders. In *Encyclopedia of the human brain*, (ed V. S. Ramachandran) Vol. 2, pp. 37–49. Elsevier, Amsterdam.

Charcot, J. M. (1886–1890). Oeuvres Completes de J.-M. Charcot. A. Delahaye et E. Lecrosnier, Paris.

Dieber, M. P., Ibanez, V., Sadato, N., and Hallet, M. (1996). Cerebral structures participating in motor preparation in humans: a positron emission tomography study. *Journal of Neurophysiology*, **75** (1), 233–47.

Dove, A., Pollmann, S., Schubert, T., Wiggins, C. J., von Cramon, D. Y. (2000). Prefrontal cortex activation in task switching: an event-related fMRI study. *Brain Research Cognitive Brain Research*, **9**(1), 103–9.

DSM-IV (1994). *Diagnostic and statistical manual of mental disorders*, 4th edn. American Psychiatric Association, Washington, DC.

Frith, C. D. and Dolan, R. J. (1998). Images of psychopathology: review. *Current Opinion in Neurobiology*, **8**, 259–62.

Frith, C. D. and Frith, U. (1999). Interacting minds—biological basis. *Science*, **286**, 1692–5.

Frith, C. D., Friston, K., Liddle, P. F., and Frackowiak, R. S. (1991). Willed action and the prefrontal cortex in man: a study with PET. *Proceedings of the Royal Society of London, B: Biological Sciences*, **244**, 241–6.

Gallagher, H., Jack, A., Roepstorff, A., and Frith, C. D. (2002). Imaging the intentional stance in a competitive game. *NeuroImage*, **16**, 814–21.

Goldman-Rakic, P. S. (1998). Topography of cognition: parallel distributed networks in primate association cortex. *Annual Review of Neuroscience*, **11**, 137–56.

Halligan, P. W., Athwal, B. S., Oakley, D. A., and Frackowiak, R. S. J. (2000). Imaging hypnotic paralysis: implications for conversion hysteria. *The Lancet*, **355**, 986–7.

Halligan, P. W., Bass, C., and Marshall, J. C. (eds) (2001). *Contemporary approaches to the study of hysteria: clinical and theoretical perspectives*. Oxford University Press, Oxford.

Kjaer, T. W., Nowak, M., Kjaer, K. W., Lou, A. R., Lou, H. C. (2001). Precuneus-prefrontal activity during awareness of visual verbal stimuli. *Consciousness and Cognition*, **10**(3), 356–65.

Konishi, S., Nakajima, K., Uchida, I., Kikyo, H., Kameyama, M., and Miyashita, Y. (1999). Common inhibitory mechanism in human inferior prefrontal cortex revealed by event-related functional MRI. *Brain*, **122**, 981–91.

Krams, M., Rushworth, M. F., Deiber, M. P., Frackowiak, R. S. J., and Passingham, R. E. (1998). The preparation, execution and suppression of copied movements in the human brain. *Experimental Brain Research*, **120**, 386–98.

Lee, T. M., Liu, H. L., Tan, L. H., Chan, C. C., Mahankali, S., Feng, C. M., Hou, J., Fox, P. T., and Gao, J. H. (2002). Lie detection by functional magnetic resonance imaging. *Human Brain Mapping*, **15**, 157–64.

Leichnetz, G. R. (2001). Connections of the medial posterior parietal cortex (area 7m) in the monkey. *Anatomical Record*, **263**, 215–36.

Lewis, J. W. and Van Essen, D. C. (2000). Corticocortical connections of visual, sensorimotor, and multimodal processing areas in the parietal lobe of the macaque monkey. *Journal of Comparative Neurology*, **428**, 112–37.

Macaluso, E., Frith, C. D., and Driver, J. (2002). Supramodal effects of covert spatial orienting triggered by visual or tactile events. *Journal of Cognitive Neuroscience*, **14**, 389–401.

Marshall, J. C., Halligan, P. W., Fink, G. R., Wade, D. T., and Frackowiak, R. S. J. (1997). The functional anatomy of a hysterical paralysis. *Cognition*, **64**, B1–B8.

McConkey, K. M. (2001). Hysteria and hypnosis: cognitive and social influences. In *Contemporary approaches to the study of hysteria: clinical and theoretical perspectives* (eds. P. W. Halligan, C. Bass, and J. C. Marshall), pp. 203–15. Oxford University Press, Oxford.

Nagahama, Y., Okada, T., Katsumi, Y., Hayashi, T., Yamanchi, H., Sawamoto, N., Toma, K., Nakamura, K., Hanakawa, T., Konishi, J., Fukuyama, H. and Shibasaki, H. (1999) Transient neural activity in the medical superior frontal gyrus and precuneus time locked with attention shift between object features. *Neuroimage*, **10**(2), 193–9.

Nimnuan, C., Hotopf, M., and Wessely, S. (2000). Medically unexplained symptoms: how often and why are they missed? *QJM*, **93** (1), 21–8.

Nimnuan, C., Rabe-Hesketh, S., Wessely, S., and Hotopf, M. (2001). How many functional somatic syndromes? *Journal of Psychosomatic Research*, **51** (4), 549–57.

Oakley, D. A. (1999). Hypnosis and conversion hysteria: a unifying model. *Cognitive Neuropsychiatry*, **4**, 243–65.

Oakley, D. A. (2001). Hypnosis and suggestion in the treatment of hysteria. In *Contemporary approaches to the study of hysteria: clinical and theoretical perspectives* (eds P. W. Halligan, C. Bass, and J. C. Marshall), pp. 312–29. Oxford University Press, Oxford.

Passingham, R. E., Toni, I. and Rushworth, M. F. (2000). Specialisation within the prefrontal cortex: the ventral prefrontal cortex and associative learning. *Experimental Brain Research*, **133**(1), 103–13.

Price, C. J. and Friston, K. J. (1997). Cognitive conjunction: a new approach to brain activation experiments. *NeuroImage*, **5**, 261–70.

Rushworth, M. F., Krams, M. and Passingham R. E. (2001). The attentional role of the left parietal cortex: the distinct lateralization and localization of motor atttention in the human brain. *Journal of Cognitive Neuroscience*, **13**(5), 698–710.

Shallice, T. (2001). 'Theory of mind' and the prefrontal cortex. *Brain*, **124**, 247–8.

Shor, R. E. and Orne, E. C. (1962). *Harvard Group Scale of hypnotic susceptibility: Form A*. Consulting Psychologists Press, Palo Alto, CA.

Spence, S. A. (1999). Hysterical paralyses as disorders of action. *Cognitive Neuropsychiatry*, **4**, 203–6.

Spence, S. A. (2001). Disorders of willed action. In *Contemporary approaches to the study of hysteria: clinical and theoretical perspectives* (eds P. W. Halligan, C. Bass, and J. C. Marshall), pp. 235–50. Oxford University Press, Oxford.

Spence, S. A., Brooks, D. J., Hirsch, S. R., Liddle, P. F., Meehan, J., and Grasby, P. M. (1997). A PET study of voluntary movement in schizophrenic patients experiencing passivity phenomena (delusions of alien control). *Brain*, **120**, 1997–2011.

Spence, S. A., Crimlisk, H. L., Cope, H., Ron, M. A., and Grasby, P. M. (2000). Discrete neurophysiological correlates in prefrontal cortex during hysterical and feigned disorder of movement. *The Lancet*, **355**, 1243–4.

Stephan, K. M., Fink, G. R., Passingham, R. E., Silbersweig, D., Ceballos-Baumann, A. O., Frith, C. D., and Frackowiak, R. S. J. (1995). Functional anatomy of the mental representation of upper extremity movements in healthy subjects. *Journal of Neurophysiology*, **73**, 373–86.

Toni, I., Shah, N. J., Fink, G. R., Thoenissen, D., Passingham, R. E., and Zilles, K. (2002). Multiple movement representations in the human brain: an event-related fMRI study. *Journal of Cognitive Neuroscience*, **14** (5), 769–84.

Tiihonen, J., Kikka, J., Viinamaki, H., Lehtonen, J., and Partanen, J. (1995). Altered cerebral blood flow during hysterical parasthesia. *Biological Psychiatry*, **37**, 134–7.

Vuilleumier, P., Chicherio, C., Assal, F., Schwartz, S., Slosman, D., and Landis, T. (2001). Functional neuroanatomical correlates of hysterical sensorimotor loss. *Brain*, **124**, 1077–90.

Section 7

Disability analysis and insurance medicine

22 Origins, practice, and limitations of Disability Assessment Medicine

Mansel Aylward

Abstract

The primary function of the practitioner in Disability Assessment Medicine in the United Kingdom is to assess impartially how a person is affected by disease or disability and to relate this to policy, legislative requirements, insurance products or specific issues raised by decision makers who determine eligibility for cash and other benefits under these various schemes. A fundamental difference separates the role of doctors engaged in this specialty and their peers involved in health care delivery. The development of this specialty, which recognizes the importance of distinguishing clearly between symptoms and disability in clinical practice and as a basis for sick certification and social security benefits, has been driven by dramatic increases in sickness and incapacity for work associated with musculoskeletal disorders, mental health problems, and 'subjective health complaints' in Britain and other more developed democracies. A biological explanation for these observed increases in chronic disability is hard to adduce, set against a background of improvement in most objective measures of health. How more objective standards are achieved by which disability can be judged and 'malingering' defined, offering security to the vulnerable while protecting public funds on behalf of the taxpayer, poses a significant social policy dilemma in the twenty-first century. Disability Assessment Medicine has offered some tools for a more robust and expert advisory service for decision makers. However, new conceptual frameworks, methodologies, and reasoned professional judgements based upon biopsychosocial models of disability have moved the discipline away from its foundation on the biomedical model to address complex analysis of inappropriate illness behaviours and to seek out reasons for discrepancies between functional capacity and performance.

Introduction

Disability Assessment Medicine is the specialty concerned with the assessment of people with disabilities that provides impartial medical advice and reports for decision makers in the United Kingdom (Aylward and Sawney 1999). Many such decision makers work for the Department for Work and Pensions in Great Britain and their job is to determine eligibility for a range of state incapacity and disability related benefits. Others are employed as 'finders of fact' in insurance companies, appeals tribunals, and courts of law. A comprehensive list of decision makers is provided in Table 22.1 which also describes the cardinal features that decision makers expect in a

Table 22.1 Decision makers in disability assessment

Who is a decision maker?
The decision maker is usually the 'finder of fact' who decides a question by weighing the available evidence in accordance with the relevant legislation or policy specification
Benefit adjudicator
Insurance officer or claims assessor
Insurance ombudsman
Employer
Pension adjudicator
Personal employment adviser
Courts and tribunals
Local authority officer
What decision makers expect from a medical report
The following elements are considered essential:
Legibility
Absence of medical jargon
Consistency—do the doctor's comments justify the conclusions drawn, especially when they differ from the client's?
Based on evidence—opinion alone may be persuasive but it can never take precedence over opinion based on factual evidence

medical report to make it 'fit for purpose'. Disability Assessment Medicine also plays a key role in advising employers in relation to the Disability Discrimination Act (1995), and local authorities in their provision of community care services.

In the practice of disability assessment medicine, doctors act as specialist disability analysts. There is, however, a fundamental difference between the roles, objectives, and practices of doctors engaged in this specialty and their peers involved in the traditional delivery of health care and therapeutic management. The former doctors' primary function is to assess how a person is affected by disease or disability and to relate this to the relevant policy, legislative requirements, and/or specific issues raised by decision makers. It necessarily follows that the disability analyst will also need to be satisfied that the symptoms, functional limitations, and restrictions which a person reports are adequately explained by a medically recognized disease or definitive neurobiological or psychological dysfunction. Moreover, disability assessment medicine encompasses more than just an evidence based evaluative and assessment role for its practitioners; it also has an important part to play in educating health professionals, employers, politicians, and the public at large about disability issues and awareness. In addition, it also provides a conceptual framework for: (a) setting and pursuing research agendas aimed at the development and validation of more objective methods for assessing functional restrictions and limitations; (b) for the incorporation of evidence-based examination and assessment protocols in day-to-day practice; and (c) it attempts to devise and evaluate methodologies which help distinguish volition and intent from established or putative pathological biopsychosocial variables in abnormal illness behaviour and medically unexplained symptoms.

Impairment and disability

The development and practice of Disability Assessment Medicine to date has been based very largely on a precise understanding of the conceptual differences between impairment and disability. To that end, the specialty resides firmly within the compass of the modern biomedical (disease) model (Allan and Waddell 1989; Aylward and LoCascio 1995; Hadler 1995).

The International Classification of Impairments, Disabilities and Handicaps (ICIDH) defines impairment as 'any loss or abnormality of anatomical, physiological or psychological structure or function' (World Health Organization 1980). In a similar vein, the American Medical Association defines impairment as 'a loss, loss of use, or derangement of any body part, organ system or organ function' (Cocchiarella and Andersson 2000). These biological or medical definitions require some form of measurement (preferably an objective one) to demonstrate qualitative or quantitative differences from normal variation. This works well for clear-cut physical pathology such as amputation, blindness, reduced lung volumes, and spirometric tests, etc. However, strict adherence to these measures for restricted or limited function provides very little information on how a particular individual's activity and performance are restricted or limited. Moreover, both definitions stress that physical impairment may result either from *pathological or anatomical loss* or *abnormality of structure* or *physical loss or limitation of function,* or indeed some combination of both types of physical impairment. This is equally applicable to mental impairment since the medical disease model assumes that this follows from structural and functional changes that originate primarily in the brain.

Drawing upon several studies of assessed physical impairment albeit in patients with low back pain, Waddell *et al.* (1992) and Moffroid *et al.* (1992, 1994) demonstrated that there is frequently no clinical or radiological evidence of permanent anatomical or structural damage; that clinical examination merely provides one measure of physiological impairment or functional limitation associated with the subjective complaint of pain; and clinical assessments are principally measures of performance and are highly dependent on patient effort. Physiological loss of function rather than persisting physical damage is thus likely to be the main determinant of impairment in the context of pain. It follows that measures of impairment by clinical examination may be unable to distinguish between capacity and performance. Demonstrable functional limitations in the context of pain, and arguably in fatigue, could be attributed to physiological impairment or, indeed, to observed performance.

Disability, on the other hand, is defined as 'any restriction or lack (resulting from impairment) of ability to perform an activity in a manner or within the range considered normal for a human being' (World Health Organization 1980). In some UK social security definitions (Aylward and LoCascio 1995) this is supplemented by reference to 'normal ranges for a person of the same age and gender'. This concept of disability resting on subjective accounts of 'can do' or 'can't do' poses challenges to accurate, impartial, and equitable assessment. As a consequence, disability assessment medicine recognizes that reported and observed activity and performance may be due to the interaction of a variety of factors: (a) actual loss of function; (b) restrictions of function; (c) premature termination of activity; (d) sub-optimal performance; (e) environment; and (f) motivation and attitude. In many of these pain or fatigue states *per se*, expectations of pain or fatigue and indeed other perceived adverse effects of an activity can act to limit function, restrict activity and thus performance.

Disability Assessment Medicine: origins and practice

Aylward and LoCascio (1995) believed that the observed increase in the number of recipients of Invalidity Benefit in the United Kingdom and Long-term Disability benefits in the United States were due primarily to a cultural shift in medical practice in both countries. They held that the indiscriminate acceptance of subjective health complaints by many in the medical profession as the sole manifestation of a variety of ill-defined medical conditions reflected a significant change from past practices which had been reluctant to accept subjective complaints as the sole or necessary basis for diagnosis, chronic disability, and incapacity for work. Furthermore, they

Table 22.2 The components of functional capacity assessment and their definitions (from Aylward and LoCascio 1995)

Functional impairment	The reduction of function in, or loss of, a body part, organ or system
Functional limitation	What a person cannot do because of illness, disease, or injury
Functional restriction	What a person should not do because of risk of recurrence, delayed healing or injury to self or others
Functional capacity	The ability (mental, physical, or sensory) to perform a particular task or activity

argued that 'insidious medicalization' (Halligan, personal communication) of a growing numbers of syndromes and disorders defined in terms of symptoms rather than pathology had confused, rather than clarified, a reasoned approach to disability analysis considered within the biomedical model of illness. The advent of new psychiatric diagnoses such as factitious and somatoform disorders, and the confusing terminology represented by 'functional overlay' and 'illness behaviour', etc., further impeded the distinction between illness deception and behaviours which may well depend on underlying disease processes. Against this background, Aylward and LoCascio (1995) were among the first to advocate and define a structured approach to disability analysis which has subsequently evolved into disability assessment medicine. The successful application of this approach critically depended upon the adoption of a standard terminology for functional capacity assessment; the elements of which are listed and defined in Table 22.2.

How then does the practitioner of disability assessment medicine reach a reasoned opinion on which factors predominate among the spectrum of influences which may be affecting a person's performance? When self-reported limitations on activity and performance are at odds with clinical findings and the expectations which flow from a particular diagnosis, or indeed in the absence of recognizable pathology, how should the practitioner interpret these inconsistencies? Within the biomedical model consistency of behaviour across functional capacities is a well-established clinical principle (Waddell and McCulloch 1980) when account is taken of known variability and fluctuation, and currently is a cardinal feature of disability analysis. Impairment of any kind should demonstrate some consistency of effect regardless of the setting. But people with similar impairments have very different degrees of restricted activity (i.e. disability). In order to explain the variation in performance and activity among people who, within the limits of measurement, have identical impairments there must be a search for causes.

The principle of consistency adopted throughout psychometric testing can be applied with equal merit to functional analysis. It is important to note, however, that lack of consistency must be distinguished from exacerbation and remission in disease and must be cautiously interpreted in these conditions where variability and fluctuation in bodily functions are well documented. In such conditions, variability of symptoms and performance are almost invariably associated with corresponding variations in objective findings. The challenge to the disability analyst is therefore one of pattern recognition.

Aylward and LoCascio (1995) argue that consensus in the setting of functional analysis is founded on agreed expert opinion which is not always available. The disability analyst can only feel confident that impairment and disability are present despite the absence of demonstrable pathology if medical science has exhaustively explored all reasonable and diagnostic avenues and that volition and intent have been addressed.

The disability analyst's task is to formulate the likely reasons. And here the most difficult challenge which confronts disability analysis is manifest: inconsistency between expected and observed performance and the spectre of illness deception and malingering. When inconsistencies raise suspicion of deception, these have to be interpreted with great caution. Inconsistencies are not confined to people who might intentionally feign symptoms in pursuit of a consciously desired end (Rogers and Cavanagh 1983); non-organic physical signs characterize inappropriate chronic illness behaviour (Waddell and McCulloch 1980), and confusion about what constitutes malingering is a formidable barrier to the adoption of a coherent and robust stance when deception is suspected.

Attempts to rationalize symptoms and syndromes which occur either in the absence of a discernible abnormality of body and/or mind functions, or are inadequately explained by demonstrable pathology or disturbed psychological functioning, draw upon a series of conceptual models. What do these models offer to the disability analyst delving for the reasons which might account for the variation in performance inexplicable on the basis of known pathology, medically unexplained symptoms, and subjective health complaints?

Conceptual models

The biomedical model

The biomedical model, to which reference has already been made, (see Chapter 1) views physical injury to or dysfunction in an organ or body system as the cause of impairment and any consequent disability. There is also an expectation of 'cure' or residual disability. The latter, nonetheless, can be explained as a simple continuation of the effects or consequences of the disease or injury. This model is however limited in offering an explanation for 'subjective health complaints', which in the main are non-specific bodily symptoms that affect most people; yet in the form of pain, fatigue, or lapses of concentration commonly feature as manifestations of many enigmatic conditions for which no adequate physical pathology is demonstrable. By the same token, the biomedical model assumes that mental disorders result from structural and functional changes affecting the brain. Medically unexplained symptoms, whether these are subjective health complaints or more gross examples of illness-like behaviour, are difficult to accommodate within this medical model. At one extreme, the explanation could be malingering, at the other, the elaboration of new not yet fully understood functional diagnoses, principally psychiatric, on the assumption of functional disturbances of the nervous system (Sharpe and Carson 2001).

The magnitude of the problem posed by subjective health complaints, and thus the inadequacy of the biomedical model in accommodating them, is well illustrated by the findings in patients presenting to a US internal medicine department: only 16 per cent had any discernible underlying physical pathology, a psychiatric aetiology was favoured in 10 per cent, but 74 per cent had no identifiable medical explanation (Kroenke and Mangelsdorff 1989). These are not isolated findings. In Norway, more than 50 per cent of sick certification is based on subjective health complaints, predominantly of a musculoskeletal nature (Ursin 1997).

By their very nature, subjective health complaints depend on self-report. For the disability analyst, this raises several major challenges: external consistency compared with objective findings and clinical diagnosis; internal consistency compared with medical history, therapy, and management, and sickness absence record; psychosocial factors and, of course, credibility. Trends in social security statistics in Great Britain reveal very substantial increases in subjective health complaints during recent years (Aylward 2002). Non-specific low back pain is one of the most common reasons for chronic disability and incapacity for work in people of working age. Yet there is no evidence that low back pain is more severe and common than it has always been (Allan and Waddell 1989; Office of National Statistics 1993–98; Leino 2001). A biomedical explanation cannot be justified for the epidemic of chronic disability attributable to low back pain which has been witnessed in the social security systems of most industrialized countries in the past few decades. It has been argued that this 'epidemic' may owe much of its explanation to social and cultural phenomena that reflect changed understanding and management of low back pain and disability (Croft 2000; Waddell *et al.* 2002). The biomedical model is thus not only inadequate in providing an understanding of subjective health complaints and their growth in recent years, but fails as a conceptual framework to offer a viable explanation for trends in social security statistics.

The social model of disability

Although the social models of disability (Finkelstein 1996; Rowlingson and Berthoud 1996; Duckworth 2001) have emerged largely to articulate the needs and rights of people with disabilities and as a reaction to the medical model, they too imply that the disabled person has a passive role and bears little responsibility for his or her incapacity or recovery. These models assume that the restrictions imposed on disabled people rest not with the person's functional limitations but are a consequence of the way in which society is organized for able-bodied persons (Finkelstein 1996; Duckworth 2001). With their emphasis on the personal perspectives of disabled people, the social models endorse powerful and political social oppression models. 'The Social Model' of Rowlingson and Berthoud (1996), for example, sees the need for social action by society at large. In contrast to the biomedical model, disability is a sociopolitical rather than a medical issue. Along with other disadvantaged groups in society, equal opportunities, and rights have to be asserted by and on behalf of disabled people. Emphasis on the environmental and social context neglects an intellectual pursuit of other factors which are involved in the occurrence of medically unexplained symptoms and subjective health complaints. Rowlingson and Berthoud (1996) compared the medical and social models of disability. Their comparison, however, permits no middle ground between the extremes of a medical model with medical solutions and a social context with social solutions (Table 22.3). Neither model in the comparison focuses on the roles of disabled people themselves in either context. The social model reflects the perceptions, experiences, and observations of disabled people. Though it is lacking by way of scientific justification and impartiality, it nonetheless possesses powerful social and political arguments that have to be

Table 22.3 Comparison of the medical, social, and economic models of disability

Medical model	Social model	Economic model
Disabled people are disadvantaged directly by their impairments	Disabled people are disadvantaged by society's failure to accommodate everyone's abilities	Social security benefit trends reflect economic pressures and incentives more than actual disability
Disabled people are pitied as the victims of personal tragedy (accident or disease)	Disabled people are oppressed by current social and economic institutions	Recipients of benefits are advantaged by the social security system, at a high cost to society and the taxpayer
Disability is best overcome through medical treatment and rehabilitation	Disadvantage is best overcome by society adapting itself to everyone's abilities	Current social security trends are best overcome by adjusting the incentives and control mechanisms of the social security system
Both these models imply that the disabled person is the passive victim and bears little responsibility for his or her incapacity or recovery		This model implies that social security trends are a matter of economic forces and individual choice

recognized and addressed in the context of disability analysis. Disability is characterized as a political rather than a medical issue.

The economic model

This model stresses the motivational influences exerted by incentives of sick pay, social security, and workers' compensation when the worker is sick or disabled. These incentives and influences can assume greater or equal importance to the financial and social advantages brought by remunerative work. Waddell and Norlund (2000) have quite rightly pointed out that in this model incentives and risks are not entirely financial. Their analysis of social security trends in Sweden lend considerable support to the view that self-interest and personal gain should not be perceived as manifestations of selfishness or greed.

In support of this conceptual framework, various strands of evidence are advanced. A biological explanation for the dramatic increases in recipients of disability and incapacity-related benefits in the last 30 years is hard to adduce, but during this time more generous benefits have become more widely available. However, evidence is lacking for a causal effect here. In the United Kingdom, a close link has been demonstrated between age-adjusted receipt of sickness and disability benefits and unemployment rates for men (though it is weaker for women). Regression analysis implies that more than half of the variance in claims for incapacity-related benefits is associated with the local unemployment rate in some geographical areas (Department for Work and Pensions, unpublished data). Yet again this does not establish cause and effect; this variance in common could be due to shared causes or trends. Moreover, in their analysis of social security trends in Sweden compared with other European countries, Waddell and Norlund (2000) concluded that the structure and mechanisms of social security systems and the ease or difficulty of access to benefits or compensation had a greater impact on the number of claims and the number and duration of benefits paid. An empirical economic model to explain apparent increases in the numbers of people claiming and receiving social security benefits is limited by focusing predominantly on financial incentives and deterrents at the expense of exploring other factors. Furthermore, if the hypothetical 'economic man' is driven in this model by the balance of incentives and risks in the choice of worklessness and a life on benefits, then volition and intent in the pursuit of personal advantage assume particular importance. Viewed in this way, conscious adoption of the sick role, whatever the mitigating circumstances, represents a conflict between personal and social values.

The cultural model

The normal limits of human behaviour are by definition very largely set by a particular society's tolerance of what is acceptable. What determines that tolerance? Behaviour that threatens the life and well-being of the individual within a society, or the integrity of the society itself, can be seen to be unacceptable even to a member of an alternative social system which does not share the norms and beliefs of the observed society. The sick or disabled role is a social status adopted by the individual and sanctioned by other members of society (Parsons 1951). It is therefore subject to social rules, beliefs, attitudes, influences, and acceptable behaviours that predominate in a particular society at a particular time: it has to conform and be acceptable to the culture of the social group (see Prior and Wood, Chapter 9). The medical, social, and economic models described above reflect different cultures. Some elements of each may co-exist but the social models advanced by groups representing disabled people and disabled people themselves represent a culture which is diametrically opposed to that which espouses the empirical economic model.

Table 22.4 Social influences on low back pain and disability

Social issues	
Culture	Unemployment
Family	Retirement
Social class	Sickness and incapacity benefit
Job satisfaction and psychosocial	Compensation and litigation
Aspects of work	

The above social issues can all affect	
Reporting of low back pain	Pain behaviour
Disability	Health care and sick certification
Sickness absence	Early retirement

Summarized from Waddell and Waddell (2000).

Waddell and Waddell (2000) reviewed 470 studies of social influences on low back pain and disability. Table 22.4 lists the social influences for which these authors provide extensive evidence. These social influences are complex and interact with considerable variability in the strength of association and magnitude of effect, but they nonetheless identify the spectrum of social issues which may well be important in promoting or perpetuating illness and/or disability related behaviours.

Berthoud (1998) has proposed that trends in disability benefits are set in a broader social context in which behaviour among employers has changed as a result of the rapid expansion of supply of labour over demand with greater choice of workers, leaving disabled people disadvantaged and excluded. Additionally, Berthoud (1998) suggests that the culture has changed to one in which society more readily accepts that people with work-limiting health problems need not work and are entitled to society's support in the form of social security benefits. But who or what decides which health problems are sufficiently work-limiting to justify society's tolerance of an increasing burden brought by a proliferation of people in receipt of social security benefits? Manifestations of physical disease or injury which limit or restrict an individual's full participation in society are quite rightly not only well understood by society but justify society's support and accommodation for that individual. Manifestations of psychiatric illness are generally understood and tolerated by most societies, albeit set against a background that the behaviour is beyond the control of the affected individual, that it results from some disturbance of the mind, and that there should be health-focused and social interventions to address the abnormality of behaviour, thoughts, and attitudes.

Human illness and disability are expressed as social phenomena. If, however, there is no explanation that can be understood on the basis of a discernible abnormality of functions of the body and/or mind, who or what sets the limits by which society gauges, tolerates, accommodates, and supports that qualitative difference from normal variation? This has largely been left to the medical and allied professionals. The risk today is that medicine and society at times may sanction some forms of illness behaviour by at best marginalizing and at worst ignoring the role played here by volition and intent (see Halligan *et al.*, Chapter 1).

Biopsychosocial models

None of the above models on its own succeeds in taking account of the range of factors which can influence the nature and extent of physical or psychological dysfunction. They all fail in one way or another to acknowledge attitudes and beliefs, psychological distress, social, and cultural influences, and personal experiences brought to greater or lesser extent by an individual person to the display of functional limitations and restrictions in its social context. A better understanding of chronic low back pain and disability, and management, is best provided by a biopsychosocial model which considers all the physical, psychological, and social factors which may be involved (Engel 1977; Waddell 1987; Mendelson, Chapter 17). Many patients with medically unexplained symptoms do not have psychiatric disorders; these may be the result of minor pathology, physiological perceptions, and other factors including previous experience of illness (Nimnuan *et al.* 2000).

According to the attractive biopsychosocial model developed by Waddell (1998) and Main and Spanswick (2000), an initiating physical problem or perception, when filtered through the affected individual's attitudes, beliefs, coping strategies, cultural perspectives, and social context, may be experienced as magnified or amplified and predispose to illness behaviour. Thus, the development and maintenance of chronic pain and fatigue, chronic disability and, indeed, long term incapacity for work, particularly in the context of low back pain and chronic fatigue states, rests more on psychological and psychosocial influences than on the original benign and mild forms of physical or mental impairments.

Waddell (1998) further argues that disability is not static but a dynamic process which evolves through distinct phases over time: the relevant model of disability may be different at various stages of this process. Waddell (2002) argues that the medical model may well be the most appropriate for most patients in the immediate aftermath of a physical injury, acute illness or disease. But within a few short weeks psychosocial issues start to predominate, and following the lapse of 1 or 2 years the initiating physical or psychological dysfunction will bear little, if any, relevance to the manifest illness behaviour. Psychosocial factors, expectations, and behaviours are thus very different at the acute, sub-acute, and chronic stages in the development of chronic disability. Capacity for work deteriorates and the chances of effective rehabilitation and return to work recede. Social Security statistics also demonstrate that some 40 per cent of new claimants for incapacity benefits return to work within 6 months, but those on benefit at 6 months have a very strong likelihood of remaining on benefit for years. Of those beginning a claim in 2000 around 30 per cent will be on benefit for at least 4 years (Aylward 2002).

Illness behaviour itself is not considered to be a formal diagnosis but is a melange of an affected individual's observable activities, conduct and performance to express, and to transmit to others, his/her self-perception or interpretation of an altered state of health. Nor should it be defined in terms of a continuum of pathology. The manifestations of illness behaviours according to this model do not necessarily provide information about the initiating biomedical stimulus whether this be pain, fatigue or psychological distress. Nonetheless, in keeping with the traditional medical model, the biopsychosocial model recognizes that psychological and behavioural change are secondary to pain, fatigue or some other distressing complaint that most frequently has its origins in musculoskeletal and neurophysiological processes. As pointed out by Sharpe and Carson (2001), biopsychosocial models offer the potential (and indeed a danger) for an explanation and re-medicalization of unexplained symptoms around the notion of a functional disturbance of the nervous system. A paradigm shift indeed, or just a return to some of the competing theories offered to explain neurastheria in the nineteenth century (Aylward 1998)?

Is there any place for volition and or intentionality within the constraints of biopsychosocial models of disability? (See Halligan *et al.*, Chapter 1, and Malle, Chapter 6.) For the most part, the assumption is that 'patients cannot help how they react to pain'. Emotions are outside our conscious control and most illness behaviour is involuntary. Our professional role is not to sit in judgement but to understand the problem with compassion to provide the best possible management for each patient' (Waddell 1998). This view reflects the philosophy that humans are not freely determined creatures: thought, behaviour, actions, and apparent free will are determined by factors beyond the individual's control. And yet, if evolutionary psychology defines the human as the moral

Table 22.5 Biopsychosocial elements in disability

Bio	Psycho	Social
Permanent physiological or psychological impairment	Attitudes and beliefs Psychological distress	Occupational demands (physical and psychological)
Function	Coping strategies Illness behaviour	Economic incentives and controls
	Motivation, effort, and performance	'Cultural' attitudes Behaviour

From Waddell (2002).

animal endowed with a capacity to make value-driven choices and an intentional approach to life then the emergence of a moral sense in human consciousness drives us away from genetically programmed behaviour, instinctive responses and the overriding effect of emotion. No doubt, we are creatures who are in conflict with ourselves; creatures in whom the life-force has started observing itself (Holloway 2001). Frankl (1963) called this our 'ultimate freedom'—the potential freedom to exercise individual choice about one's attitudes, behaviours, and responses to a given situation (see Halligan *et al.*, Chapter 1).

The recent International Classification of Functioning, Disability and Health (ICFDH) (World Health Organization 2000) no longer focuses solely on people with disabilities, but by attempting to describe functional states associated with health conditions is applicable to all. The limitations of the medical model are recognized and thus assumptions on cause and effect are avoided. Functional states are classified across three dimensions. Disability encompasses all of these inter-related and interacting biopsychosocial dimensions. According to a biopsychosocial model a person's functioning or disability in the social context is affected by complex interactions between their health condition, environmental, social and personal factors (Table 22.5). Activity limitations (equivalent to disability) are no longer required to be described as 'resulting from an impairment'. The biopsychosocial model is triumphant; aetiology no longer features in the equation.

Illness behaviours

To return to illness behaviours and the disability manifested in them. Are all illness behaviours explicable within a medical or biopsychosocial model?

Illness deception does occur (Boden 1996; LoPiccolo *et al.* 1999). However, data on the prevalence of illness deception is meagre and difficult to find. Moreover, the identification of illness deception and its distinction from psychosocial factors lacks empirical discriminative and investigative tools in disability assessment medicine (Aylward and LoCascio 1995).

Biopsychosocial models provide powerful conceptual frameworks to better understand and manage illness behaviours, subjective health complaints, and unexplained symptoms. But their apparent failure to acknowledge that illness behaviours may also be driven by the subject's choice and intent is a formidable barrier to the adoption of a coherent and robust stance by the practitioner of disability assessment medicine when deception is strongly suspected.

Furthermore, if the beliefs, attitudes, and coping strategies that influence the development of chronic disability in an individual are founded on a rejection of social moral values or a compliance with cultures which deviate from value-driven society is there evidence that these are outside conscious control? If not how should society accommodate them? The biopsychosocial model also lends itself to interpretation as an implicit medical alternative to the limitations of the traditional medical model: the paradigm shift proposed by Sharpe and Carson (2001) in which unexplained symptoms are re-medicalized as qualitatively different from but nonetheless consequent to some as yet unrecognized dysfunction in an organ or body system supports this view. Is there a further paradigm shift around the corner—the concept of 'biopsychosocial illness'? Psychosocial factors do not only operate in perpetuating chronic disability in what might be called inappropriate illness behaviour (i.e. in which magnified perceptions accompany affective illness-like behaviour) but may be equally important as determinants of chronicity in people affected by recognizable disease where aetiology and significant impairment are not in doubt. In the latter, psychosocial influences are not dismissed and optimum treatment plans would attempt to recognize and address them.

In general, the nature and range of psychosocial factors which impact on chronic disability due to demonstrable diseases are unlikely to differ significantly from those that perpetuate the chronic disability of inappropriate illness behaviour. Save perhaps in one respect: iatrogenic psychological distress generated by a concern that 'doctors can't find out what's wrong with me' is likely to be a common feature in many with inappropriate illness behaviours. Biopsychosocial influences which perpetuate disability and deter optimum functional recovery are important in illness behaviours irrespective of aetiological considerations. What then distinguishes illness behaviours which are explicable almost exclusively on the basis of complex constitutional beliefs and psychosocial determinants from those which have a substantial pathological component contributing to the observed disability? If most illness behaviour is assumed to be involuntary (Waddell 1988) what sets it apart from psychiatric disorders? In the absence of any demonstrable, or even putative, structural or functional abnormality of the nervous system, and even allowing for gate control theories of pain (Main and Spanswick 2000), the dismissal of consciously motivated intent from the equation leads ineluctably to a consideration of the following legitimate frameworks for exploring abnormal illness behaviours:

(1) that there could be functional or structural lesions which have yet to be identified and elaborated; or

(2) that psychosocial influences on behaviour are so powerful that they preclude the exercise of any significant conscious control.

The re-medicalization implicit in proposition (1) is compatible with the medical and biopsychosocial models; though in the latter the biomedical component would predominate. Proposition (2), however, provides a challenge principally for all of us. There is a pressing need to search for the reasons for, as well as the causes of, why people behave in this way; to ascertain the internal motivations, reasons, and intentions that characterize a mental state that generates the altered behaviour; and to define more precisely how exposure to psychosocial factors disturbs the affective, cognitive, behavioural, and conscious components of the mind. A gargantuan task indeed, but without research and investigation along these lines the unravelling of the enigma of illness behaviours will remain a forlorn hope. Equally important, the execution of a structured programme of research of this kind would have to confront alternative explanations for some illness behaviours on the bases of volition and the adoption or rejection of social moral values.

Is Disability Assessment Medicine up to meeting the challenge?

Disability Assessment Medicine, founded upon the modern biomedical model (Aylward and LoCascio 1995), has had to move on to consider the limitations imposed on its original concepts and practices embedded in the biomedical model. That model's failure to account for subject-ive health complaints and unexplained symptoms and syndromes limits the claims that this new specialty can provide an accurate, impartial, and equitable process of disability analysis. The intro-duction of new conceptual frameworks, methodologies, and reasoned professional judgements based on biopsychosocial models of disability have gone some way to address complexities in the analysis of inappropriate illness behaviours and to seek out reasons for discrepancies between functional capacity and performance (Aylward and Sawney 1999). Further progress, however, is impeded by an understandable reluctance by many protagonists of the biopsychosocial philosophy openly to debate and critically explore the possibility that some illness behaviours may be driven by choice and conscious intent.

This failure to acknowledge that in some cases medically unexplained symptoms are outside conscious control frustrates progress towards a proper, concerted, and structured evaluation of the reasons why some people behave in a particular way under the influence of psychosocial factors. It encourages a creeping medicalization of ill-defined syndromes of questionable aetiology by cultivating a proliferation of descriptive psychiatric diagnoses of uncertain scientific validity. Most importantly, perhaps, it perpetuates a deterministic culture which very substantially diminishes an individual's capacity to make value-driven choices. That in itself surrenders to other people and to imposed circumstance an individual's unshackled participation in society.

Despite these limitations, with evidence provided by existing tools and the structured approach to disability analysis the practitioner of disability assessment medicine can still offer a robust and expert advisory service to decision makers. At the heart of which is the construction of convincing opinions and arguments to convey degrees of consistency between observed performance and activity, self-reported functional limitations and restrictions, and reasoned judgements of expected functional capacity. Documentation of intent, however, can rarely be provided. Even so, disability analysis now has the much firmer scientific base that it has long lacked. Until the sensitivities and ambiguities surrounding the attribution of malingering and illness deception are robustly confronted and resolved the practice of this new discipline will not work as well as it should. Moreover, unless there is clarification of the ambiguities about the relative contributions to the provocation and perpetuation of illness behaviours by volition and intent on the one hand and biopsychosocial influences on the other, there can be little further progress. But it is disability assessment medicine itself that offers the intellectual framework within which fruitful debate and dedicated research should be encouraged to flourish.

References

Allan, D. B. and Waddell, G. (1989). An historical perspective on low back pain and disability. *Orthopedica Scandinavica*, **60** (Suppl 234), 1–23.

American Medical Association (1993). *Guides to the Evaluation of Permanent Impairment*, 4th edn, pp. 94–138. American Medical Association, Chicago, IL.

Aylward, M. (1998). Chronic fatigue and related syndromes: historical perspectives. In *Proceedings of the 12th International Congress*, 5–6 June 1998. EUMASS, London. (www.eumass.com/CFS2.htm)

Aylward, M. (2002). Health and welfare government initiatives and strategy, and developing trends in incapacity-related benefits. In *Trends in health*, Chief Medical Officer's Report. UNUM Provident, London.

Aylward, M. and LoCascio, J. (1995). Problems in assessment of psychosomatic conditions in social security benefits and related commercial schemes. *Journal of Psychosomatic Research*, **39**, 755–65.

Aylward, M. and Sawney, P. (1999). Disability assessment medicine. *British Medical Journal* (Classified), 2–3.

Berthoud, R. (1998). *Disability benefits. A review of the issues and options for reform*. Joseph Rowntree Foundation, York.

Boden, L. I. (1996). Work disability in an economic context. In *Psychological aspects of musculo-skeletal disorders in office work* (eds. S. Moon and S. L. Sauter), pp. 287–94. Taylor and Francis, London.

Cocchiarella, L. and Andersson, G. B. J. (eds) (2000). *Guides to the evaluation of permanent impairment*, 5th edn. American Medical Association, Chicago, IL.

Croft, P. (2000). Is life becoming more of a pain? *British Medical Journal*, **320**, 1552–3 (editorial).

Duckworth, S. (2001). The disabled person's perspective. In New beginnings: a symposium on disability. UNUM, London.

Engel, G. L. (1977). The need for a new medical model: a challenge for biomedicine. *Science*, **196**, 129–36.

Finkelstein, V. (1996). Modelling disability. http://www.leeds.ac.uk/disability-studies/archiveuk/finkelstein/models/models.htm

Frankl, V. E. (1963). *Man's search for meaning*. Washington Square Press, Simon and Schuster, New York, NY.

Hadler, N. M. (1995). The disabling backache: an international perspective. *Spine*, **20**, 640–9.

Holloway, O. (2001). Doubts and loves. What is left of Christianity. Canongate, Edinburgh.

Howard, M. (1998). Disability dilemmas: welfare to work for early retirement. In *Welfare in working order* (eds C. Openheim and J. McCormick). Institute for Public Policy Research, London.

Kroenke, K. and Mangelsdorff, D. (1989). Common symptoms in ambulatory care: incidence, evaluation, therapy and outcome. *American Journal of Medicine*, **86**, 262–6.

Leino, P. L., Berg, M. A., and Puschka, P. (1994). Is back pain increasing? Results from national surveys in Finland. *Scandinavian Journal of Rheumatology*, **23**, 269–74.

LoPiccolo, C. J., Goodkin, K., and Bacdewicz, T. T. (1999). Current issues in the diagnosis and management of malingering. *Annals of Medicine*, **31**, 166–74.

Main, C. J. and Spanswick, C. C. (2000). *Textbook on interdisciplinary pain management*. Churchill Livingstone, Edinburgh.

Moffroid, M. T., Haugh, L. D., Henry, S. M., and Short, B. (1994). Distinguishable groups of musculoskeletal low back pain patients and asymptomatic control subjects based on physical measures of the NIOSH low back atlas. *Spine*, **19**, 1350–8.

Moffroid, M. T., Haugh, L. D., and Hodous, T. (1992). Sensitivity and specificity of the NIOSH low back atlas. NIOSH Report RFP 200–89–2917 (P) pp. 1–71. National Institute Occupational Safety & Health, Morgantown, WV.

Nimnuan, C., Hotopf, M., and Wessely, S. (2000). Medically unexplained symptoms: how often and why are they missed? *Quarterly Journal of Medicine*, **93** (1), 21–8.

Office of National Statistics (1993, 1996, 1998). Omnibus survey back pain module 1993, 1996, 1998. Department of Health, Statistics Division 3, London, http://www.doh.gov.uk/public/backpain.htm

Parsons, T. (1951). The social system. Free Press, New York, NY.

Rogers, R., and Cavanaugh, J. L. (1983). "Nothing but the truth. . ." A re-examination of malingering. *Journal of Law and Psychiatry*, **11**, 443–60.

Rowlingson, K. and Berthoud, R. (1996). Disability, benefits and employment. Department of Social Security Research Report No. 54. HMSO, London.

Sharpe, M. and Carson, A. (2001). 'Unexplained' somatic symptoms, functional syndromes, and somatization: do we need a paradigm shift? *Annals of Internal Medicine*, **134**, 926–30.

Ursin, H. (1997). Sensitization, somatization, and subjective health complaints: a review. *Internal Journal of Behavioural Medicine*, **4**, 105–16.

Waddell, G. (1987). A new clinical model for the treatment of low back pain. Spine, **12**, 632–44.

Waddell, G. (ed.) (1998). *The back pain revolution*. Churchill Livingstone, Edinburgh.

Waddell, G. (2002). *Models of disability using low back pain as an example*. The Royal Society of Medicine Press Ltd, London.

Waddell, G., Aylward, M., and Sawney, P. (2002). *Back pain, incapacity for work and social security benefits: an international literature review and analysis*. The Royal Society of Medicine Press Ltd, London.

Waddell, G. and McCulloch, O. (1980). Non organic physical signs in low back pain. *Spine*, **5**, 117–18.

Waddell, G. and Main, C. J. (1998). A new clinical model of low back pain and disability. In *The back pain revolution* (ed. G. Waddell), pp. 223–40. Churchill Livingstone, Edinburgh.

Waddell, G. and Norlund, A. (2000). A review of social security systems. In *Neck and back pain: the scientific evidence of causes, diagnosis and treatment* (eds A. Nachemson and E. Jonsson), pp. 427–71. Lippincott, Williams & Wilkins, Philadelphia, PA.

Waddell, G., Sommerville, D., Henderson, I., and Newton, M. (1992). Objective clinical evaluation of physical impairment in chronic low back pain. *Spine*, **17**, 617–28.

Waddell, G. and Waddell, H. (2000). A review of social influences on neck and back pain and disability. In *Neck and back pain: the scientific evidence of causes, diagnosis and treatment* (eds A. Nachemson and E. Jonsson), pp. 13–55. Lippincott, Williams & Wilkins, Philadelphia, PA.

World Health Organization (1980). *WHO international classification of impairments, disabilities and handicaps (ICIDH)*. World Health Organization, Geneva.

World Health Organization (2000). *WHO international classification of functioning, disability and health (ICFDH)*. World Health Organization, Geneva.

23 Malingering, insurance medicine, and the medicalization of fraud

John LoCascio

Abstract

Malingering is a concept that spans law and medicine and has important societal consequences. Disability-related programmes in both the public and private sectors are faced with increasing numbers of disability claims despite improved health care and job design (the disability paradox). As a result, medical providers face questions of malingering and related issues with increasing frequency. However, there is a paucity of data as to the demographics and exact magnitude of the problem. Changes in medical technology, confusion between medical and legal concepts, and unrecognized clinical assumptions make malingering difficult to analyse and document, and may result in risk to unskilled analysts. To be most effective, the analyst must: distinguish malingering from fraud; understand the difference between the clinical and analytical role; know the limits of medical data; and apply functional concepts in a disciplined manner.

In perspective

Malingering is viewed medically by medical practitioners and legally by legal practitioners. Each has something to contribute, and insurance companies may obtain both medical and legal advice when questions of malingering arise. But insurance companies cannot treat malingering as an isolated medical or legal technicality. The insurance industry is neither medically nor legally driven. It is driven by societal imperatives. Commercial insurance sells products into society via the commercial marketplace. And, despite the absence of an obvious profit motive, governmental programs respond to a political 'marketplace' following analogous laws of supply and demand. Medicine and the law are like the blind men describing the elephant; each has an important part of the truth, but neither sees the issue in societal perspective.

In this chapter, I will consider malingering in the context of commercial disability insurance, which in the United Kingdom is also known as Permanent Health Insurance (PHI). Analogous governmental programmes are Social Security Disability (in the United States) and Incapacity Benefit (in the United Kingdom). All such programmes somehow insure the continuance of income of individuals and, indirectly, of others in the society. Viewed in this way, societies have an interest in maintaining the health of insurance programmes which are, therefore, highly regulated. In other words, insurance is not regulated solely for the protection of the consumer. It is also regulated to insure the stability and health of the industry and the greater society. Thus, all such programmes have a two-fold charge: to pay valid claims promptly and fairly, and to simultaneously avoid the depletion of a necessary resource by identifying claims that are not valid.

This charge has grown increasingly difficult as law, medicine, and the workplace evolve: as work becomes less physical and more intellectual; as claims for benefit become less 'objective' and more 'subjective'. As a result, insurers are faced with a disability paradox: an increasingly healthy society; safer and less physically demanding workplaces; but more reported disability (Aylward and LoCascio 1995; see also Baron and Poole, Chapter 19).

This has awakened the modern interest in malingering. Thus, the object of this chapter is to consider some of the ways medicine relates to law and insurance in questions of malingering, and how medical providers can most effectively present this knowledge to insurers and to the greater society.

Defining the problem

There is no reliable data on the incidence and cost of malingering *per se*. However, malingering is a phenomenon that: (a) affects insurance programmes with high medical content;[1] and (b) is included in the wider concept of 'fraud and abuse'.[2]

'High medical content' refers to the fact that certain insurance products (and their governmental equivalents) base the award of benefit on the provision of medical care or its outcome. Classic 'health insurance' first comes to mind, by which is meant indemnity or managed care programmes that provide patients with financial or other access to care and treatment. An example of this type of programme in the United Kingdom is the National Health Service (NHS). In the United States, managed care programmes, such as Preferred Provider Organizations (PPOs), are more familiar. The NHS provides benefit 'in kind', and the PPO 'in cash' after service has been provided. In order to manage (or 'quality assure') such a programme, one must obtain and evaluate large amounts of direct care documentation. In contrast, a product with 'low medical content' is Life Assurance because it is contingent only upon proof of death, often regardless of the cause of death, or type or extent of medical care associated with the death.

Programmes that provide protection for the 'disabled'[3] constitute the second most medically intensive class of insurance products because they are usually contingent on a medical cause of inability to work. In the United States, such programmes are actually classified as part of the health insurance industry (Life Office Management Association 1999), a structure that is reflected in the UK classification of PHI.[4] For this reason, data on fraud and abuse in health insurance programmes are an indicator of malingering.

Dearth of data

Data on fraud and abuse are difficult to obtain. The General Accounting Office (GAO) of the US Congress has proven to be the best source; the result of national scope and an excellent website.[5] Conversely, the absence of data from other sources is worthy of discussion.

Obstacles to gathering and sharing data on fraud and abuse include the following.

[1] See GAO/HRD-92-69, p. 1, a document available from the General Accounting Office (GAO), the investigative branch of the US Congress. See also footnote 4.

[2] Fraud and abuse is a term-of-art used by investigators to refer to overpayments due to errors in the processing of claims which result from the provision of deceptive or distorted information.

[3] For purposes of this discussion, *disability* is defined as the inability to perform a task necessary to some defined occupation. Disability can also be defined in terms of the inability to perform any relevant societal function, as it is in the World Health Organization (WHO) *International Classification of Impairments, Disabilities and Handicaps* (ICIDH).

[4] Other European regulation, however, may classify disability programmes under the umbrella of Life Assurance.

[5] The GAO website (www.gao.gov) is easily searchable with little practice. The naming convention of reports is *GAO/GGD-96-1* where the initial GAO refers to the site, and the terminal alpha-numeric combination will directly access the report. Reports can also be researched by title or class.

Limitation of available data

Governmental programmes report data but often limit the type of data they gather. This may be the result of past controversy, including the perception of discrimination. On the other hand, commercial sources may not report data because they consider it to be proprietary and are concerned that its unilateral release may result in competitive disadvantage. The anonymous release of pooled data would 'level the playing field', but anti-trust concerns prohibit commercial pooling and there is no national database in the United States that can receive and distribute the information. Another option, the release of information about specific cases, may result in the identification of a particular individual and involves other legal risks (*GAO/HRD-92-69*, p. 16).[6]

The hidden nature of fraud and abuse

This refers to the reluctance of individuals to draw attention to the fact that they may have obtained benefit in a way that is in whole or in part invalid. The implications for the study of malingering are obvious; if we are unaware of the majority of such claims, how can we judge the true extent of the problem? As the cross-examining barrister might ask: 'Doctor, can you tell me how many times you have failed to detect a lie?' (Ziskin and Faust 1988).

Lack of a standard definition of fraud and abuse

Not all fraud is *hard fraud*; that is to say, a deceptive act which is premeditated from the outset for the clear purpose of obtaining benefit. What might be called *soft fraud* can occur when patients with known conditions give up employment but later discover that their impairment is not severe enough to qualify for benefit, leading them to consciously exaggerate existing symptoms. *Opportunistic fraud* may result when a valid claim is paid, subsequent recovery occurs, but the patient continues to report symptoms he or she has learned are difficult to assess.

The cost of prosecution

The hardest definition of hard fraud is a guilty verdict in a court of law. However, the successful pursuit of such a case is costly. No detailed and comprehensive accounting of the costs of fraud litigation across the United States is available. However, some idea may be gained from the criteria of the US Federal Prosecutor's office (*GAO/HRD-92-69*, pp. 4, 20). Cases with a potential value of less than US$ 100 000.00 are usually not pursued. Of those pursued, many are not prosecuted because: there is a lack of evidence, benefits are terminated without challenge, or a settlement is reached.

Estimating the cost of fraud and abuse

These problems notwithstanding, the growing interest of insurers in malingering mirrors a growing awareness of the cost of fraud and abuse. For example, Medicare is a US Federal programme that provides health care insurance for persons over 65 years of age. *GAO/HRD-92-1* estimates 1991 Medicare payments at US$ 115 billion. But Medicare accounts for only a fraction of health care expenditures in the United States. *GAO/HRD-93-8* estimates total health care expenditures

---

[6] An excellent source of background information is also available to the reader in *GAO/GGD-96-101*.

(commercial plus governmental) for 1991 to be in the range of US\$ 800 billion. And *GAO/HRD-92-69* (p. 1) estimates losses to fraud and abuse at 10 per cent of total expenditures or approximately US\$ 70 billion. *GAO/HRD-96-101* estimates 1995 losses at US\$ 100 billion.

More recent estimates vary widely. In the *Health Care Fraud and Abuse Control Program Annual Report for FY 1998*, the US Department of Health and Human Services (DHHS) and the Department of Justice (DOJ) estimate rates of Medicare overpayment due to fraud and abuse of 14 per cent in 1996, 11 per cent in 1997, and 7.1 per cent in 1998 (available at www.usdoj.gov). However, these estimates appear to be based on anecdotal evidence of the success of stepped-up enforcement efforts. While the GAO estimate of 10 per cent may also be criticized, data was gathered from a broader range of governmental and commercial organizations.

In summary, it seems reasonable to assume that approximately 10 per cent of expenditures in health and disability programmes are lost to fraud and abuse, of which malingering accounts for a substantial portion. Barring fundamental changes in societal outlook, legislation, or the structure of benefit programs, this estimate is unlikely to change.

Fraud and malingering

> The question of disease—that and nothing more—is the one for the physician to determine.
>
> (Drewy 1896)

Increasing claim numbers, the disability paradox, and growing awareness of the cost of fraud and abuse have caused insurance administrators to consult medical providers with increasing frequency. In response to questions of fraud or malingering, too many clinicians paraphrase former US Supreme Court Justice Potter Stewart, stating (in effect) 'although I can't define it, I know it when I see it.' Elsewhere in this volume, the data presented by Vrij and Mann (Chapter 27) underscore the difficulties of this assumption and complement the prior work of Faust (1995). Clearly, such questions require more than a clinical opinion; they require a forensic argument, where 'forensic' means 'pertaining to or used in courts of law or public debate'. In the broadest sense this means, 'effective, reasoned, and defensible'. In questions of malingering, it can ultimately require effectiveness in the context of Civil or Criminal Law (see Sprince, Chapter 18).

When posed, such questions appear to be medical in nature. However, they are strongly influenced by contractual or other considerations unfamiliar to the medical provider. In addition, business personnel are seldom medical or legal professionals and may use the terms 'fraud' and 'malingering' interchangeably. This is also a common clinical mistake and increases the likelihood of vague and ineffective responses which can expose both questioner and provider to legal risk.

The first requirement in addressing questions of malingering is to recognize that malingering and fraud are related but distinct. That is, they share crucial elements but contain critical differences. Fraud is a purely legal concept; malingering is a related concept with a medical context. It might be said that malingering is the 'medicalization' of fraud.

The risk of confusion is explicitly recognized by the DSM-IV (American Psychiatric Association 1994):

> When the DSM-IV categories, criteria, and textual descriptions are employed for forensic purposes, there are significant risks that diagnostic information will be misused or misunderstood. These dangers arise because of the imperfect fit between the questions of ultimate concern to the law and the information contained in a clinical diagnosis.

Note the DSM does not define malingering as an Axis I or II diagnosis, but as a 'V code' or 'other condition that may be a focus of medical attention' (American Psychiatric Association

1994, p. 675). This contrast, so clear to Dr Drewy over a century ago, is ironically blurred by the complexities of modern law and medicine.

To be fair, the definitions of 'malingering' and 'fraud' overlap in such a way that even standard texts may confuse the two. *Black's Law Dictionary* devotes two full pages to fraud, but for our purposes we may consider fraud to be:

> A knowing misrepresentation of the truth or concealment of a material fact to induce another to act to his or her detriment.

On the other hand, the DSM-IV describes malingering (V65.2) as follows:

> The essential feature of Malingering is the intentional production of false or grossly exaggerated physical or psychological symptoms, motivated by external incentives such as avoiding military duty, avoiding work, obtaining financial compensation . . . etc.

In essence, both fraud and malingering provide some sort of desired return and require the demonstration of intent. Malingering, however, also requires a medical context.

Elsewhere in this volume Mendelson (Chapter 17) concludes:

> Thus, malingering does not fall within the lexicon of the diagnostician, but is a form of behaviour to be assessed or evaluated on the basis of facts.

The lesson is that the clinician, when presented with a question of malingering, should exercise thoughtful caution, carefully consider the likelihood of malingering, and avoid an allegation of fraud.

Intent versus motive

Let us consider one of the 'imperfect fits' between medical and legal data.

Medical records may suggest 'motive', but motive is not intent. Suppose someone in financial need seeks benefit but fails to qualify. We may infer a motive to obtain benefit but such circumstances alone do not prove that the person intends to deceive. Put another way, intent predicates motive but motive does not predicate intent. In many ways the distinction between motive and intent is analogous to the clinical distinction between factitious disorder and somatization disorder.

Suppose that the medical records reasonably demonstrate that the patient understood the questions asked, the answers given, and the plan of care. Suppose further that other medical records demonstrate that the patient's behaviour consistently contradicts the history (e.g. a person limps in public view but not when distracted or outside of public view as recorded on CCTV). One may conclude that this is suggestive of, or most consistent with, intent and that there is a medical likelihood of malingering. However, it is difficult to exclude all alternative explanations on the basis of the medical record alone. Here, difficulties arise because the concepts of motive and intent are distinct in the law but closely related and otherwise easily confused. Demonstration of the medical likelihood of malingering significantly contributes to a legal analysis of fraud, but the final analysis of intent, and therefore of fraud or malingering, is best left to legal professionals.

Remember: medical records can suggest that malingering is the most likely explanation of a pattern of behaviour, but they rarely can prove fraud for the simple reason that medical data seldom contain statements of intent.[7] Stating the likelihood of malingering is well within the sphere of expertise of a medical resource. Stating the certainty of malingering is much more difficult.

---

[7] Some would point to symptom validity testing in neuropsychological batteries as an exception to this rule (see Frederick, Chapter 25).

And asserting intent on the basis of medical records alone is usually problematic and fraught with risk. If asked to comment on fraud or to prove intent, the medical consultant should engage the poser in full and frank discussion including reasonable consideration of legal guidance.

In the next sections we will consider concepts, tools, and approaches to better document cases of suspected malingering.

Clinical analysis differs from functional analysis

Functional analysts begin their carriers as clinicians, and clinicians use certain, understandable and appropriate assumptions in their daily work: for example, until proved otherwise, clinicians assume that patient's histories are accurate and that the patient has strong conscious and unconscious drives to recover. These assumptions are appropriate to the overwhelming majority of patients seen in practice. They are also necessary; without them medical practice would be impossibly cumbersome and inefficient. Imagine having to verify every history, especially when experience teaches that the vast majority of clinical work is accurate and successful. However, think how poorly adapted such assumptions are to the detection of malingering.

When the medical resource becomes a functional analyst, it is necessary to recall that the cases that are referred for disability benefit are not the rule of clinical practice, but the exception. That is to say, they are in the minority of cases that, despite the best efforts of the medical system, fail to improve enough to resume normal life activities, including gainful employment. When such a case also lacks objectification, especially in this day of advanced chemical, imaging, and histological techniques, they are part of an even smaller minority.[8] In other words, they are the clear exceptions to the clinical rule.

What assumptions should the functional analyst use to produce a more forensic report? First, no statement should be assumed to be either valid or invalid. Everything must be interpreted in the broader context of the case in question (which may include so-called 'non-medical' data[9] such as video surveillance, reports of employment evaluations, school attendance, and records of other activities). Second, the analyst must recognize that assumptions, by their nature, are unspoken, and guard against the unconscious adoption of a mode of thought which they might naturally employ in the clinical role. Third, we must recognize that clinical assumptions place natural limits on the structure and content of medical records, but that these limits can be addressed by the gathering of a wide range of medical records and by the use of para-medical data.

Functional documentation and analysis

Providing a comprehensive treatise on all aspects of functional analysis is beyond the scope of this chapter. However, in view of the characteristics of malingering, the analyst should keep three questions in mind:

- Did the patient understand the medical issues?
- Are the reported and actual behaviours consistent or inconsistent through time and across observers?
- Are the functional capacities in question well defined?

---

[8] In the particular case of malingering, DSM-IV, V65.2, p. 683, notes four qualities: medicolegal context; *discrepancy between claimed disability and objective findings*, lack of cooperation, and presence of antisocial personality disorder (author's emphasis).

[9] I prefer to label such data as 'para-medical' in that it is often gathered by a non-medical resource, but provides direct or indirect observation, one of the most basic types of medical data.

Did the patient understand the medical issues?

The point here is simple but seldom articulated. It is helpful to note the degree to which the patient is physically, psychiatrically, and intellectually capable of understanding the questions asked, of answering those questions, and of following the treatment plan. Depending on the medical orientation of the specialist, one of the first two issues may be addressed. However, in questions of malingering, it is most helpful for the analyst to note whether the questions are asked and directions given in a manner appropriate to the patient's training, education, and experience (as far as these are known or may be estimated).

Are the reported and actual behaviours consistent or inconsistent?

Clinical providers recognize the strengths of clinical data, but seldom its weaknesses. One weakness is the limited availability of old records. This is a practical reality. Older records seem less relevant to modern, technically oriented practitioners, practitioners do not want multiple copies of similar data, and record gathering is limited by time and cost.

The situation for the forensic analyst is the reverse. Old records are especially important in complex cases with symptoms in excess of findings, and multiple caregivers over extended periods of time.

Quantity of data collected

Forensic arguments can be fashioned from clinical data, but this requires more extensive records than the clinician usually obtains. Like the clinician, the functional analyst obtains records to establish a baseline, but there is often an additional need to observe patterns of behaviour over time and across caregivers. Therefore, insurance companies expect and are better equipped to gather records more extensively in order to analyse patterns of behaviour.[10] Nowhere is the comparison of actual to reported behaviour more important than in the analysis of malingering. As a result, one of the skills most valued by an insurer is the ability to quickly identify and obtain large quantities of pertinent data without wasteful duplication.

Once data is obtained, it must be analysed, and to this end certain basic concepts are invaluable.[11] In brief, it is important to keep the following in mind.

Functional concepts

Diagnosis does not equal disability. A well-established diagnosis allows for easier documentation but does little to validate or invalidate claims of functional impairment.

Impairment does not equal disability. Impairment simply means a diminution of function from a baseline.[12] That baseline may be high or low, the diminution great or small, and the result may

---

[10] Unfortunately, in the author's experience, governmental programmes are seldom equipped to do so. The clear exception to this rule is the first Federal appeal level of US Social Security Disability, where the Administrative Law Judge gathers extensive old records and produces a standard analysis.

[11] The reader may recognize similarities between this terminology and that of the WHO (1980, p. 11). Diagrammatically, these concepts are a detailed explosion which reads:

disease → diagnosis → impairment → limitation/restriction → (residual) functional capacity → disability → handicap

where the underlined terms are those added in this text (see also, Aylward and LoCascio 1995).

[12] The definition given derives from the American Medical Association (AMA) *Guides to the Evaluation of Permanent Impairment.* Some confusion exists when older insurance contracts or the language in an Act equates impairment with disability. The AMA definition is preferable in the author's opinion.

or may not preclude the patient from performing any particular task. Diminution of function, however, can result in either restriction or limitation.

Limitation is the physical inability, as a consequence of illness or injury, to perform a certain act or skill. As such, limitation is more subject to measurement or objectification. In many cases, this is accomplished by examination, laboratory studies, or imaging. A less commonly used means of objectifying subtle, physical limitation is provided by special procedures such as formal functional capacity evaluation. Psychiatric limitation is more challenging. It is usually documented by history or by behavioural observation, and can be partially objectified by formal psychometric or neuropsychological testing.

Restriction is what a patient is reasonably told not to do because of an unacceptable risk of harm to self or others. By definition, this means that the person must be capable of performing the skill or action (that is, they must not be *limited* from it). The classic example of medical restriction is a driving prohibition after recovery from a documented seizure.[13]

The distinction between limitation and restriction is intellectually clear to clinicians, but is not vital to the provision of care. Do not expect to find it clearly drawn in the medical record. However, it is critical to the functional analyst, and it is most important to bear in mind when questioning a claimant, a physician caring for a claimant, or when evaluating observational data. If a person is observed performing an act from which he or she is said to be constantly limited, a clear contradiction is demonstrated. However, if a person is seen to perform an act from which they are restricted, what is demonstrated is disregard of medical advice. The latter is helpful, but the former is the most powerful demonstration of a contradiction of the medical data.

Functional Capacity (FC) is the most important of all the functional concepts. A functional capacity is a defined task: physical tasks such as walking, lifting, and reading; but also psychological tasks such as impulse control, memory, multiple simultaneous attention, and calculation. FCs are complex, requiring the participation and coordination of multiple systems.

Although most clinicians do not focus on the concept, FC is the unrecognized starting point of almost all patient visits. Patients do not walk into a consulting room and announce they have multiple sclerosis (a diagnosis) producing bilateral optic neuritis (an impairment) with acquired loss of colour vision (a limitation). Rather, the patient announces that they are concerned because they can no longer match colours as a printer's assistant (an FC). The patient does not announce that they have a history of steroid therapy with secondary proximal muscle weakness of the hip extensors (an impairment) with a 50 per cent loss of power (a limitation). Rather, they say they can no longer stand without the use of their arms (an FC).

Consistency

Finally, it is important to remember that a limitation or restriction usually affects more than one FC, and must do so in a consistent manner. The person who is limited to typing for 20 min by virtue of forearm pain but can play piano for an hour may seem a *reductio ad absurdum*, but such cases are not unheard of in the industry. The point is that the intellectual construct of restriction and limitation as higher-level concepts that include multiple FCs finds its corollary in the real world of medical observation and functional analysis. For example, much of the analysis of validity which is incorporated in formal functional capacities evaluation for physical impairment utilizes this concept.

Claims personnel, as well as medical personnel, should be taught to focus on FC in their interviews. Lack of reference to loss of a well-defined FC across a mass of medical records

---

[13] During a seizure the person is *limited* from driving. After recovery and stabilization on medication, the person is *restricted* from driving until certain criteria are met. By definition, a person cannot be simultaneously limited and restricted from an activity.

should arouse attention.[14] The obverse; clear definition of pertinent FCs, allows the medical consultant to best gather data; demonstrate functional consistency (or the lack thereof); and best obtain an independent medical examination (IME) in case of dispute.

Pattern of impairment

Every medical student is drilled in the fundamentals of history taking (What can't you do? Why can't you do it? What makes it better? Worse? How often is it like that?) Is it not remarkable that a clear pattern of symptoms is so seldom found in the medical records supporting an insurance claim? In such cases, it is left to the medical consultant to define a pattern as clearly as possible, and careful note should be taken of any difficulties encountered. There are many ways to this; often a diary is recommended. I favour a series of three questions: 'Please describe a bad day. Please describe a good day. Please tell me how many good days and bad days you have in an average week.' Armed with this knowledge about any particular symptom and the corresponding reduction in an FC, the medical resource can proceed to analyse the consistency of the history against the medical or observational data.

Documentation

In conclusion, the most important product of the medical consultant is clear, credible, and defensible documentation. Such documentation requires familiarity with contractual (or regulatory), medicolegal, and societal context. Beyond the DSM-IV criteria, how can you best document the case for or against malingering?

- Discover sufficient medical and observational records through time and across observers.
- Demonstrate the likelihood that the patient understood the medical questions and instructions.
- Define limitation or restriction and the reported pattern of reduction in specific FC.
- Document, with specific allusion to existing records, any lack of consistency of reported to actual FC.
- Defer the final demonstration of intent to your legal or other colleagues.

Future direction

This volume compiles many stimulating perspectives and approaches in a newly invigorated field. Some of us are compelled by the structure of our work to analyse the individual's behaviour, others the behaviour of groups. Perhaps one day a technician will directly address questions of intent through a practical method of 'lie detection' (see Craig and Hill, Chapter 26). But remember our starting point:

> Medicine and the law are like the blind men describing the elephant; each has an important part of the truth, but neither sees the issue in societal perspective.

Beyond success or failure in any particular avenue of inquiry lies the greater challenge of usefulness. Will practical 'lie detection' eliminate problems of data or definition, like those of concern

---

[14] Sherlock Holmes draws the attention of the owner of *Silver Blaze*, '... to the curious incident of the dog in the night-time'. 'But the dog did nothing in the night-time', is the reply. 'That is the curious incident', replies Holmes. In much the same way, a question not asked, a test not done, or an opinion not sought, may be an important source of insight.

to the DSM, where we are told:

> ... dangers arise because of the imperfect fit between the questions of ultimate concern to the law and the information contained in a clinical diagnosis (?)

To this end we cannot do better than to consider the thoughts of Byrne and Stokes (Chapter 4), whose monkeys, ironically, prove to be most thoughtful:

> Ideally, perhaps, preventive measures should take no account of intentionality, and simply aim to reduce the overall frequency. ... it may be better simply to change the payoff matrix in such a way that it discourages malingering.

But 'changing the payoff matrix' is not the province of medicine or of the law. It is the province of the society; through legislation, regulation, and the design of innovative commercial products. I, for one, believe that the question of malingering is not so much a problem to be solved, as a reflection of the human condition. Each of the several approaches will continue to play its part, and both the successes and failures of each of us who contributed to this volume (and many kindred spirits) will better define that condition, day by day.

References

American Psychiatric Association (1994). *Diagnostic and statistical manual of mental disorders*, 4th edn (DSM-IV), p. xxiii, American Psychiatric Association, Washington, DC.

Aylward, M. and LoCascio, J. (1995). Problems in the assessment of psychosomatic conditions in social security benefits and related commercial schemes. *Journal of Psychosomatic Research*, **39** (6), 755–65.

Drewy, W. F. (1896). *Journal of the American Medical Association*, **27**, 798–801.

Faust, D. (1995). The detection of deception. *Neurology Clinics*, **13** (2), 255–65.

Life Office Management Association (LOMA) (1999). *Principles of insurance: life, health, and annuities*, 2nd edn, p. 10. LOMA, Atlanta, GA.

World Health Organization (WHO) (1980). *International classification of impairments, disabilities and handicaps* (ICIDH). WHO, Geneva.

Ziskin, J. and Faust, D. (1988). *Coping with psychiatric and psychological testimony*, 4th edn. Law and Psychology Press, Los Angeles, CA.

Section 8

Deception detection

24 Investigating benefit fraud and illness deception in the United Kingdom

Richard Kitchen

Abstract

This chapter will consider the issues that a benefit fraud investigator needs to establish when investigating illness deception as a criminal offence. It will not seek to explain the intricacies of the British welfare system, in which the investigator works, or attempt to provide a comprehensive overview of the English Criminal Justice system where benefit fraud is alleged (see Jones, Chapter 16 and Sprince, Chapter 18). The main purpose is to consider the extent to which illness deception contributes to alleged fraud within the UK benefit system.

The chapter sets out to describe the purpose of the UK Department for Work and Pensions (DWP) in relation to illness or disability benefits. It will also outline the relevant issues for an investigator charged with countering fraudulent claims to such benefits. This will involve considering the relevance of malingering and illness deception in the context of frauds tackled by investigators from the DWP and a review of the evidence required in criminal courts for frauds where illness deception is alleged. Finally, the chapter will highlight some of the constraints placed on investigators, including regulatory and practical considerations and will attempt to locate the evidence that can be provided in criminal courts by expert witnesses in illness deception.

The UK Department for Work and Pensions

The UK DWP was formed in 2001. It took over some of the work previously carried out by the Department of Social Security and the Department for Education and Employment. The new Department manages a programme spend in welfare benefits in excess of £100 billion per annum. Its customers are, for all practical purposes, the total population of Great Britain; all of whom are at some time beneficiaries of income from the State, whether it be support while they are out of work or in relation to child benefit or pensions.

The Department administers welfare benefits for pensioners, for children and for people of working age. All of these benefits are subject to fraudulent claims (as is any financial system that is open to a wide group of clients) but this chapter will concentrate on those of working age, and specifically on one of the disability benefits claimed by them: Disability Living Allowance (DLA). The characteristics of this benefit facilitate an in-depth examination of the relationship between malingering and the criminal law fraud.

DLA is a tax-free, non-contributory benefit for those needing help with everyday living. It is intended to help people get around or with their personal care, or both. DLA is not based upon the nature of the disability, but on the effects of it, as reported by the claimant. The patient's assessment is frequently supported by other evidence, including reports from the claimant's General practitioner (GP), or following examinations undertaken by approved examining medical practitioners. In awarding DLA the Department may take account of medical advice in conjunction with the claimant's description of the impact of the disability.

DLA is payable to people with degrees of care needs or mobility requirements that result from physical and/or mental disabilities. These care needs are a fertile area for exaggeration or even complete fabrication by those who would engage in fraud. For example, a recent case in the North East of England concerned a married couple, each of whom was claiming DLA (and related benefits) and naming the other as their carer. The case came to light when the husband's car was stolen while he was jogging on the beach. He turned up at the Crown Court to plead not guilty to fraud in a wheelchair and wearing a neck support. He claimed to suffer from osteo-arthritis, sciatica, vertigo, blackouts and said that he was losing his sight. His wife said that she had angina, suffered from breathlessness, and could not walk more than 30 yards. During the investigation, it transpired that there were no disability aids in the house, not even a handrail on the stair. Meanwhile, the husband ran two businesses and went jogging regularly. Both were convicted of their part in fraud totalling £70 000.

There are currently 2.3 million people in Great Britain claiming DLA. Of these some 400 000 people have taken up the option available to all claimants to have a subsidized motor vehicle (adapted to take account of their disability if necessary) paid for out of their DLA benefit. It is worth pointing out, that people awarded DLA are permitted to engage in paid work—although clearly it would raise questions if the nature of that work was incompatible with their claimed disability.

Countering fraud

Part of the function of the Department is to counter fraudulent requests for benefits that lead to a claimant receiving a benefit. It is estimated that, across the entire programme spend on welfare benefits, £2 billion is lost each year to fraud (i.e. about 2 per cent of total programme spend). This figure is calculated by reference to a statistical analysis of the Department's caseload, which is designed partly to inform deployment of investigators to the main areas of risk. Just under 15 per cent of the Department's investigation resource will be deployed against fraud in health related benefits in the current year.

Investigating fraudulent claims

In all, 5000 of the Department's 125 000 staff are directly employed in the investigation of fraud. However, every member of the Department has a responsibility for stopping fraud from entering into the Department's systems. Front-line staff receiving claimants onto the system, advisers and those involved in dealing with a claimant during the lifetime of a claim are all expected to be alert to error and take corrective action. They are supported in this task by information technology (IT) but the key task is a critical review of the information provided by the claimant. DLA presents particular difficulties for front-line staff given the potential for a client to exaggerate or fabricate their needs for care. Where there is suspicion that a claim is (or may be) false, the case will be reported to the investigation department. The front-line member of staff reporting suspicion will be expected to set out the grounds upon which the suspicion is based. The most frequent references to investigation follow from allegations received from members of the public—often neighbours who see the claimant engaged in activities incompatible with their claimed condition.

Investigators are regionally based throughout Great Britain. They work to a departmental specification that sets out the priorities for the investigation service, integrating their activities with preventive measures intended to discourage fraud and minimize error. The priority for the Department is to tackle fraud on short-term benefits such as paying benefit to people who claim to be unemployed when, in fact, they have work. The statistical caseload analysis referred to above tells us that this is where our systems are most subject to fraudulent claims. This chapter concentrates on DLA, one of the longer-term health-related benefits. Fraud on these systems forms only a small part of the investigators' task and it is here that the concept of malingering is relevant.

Malingering

It is unnecessary for the purposes of this paper to agonise over the different definitions of malingering, these are discussed in Chapters 1, 3, and 5. Even so, it is helpful to explain the limited relevance of this broad concept to welfare fraud investigators. First, it is necessary to exclude from the discussion those who are unemployed and seeking work. A person of working age who is unemployed and seeking work will usually be entitled to benefit, even if the reason given for unemployment is a false statement of ill health. The reason for his or her unemployment is not relevant to the payment of benefit. There are two questions for the Department.

The first is whether the claimant is indeed seeking work. This is a matter for those involved in benefit administration rather than for criminal law investigators, and vigorous efforts are made to help into work people who are entitled to work in the United Kingdom, whatever their background, education, ability, or history. A person who consistently declines work of which they are capable may be refused benefit, but they will not be prosecuted for fraud for that reason alone.

The second question is whether the claimant is in fact in paid employment. If the administrator handling the claim suspects that the claimant is in fact working (perhaps in the informal economy) the claim will be referred to investigators. In 'working and claiming' fraud the focus of the investigation will be on establishing whether the claimant has paid work, not on any claimed illness or disability.

This brings us to the welfare benefits that are specifically dependent on disability or incapacity. In other words: benefits that are accessible only to people with health-related needs. In these regimes, a false statement about care needs based upon an illness deception or malingering is the mechanism for making a fraudulent claim. Figure 24.1 illustrates the point.

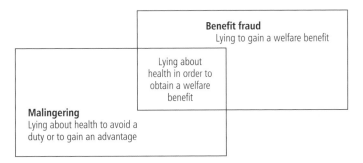

Figure 24.1   The overlap between malingering and benifit fraud.

What is fraud in the context of welfare benefits?

A simple working definition of fraud (Fig. 24.2) adequate for this chapter would be: A *dishonest intent* to obtain *financial advantage* through *a deception*.

All three elements must be proven to the criminal standard before fraud is established. It is convenient to take them in reverse order.

Deception

Deception in this context is an *act* (or omission—such as a failure to notify a change in relevant circumstances) that facilitates a fraud. This is sometimes referred to as a 'guilty act'. The type of deception will vary with the fraud. Illness deception is only one variation among the many found in benefit fraud. In order to derive benefit to which they are not entitled a person may also lie about their financial circumstances; their employment status or their family circumstances (e.g. claiming to have children who do not exist in order to obtain child-related benefits). These deceptions would require an investigator to show that the family, financial, or employment circumstances are at variance with reality. The investigator must prove that there was an act of deception—and show the link between the deception and financial advantage sought or received.

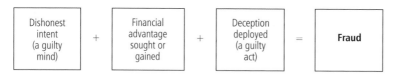

Figure 24.2 Definition of fraud in the context of welfare benefits.

Financial advantage

People deceive others intentionally and dishonestly for a variety of reasons; for example, in order to gain status or to win praise. For the most part, such social deceptions are not relevant to benefit fraud investigation but where deception is evidentially linked to financial advantage in terms of the benefit system it becomes a key ingredient of the case.

There is no requirement in law to show that the financial advantage was actually obtained. In theory, a deception that is intended to gain that advantage is sufficient, whether or not the attempted fraud is successful. In reality, there are often practical difficulties where a fraud has been stopped in its tracks and there are no arrears of benefit. Discussion of those difficulties is outside the scope of this chapter.

Dishonest intent

In proving the suspected fraud, the investigator must show that the suspect had a dishonest purpose in mind (a 'guilty mind'). In benefit fraud, the dishonest purpose is to gain income to which there is no entitlement. It is not enough to show that an error was made or even that not enough care was taken to get the facts correct. Negligence is not enough. The investigator must have evidence of the intended socially deviant purpose.

The test of dishonesty in UK law is set out in a speech given by Lord Lane in the UK Court of Appeal in 1982.[1] He said that there are 'infinite categories of dishonesty' and set out a test where there is doubt over intent. He indicated that the Jury should consider both subjective and objective tests and he illustrated these tests with an example of a man who comes from a country

---

[1] R v. Ghosh (1982) 3 WLR 10 Court of Appeal (Criminal Division).

where public transport is free. On his first day in the UK he travels on a bus and gets off without paying. Lord Lane's position was that, 'He never had any intention of paying. His mind is clearly honest but his conduct, judged objectively by what he has done, is dishonest'.

Lord Lane went on to say 'If dishonesty is something in the mind of the accused then if the mind of the accused is honest, it cannot be deemed dishonest merely because members of the Jury would regard it as dishonest'. On the other hand, a purely subjective test 'is to abandon all standards but that of the accused himself, and to bring about a state of affairs in which Robin Hood would be no robber. It is no defence for a man to say "I knew that what I was doing is generally regarded as dishonest; but I do not regard it as dishonest myself, therefore I am not guilty". .... In determining whether the prosecution has proved that the defendant was acting dishonestly, a jury must first of all decide whether, according to the ordinary standards of reasonable and honest people whether what was done was dishonest. If it was dishonest by those standards, then the jury must consider whether the defendant must have realised that what he was doing was by those standards dishonest.'

In most benefit frauds, it is unnecessary to go beyond the first (objective) test. There are very few occasions where the defendant claims that he or she did not know that it is dishonest to tell a lie that is material to the claim. Sometimes, evidence of intent is obtained through a direct admission of dishonesty. Where there is no admission, evidence of dishonesty is usually found in the behaviour of the suspect. It may be from evidence of lies told or, in illness deception, for example, it may be ostentatious use made of medical aids (that are otherwise unnecessary) when making a claim to benefit. In the example given above, the use by the jogger of a wheelchair and neckbrace was demonstrably a ruse from which dishonest intent could be reasonably be inferred. Even though there was no admission of fraud the court were content that dishonest intent was proven.

What does the benefit fraud investigator do?

The task for investigators can be simply stated. The investigator must demonstrate to the satisfaction of a court that:

- there is a normal system or process for the payment of benefit;
- that, in the case at issue, there was an abnormality in that system or process that resulted in an overpayment to an individual; and then,
- he or she (and there is a high percentage of female investigators) must establish that the cause of the abnormality was some action or inaction by the claimant taken by him with the dishonest intent of gaining the overpayment.

The starting point is to show that there is a system and demonstrate to the Court what that system is. This is the benchmark of normal process against which the allegedly abnormal claimant behaviour will be compared. In simple cases, it is unnecessary formally to bring forward evidence to show the normal process—the courts will assume (take notice of) facts that are commonly accepted. If an alleged fraud relates to obtaining entry to a sporting event without payment for example, they will accept without evidence that it is normal to pay for entry.

However, in benefit fraud cases where there is a lie about personal circumstances, we must prove that there was an obligation to honestly declare the relevant facts. To this end, evidence will be given in court by an administrator showing that he or she asks normally questions about a claimant's circumstances in order to establish whether there is entitlement to benefit. This is the starting point for considering the motivation for the claimant's false answer.

If the court is convinced that a false answer was given; and that the false answer was a deception perpetrated by the beneficiary of an overpayment of a benefit; and that the beneficiary deployed the deception dishonestly intending to obtain the overpayment, knowing that he was not entitled to that benefit—then fraud is proven.

An example of a false claim for benefit

A recent investigation concerned a painter and decorator, Mr Green, who had for 5 years claimed benefits for disability, saying that he was unable to continue his trade because of back pain. In his claim, he said he had gradually become disabled because of the pain, to the extent that he now had to use a wheelchair and live downstairs in his house. The local health authority provided him with aids for disabled living including a wheelchair and—as there was no downstairs toilet in his house—a commode. He had been claiming benefits totalling £62 000 over 5 years when information was received saying that he was self-employed supplying decorating services.

It was alleged that Mr Green was lying about his care needs in order to claim benefit and an investigation was commenced. Proving the normal system is a simple task of documenting and obtaining witness statements outlining the process for claiming benefit. Equally, proving that there was a deception was not, in the case of Mr Green, a difficult one. As alleged by the informant, Mr Green spent every working day painting and decorating at both domestic and business premises. Observations showed him carrying cans of paint, climbing ladders to paint buildings, and lifting ladders onto the top of his van. He was seen and video-taped in a variety of work-related situations showing that he was capable of activities that he had said in this claim for benefit that he was unable to perform. Checking the records of his (commercial) customers showed that he had been working as a painter and decorator for the whole period of the claim to benefit.

Proving dishonest intent in relation to his claims to health care benefits was also relatively easy, though it is necessary to do so indirectly through inference from his activities, rather than from the activities themselves. During the investigation, it was found that the medical aids in his possession, the wheelchair and commode were stored, unused for medical purposes, in his home. Questioning by the investigating officer established that he had obtained them not for their intended use but in order to add credibility to his claim that he was unable to manage for himself in his day-to-day living. It was his answers in this interview that provided evidence of dishonest intent, revealing his conscious motivation for his actions.

Evidence and proof

In the criminal courts, evidence of dishonest intent must meet the standard of proof required by law. It is well known that the criminal courts require evidence 'beyond reasonable doubt'. Often the layman will put the emphasis on doubt (indeed most defence lawyers do so) but the courts require that the 'doubt' be *reasonable*. There must be grounds for doubt, not just unreasonable prejudice against conviction. This is a matter for the Jury in criminal cases and the Judge will give them guidance on the meaning of 'reasonable doubt' but leave to the Jury a duty to consider and come to a view on guilt.

The burden of proving a case in criminal law rests on the prosecution[2] and in order to discharge that burden the prosecution must bring forward evidence to satisfy the court. There are three broad categories of evidence: (i) what the offender says; (ii) what third parties say about the offender(s); and (iii) expert testimony—including evidence from psychiatrists and clinical psychologists. Each witness may use exhibits and produce them (e.g. documents or videos) as part of their evidence.

---

[2] Though there are exceptions, as when a defendant has to prove an alibi.

What the offender says

This falls into two categories: first, what he says when making a claim to benefit, both orally and in writing. At this stage, the offender is not dealing with an investigator but with an administrator and will be expected to answer relevant questions asked to establish any entitlement.

At a later stage, there is normally an offence interview. What the suspect says in this interview will be recorded and the questions will largely seek to throw light on his motivation and intent. He will be warned[3] that he need not reply to the questions and that anything he does say may be used in evidence.

In the first of these interviews, the suspect will be seeking benefit. In order to establish entitlement a fraudster will have to lie when giving examples of care needs and providing some evidence of them. In the second, the investigator will point out to him evidence obtained in the course of an investigation. This may include video evidence of activities incompatible with the claimed care needs. The suspect will be required to provide explanations for discrepancies between his claimed care needs and the activities that he is shown to be engaged upon.

Since DLA is largely based upon a self-report by the claimant, it is likely that the claimant will seek to justify his self-report during the offence interview. The claimant will view the offence interview as adversarial and his position as a suspect will, no doubt, influence his responses. The interviewing officer will be seeking to establish whether the claimed condition has the disabling effect claimed and, if not, the reason why the claimant falsely stated the effect.

The offender will often seek to throw doubt upon the investigator's evidence—whether this is verbal evidence (e.g. by saying, 'I misunderstood the question asked when I first made a claim') or, on any evidence from observations ('I was having a good day but it was the only one that month'). This adversarial situation is not conducive to open and frank discussion and there is a clear parallel to the civil law situation of a doctor faced with a false health insurance claim. Where they diverge is in the right of a suspect in a criminal investigation to maintain his silence.

Evidence from third parties

This includes evidence from others who know the claimant and can speak about what they have seen (or what he/she has said to them). In proving an illness deception, this evidence is invaluable. Often this evidence will include video surveillance taken by investigators showing the claimant engaged in activities that his alleged disability would preclude, but that is not necessarily conclusive.

There are three reasons why video evidence may not be completely convincing to a jury. The first is the above-mentioned reference to the 'I was having a good day that day' defence. Often a disability is uneven in the effect it has on a sufferer and any single video will not be conclusive—though, of course, a series of videos showing the claimant without signs of a disability would be more convincing.

The second reason videos (even a succession of them) can be undermined is that they may not show when the improvement they illustrate had taken place. Indeed, for a long-term claim to benefit it is unlikely that they will. For example, a person claiming DLA for 5 years might now argue that the condition has improved (as shown by the video evidence) but by itself that does not prove that the condition was always overstated. There will, of course, be no video evidence available from the early years as investigators only undertake surveillance after they have accepted an allegation for investigation (and after consideration of whether the intrusion of privacy that is implicit in surveillance is justified by the circumstances).

---

[3] The full form of the caution used in English law need not be set out in this chapter.

Establishing the date from which the fraud commenced is important, not least because the financial benefit gained from fraud is one of the measures by which an assessment of seriousness is made by the Courts. A person who persists in a proven false claim over 5 years is seen in a different light to someone where the only evidence of improved physical condition relates to the last 6 weeks out of that 5 years.

The last problem with video evidence is that it shows only the actions/behaviours of a claimant—it cannot reveal his/her motivation. The complexities of proving dishonest intent have been referred to earlier in this chapter. Objectively, the video may show behaviours inconsistent with a claimed condition but the subjective test requires the Jury in any alleged fraud case to consider whether the claimant himself knew that his behaviour was dishonest, by the standards of the reasonable and honest man.

Where there is doubt this leads us to the final category of evidence, the expert witness.

Expert witness

If there is a defence argument that the defendant's mental condition is relevant a clinical psychologist or a psychiatrist may be called to provide testimony. Where there is a serious and credible debate in the medical world about conditions such as factitious disorder (and the debate is relevant to a particular case) the expert witness will refer to that controversy. The fact that there is debate in both academic and clinical psychology on these issues related to the role is therefore relevant to the practical criminal investigation.

Where prosecution guilt is dependent on proving a dishonest intent (as is always the case where fraud is alleged), disagreement by expert witnesses on the nature of the intent, judged subjectively, will always be a problem for the prosecution, judge, and jury. It is at least possible that this evidence will generate 'reasonable doubt' in all these parties regarding the intent of a person claiming benefit.

The investigator must also show that the financial benefit was the intended outcome of that deception. With factitious disorders this becomes almost impossible to prove. The following illustrates the potential for factitious disorders to confound the issues in proving *dishonest intent* in an alleged fraud:

- If a person feigns illness to avoid a social obligation and finds that this brings with it an *incidental and unintended* financial benefit, the case against him/her may fail (though, if he/she continues to claim monies that he/she is not entitled to after he/she becomes aware of the financial benefit he/she will probably be found guilty).

- If a claimant of social welfare benefits claims to be physically incapacitated by a factitious disorder (and factitious disorders are accepted by the court as a reality!) any case against him/her may fail because there will be doubt over the defendant's intent.

- If a claimant to welfare benefit was revealed to be knowingly feigning a disability (or indeed a factitious disorder) for the express purpose of making a claim, then the case against him should succeed.

In practice, there are very few defendants who would claim that they did not know it was wrong to defraud the benefit system. More often they will seek to claim that there was no deception and here the investigator only needs to use more mundane tests. Mr Green, the painter and decorator, claimed that he needed a wheelchair, and obtained one from the Health Authority in order to add credence to his claim. In fact, the wheelchair was found to be under the stairs in his house, covered in dust and clearly had not been used for months (if at all). Although the wheelchair had been obtained by him to support his claim to benefit, his lack of use of it in his everyday life became evidence of his deception.

Similarly, the commode he had obtained to support his story that he could not go upstairs to use the toilet was placed in a garden shed. There it was used both to store fishing tackle (a 'convenient' bowl in which to place hooks, line, and lead weights!). Mr Green's tale of a physical disability crumbled under the weight of evidence that he had been seen working as a painter and decorator (with videos of him engaged on that trade) and evidence of his non-use of the nursing aides he had discarded. In this case (as indeed with most), the physical evidence against a person claiming disability beyond that which is warranted by any physical cause there may be—and in Mr Green's case there was none at all—is accepted by the courts as sufficient to show an intention to deceive.

Political and social context

So far in this chapter, we have outlined the task for the investigator of a criminal fraud where there is illness deception. However, there are constraints on DWP investigators. Investigators do not work in a void and there is more work to be done than there are investigators to undertake it. Even if there were a complete match between resources and reported fraud, there are still some cases that would not be investigated. These include the following.

Attorney General's guidelines on public interest

There are guidelines on the value of fraud, discouraging prosecution where small sums of money are involved. Similarly, there are some categories of fraudster where it is recommended that prosecution would not normally be in the public interest. Examples include children and persons of advanced years (though even here aggravated cases will result in prosecution). It should also be acknowledged that the Department has priorities that may preclude investigations in some areas where it is felt that the resource can more effectively be used elsewhere.

Legal constraints (including the Human Rights Act)

The HRA and associated legislation requires that investigations are conducted with due regard to the right to privacy. This is entirely compatible with the values of the DWP and requires clear criteria in case selection to ensure that we only investigate those cases where we do not illegally intrude on a client's privacy. This precludes the use of some investigation techniques and inevitably selects some cases out for other, non-investigative action.

Working and claiming

Figure 24.2 illustrates the narrow focus of this chapter. We are concerned with people claiming benefits that have, as a condition of payment, a need for personal care because of disability or ill health. There are two categories of claimant and the two examples given in this chapter are drawn from one of these: people who are in work, claiming unemployment benefit and dishonestly boost their income by claiming care needs. These people are in effect making two categories of false claim to benefit, claiming both unemployment benefits and benefits relating to personal care.

The other category of fraudster involved in illness deception includes people who are unable to find work, despite making efforts to do so, and resort to illness deception as a means of boosting their social security income above the level to which they are entitled. There are some in this group who would work if work were available to them. The problem with this second group is in establishing the date on which the deception commenced. Was it from the date of the first claim or did a genuine condition requiring care improve over time. In other words, when did the fraud start? We have discussed this problem in relation to video evidence earlier in this chapter. In the absence of evidence, the Department sometimes is driven to restrict action to withdrawing benefit from a current date.

However, with those who are working and claiming there is a short-cut available that avoids the need to prove the duration of the illness deception. Access to employment records allows investigators to concentrate upon proving that the suspect is working without declaring it. Here the investigation can focus on obtaining evidence of deception and dishonest intent in the easier area of a false declaration that the claimant was out of work, whereas in fact he was working. In short, the investigator will concentrate on proving deception in relation to employment rather than proving an illness deception.

In working and claiming cases, the issue of intent does not depend on a feigned care need but on the lie made at the point of making a claim for benefit. The investigators can and do side-step the problem of proving health deception (and any issues of mental causation of a physical ailment) and seek to persuade the courts—to the criminal standard—that the claims to unemployment benefit are false, bringing down the claims to DLA and other health-related benefits in its wake.

Conclusions

Illness deception is a serious issue for the criminal law investigator and problems in proving intent have the ability to potentially severely handicap successful investigations. However, where a claimant is working and claiming the problems can be avoided through pursuing the false declarations about income from work rather than the false declarations about care needs. The already small overlap between benefit fraud and malingering illustrated in Fig. 24.1 is further reduced by this practical approach to proving fraud within the UK benefit system. Within the remaining area of common interest the complexities of factitious disease and the depth of academic debate is of only passing interest in the great majority of investigation cases. As the case illustrated in this chapter shows, fraud investigators are more concerned with wheelchairs and commodes than with the more arcane issue of whether factitious diseases exist. Even without the debate on factitious disorder, investigating illness deception is resource intensive, costly, and complex. This pragmatic approach used by benefit fraud investigators releases resource so they can efficiently pursue their primary purpose of using their specialist skills across the full range of benefit fraud.

25 Neuropsychological tests and techniques that detect malingering

Richard I. Frederick

Abstract

Certain classes of examinations for neuropsychological disability are likely to include feigned presentations of impairment. Clinical judgment alone is typically insufficient to discriminate true disability from malingered or exaggerated impairment. Psychological tests and techniques have been designed to improve detection of malingering. The strategy of 'symptom validity testing' involves comparing performance on tasks that require a discrimination between two choices to that which would have occurred by guessing. 'Floor effect' and 'atypical performance' strategies compare test performance with that of genuinely impaired individuals. 'Performance curve analysis' identifies how performance accuracy changes as test item difficulty changes. Criterion group designs are typically used to develop malingering tests and to compute classificatory accuracy. Criterion group contamination typically results in underestimation of test sensitivity and specificity. The author recommends modifications to the process of validating the diagnostic efficiencies of malingering tests to overcome this limitation.

Reasons why individuals feign neuropsychological problems

Some individuals who undergo evaluation of neuropsychological functioning attempt to influence the conclusions of the evaluator by demonstrating only a limited extent of their cognitive capacities, claiming inability to understand or to comprehend, feigning lowered verbal and reasoning skills, actively pretending to have compromised memory abilities, or making false claims of amnesia. Typically, such individuals are concerned with either monetary matters or criminal matters.

Monetary matters

In some litigation cases, individuals invent or exaggerate neuropsychological impairment in order to increase the likelihood decision makers (e.g. judges or juries) will conclude they are eligible for damages (if they can simultaneously demonstrate someone's actions could be construed as negligent and the source of some putative injury). Individuals in this category may have actually had some injury at the time of some action or accident caused by the defendant, but at the time of litigation perceive a need to present as currently injured. Alternatively, some individuals may choose to defraud a disability payment service (e.g. worker's compensation system or governmental or military disability system) by inventing or exaggerating neuropsychological impairment. In doing so, the individual is often constrained to present as impaired for as long as they wish to collect the disability payment.

Criminal matters

Evidence that basic cognitive capacities are intact is typically predictive of an ability to assist counsel and to appreciate one's circumstances sufficiently to contribute to decision-making. Evidence of impaired neuropsychological functioning, however, may lead to the conclusion that the defendant cannot provide the assistance the attorney requires to evaluate the completeness or accuracy of witness statements, cannot track decisions throughout the process, or cannot maintain alertness and awareness at critical moments. A finding of incompetency may result in an outcome which is favourable to a defendant, including a postponement of trial (which may lead to a lower likelihood of successful prosecution), the introduction of tenable mental state defence evidence, or even a decision not to prosecute.

Using tests to identify instances of improbability

Greiffenstein *et al.* (1994) found that 41 per cent of 106 consecutive referrals for neuropsychological evaluation of mild traumatic brain injury met two of four criteria for malingering. Rogers *et al.* (1994) polled 320 forensic mental health specialists who had an average of 14 years experience and who had completed an average of over 300 forensic evaluations. Their mean estimation of the rate of malingering in forensic examinations was 15.7 per cent. A meta-analysis by Rohling *et al.* (1995) revealed that the potential for compensation resulted in increased reports of pain and decreased treatment effectiveness (an effect size of 0.60).

Because a significant proportion of individuals choose to misrepresent their abilities when completing neuropsychological assessment, a number of procedures have been developed specifically for investigating the likelihood of malingering in neuropsychological assessment. Current developments in malingering test development can be traced to Rey (1941, 1958), Pankratz *et al.* (1975), Lezak (1983), Faust *et al.* (1988a,b) and Rogers (1988). Rey, a neuropsychologist in Geneva, described a number of procedures to identify malingered performance. Pankratz described a method to make abilities evident even when individuals were motivated to hide them. His writings on forced-choice testing led to the development of the most commonly used techniques to assess suspicious memory complaints. Lezak reported a number of Rey's procedures in her second edition of *Neuropsychological Assessment*. Prior to this, the techniques were not well known in the United States; subsequently, a number of investigations of the techniques she reported were published in American journals. Faust challenged the community of neuropsychologists to develop bona fide methods of malingering detection; he and his colleagues demonstrated that even highly skilled neuropsychologists could not reliably identify malingered performance simply by a review of responses to standard neuropsychological instruments. This led to a broad effort to develop specific tests for identifying malingering. Rogers (1988, 1990a,b) proposed a non-condemnatory model of malingering, articulated research methodologies for investigating malingering, and edited a compendium on detection of malingering of a variety of presentations (e.g. psychosis, personal distress). Foremost, Rogers concluded that the single most important purpose of tests and techniques was to identify convincing instances of improbability in presentation, only one element of the process of determining a person is malingering impairment.

Strategies for identifying improbable presentations

Rogers, *et al.* (1993) summarized a number of test and technique strategies used to assess malingered neuropsychological impairment. Four of these strategies have been investigated and reported sufficiently to warrant comment here.

Symptom validity testing (comparison to chance)

'Symptom validity testing' (Pankratz 1979) originally referred to the use of two-alternative forced-choice tasks which involve choosing a response between a target and foil, but may now be more commonly understood to refer to any process that investigates the likelihood of malingering. Generally, the forced-choice tasks referred to here require little ability or effort for consistent successful performance (i.e. they have low task demand); consequently, successful performances do not indicate any particular strengths (Faust and Auckley 1998). In these procedures, the subject's performance is compared to that expected by chance (i.e. random responding). A number of two-alternative trials constitutes a test. A response is required for each trial, by 'guessing' if necessary. The number of trials for which the target is chosen constitutes the total test score. Randomly choosing a target or foil within a test for an infinite number of tests results in a normal distribution of total scores (Siegel 1956). This allows for computation of the probability of observing any total score. For example, choosing the correct answer only 40 per cent of the time across 100 trials (a total score of 40) occurs only about 2 per cent of the time when answers are chosen randomly. It is generally agreed that when the probability of observing a total score is less than 5 per cent, the total score is referred to as an instance of 'below-chance' responding. Siegel (1956) reported the computational procedure to derive a z-score (and probability of observation) for any total score based on the number of trials and the probabilities of correct and incorrect responses (these probabilities are typically held equal to each other; i.e. both probabilities $= 0.5$). Given the generally very low probability of observing individuals with absolutely no ability to respond correctly, a below-chance performance is generally highly predictive of malingering (Frederick and Denney 1998).

A legitimate aspect of the task is to induce below-chance responding in participants who wish to deceive the examiner. Of course, for trials in which the probabilities of choosing either target or foil are equal and the subject has no capacity to correctly complete the task, the examiner cannot induce below- or above-chance responding; the subject merely chooses responses at random. But for individuals who wish to deceive the examiner and can discern the correct response, the examiner can sometimes induce below-chance responding by identifying the task as an important factor in determining whether impairment exists. During the examination, feedback after each trial about whether the response was correct or incorrect can lead deceptive subjects to believe they are doing too well, inducing them to increase their rate of delivering the wrong response. For subjects who intend to do well, such practices merely induce them to try even harder to respond correctly.

The use of this technique began with an assessment of suspicious psychophysiological complaints (Pankratz *et al.* 1975). It has been extended to investigation of suspicious complaints of memory impairment, amnesia, and lowered cognitive functioning.

Memory complaints

The strategy of comparison to chance is most commonly encountered as a digit memory test, in which a five-digit number is presented for memorization and, after an interference task of variable duration, two choices are presented for recognition. The Portland Digit Recognition Test (Binder 1990) is a well-researched two-alternative forced-choice five-digit number recognition task. The Victoria Symptom Validity Test (Slick *et al.* 1994) is a computerized adaptation of the five-digit memory task. Both these procedures, and less common digit memory tests, require up to 45 min or more to administer. The Test of Memory Malingering (TOMM; Tombaugh 1997), however, rapidly assesses the believability of memory impairment claims. Subjects are shown 50 simple line drawings at the rate of one per 3 s, then, over 50 trials, they are required to rapidly distinguish between two line drawings, identifying which was the one in original set of 50.

Only a small percentage of individuals who malinger actually perform below chance on these procedures, most likely because these tasks may not directly assess the complaint of the individual and because below-chance responding on simple tasks rather obviously reflects bad intentions. Individuals may not wish to risk being so obvious in feigning except when they have no other way to convince the examiner their complaint is real. Although forced-choice testing of memory abilities has become rather prevalent, because only a relatively small percentage of individuals score below chance, the primary strategy of detection for most of these tests has shifted from comparison to chance to a floor effect. For example, on the TOMM, this changes a potential cutoff score for a decision of feigning from less than 40 per cent correct to less than 90 per cent correct.

Amnesia complaints

Frederick *et al.* (1995) proposed a method to directly evaluate suspicious claims of amnesia (see also Denney 1996; Frederick and Denney 1998). Examiners identify a domain of information the subject claims not to know. Two-alternative forced-choice questions are generated from this domain. Questions are ordered so that feedback about performance does not influence choices on later questions. Because the choice of answers for truly amnesic subject can be influenced by antecedent probability, it is important to avoid questions in which the target answer has a low probability of being chosen by a truly amnesic individual. For example, bank robbers occasionally dress as women. Consider an accused bank robber who is alleged to have dressed as a woman, and who claims amnesia for the event. If the examiner asks 'What clothing did the police say you wore? A dress or shirt and trousers?,' the foil (i.e. 'shirt and trousers'), by antecedent probability, has a much higher probability of being the correct answer. Items which are systematically biased by antecedent probability to result in higher rates of choosing the foil create a substantial risk of misclassifying truly amnesic subjects as malingerers. Fortunately, it is easy to generate questions which are not systematically biased (Denney 1996). Even so, Frederick and Denney (1998) demonstrated that as long as the average probability of correct response is equal between target and foil across all items, there is no increased risk of misclassification of amnesic subjects. This procedure has proven to have a much higher rate of below-chance responding among malingerers than digit memory tests, most likely because it directly assesses the specific complaint of the subject.

Cognitive complaints

The Validity Indicator Profile (VIP; Frederick 1997) comprises two sub-tests, non-verbal picture matrices and word definition problems (each sub-test in a two-alternative format), 100 and 78 trials, respectively. Patients are obliged to complete all test items, guessing the answer when they cannot solve the item. Unlike most comparison-to-chance procedures, the items (trials) do not have equivalent difficulty; VIP items comprise a hierarchy of difficulty and many of the items are difficult to solve. Performances below chance are indicative of malingered cognitive impairment, but the primary detection strategy for the VIP is performance curve analysis (comparing average response accuracy across ranges of item difficulty).

Floor effect

The floor effect strategy involves observing performance on tasks or problems that concern over-learned material (e.g. stating one's identity or age, reciting the alphabet) or are typically easily accomplished by most individuals, including those with genuine impairment. That is, the strategy identifies performances below a level expected even for individuals with true impairment. The most commonly known floor effect test is the Rey 15-Item Memory Test (RMT; Rey 1958), which requires the memorization and recall of easily retained information.

Rey 15-Item Memory Test

The RMT (Rey 1958; Lezak 1983) consists of a card with five rows of three items that appear in a familiar logical sequence.

A   B   C

1   2   3

a   b   c

O   □   △

I   II   III

Instructions vary, but, following Lezak, subjects are typically told to remember all 15 items during a 10-s exposure. After the stimulus items are removed, a 10-s delay is sometimes interpolated, but more generally subjects are told to immediately reproduce the items in the correct order on a blank sheet of paper. Frederick (2002a) reported Rey's original instructions for the RMT; they differ substantially from the instructions popularized by Lezak (1983). The score consistently reported in the literature is the number of correctly recalled items (Goldberg and Miller 1986; Schretlen *et al.* 1991; Bernard *et al.* 1993; Lee *et al.* 1992; Hays *et al.* 1993; Guilmette *et al.* 1994; Arnett *et al.* 1995). Scores range from 0 to 15; lower scores are consistent with an intention to perform poorly.

Lezak (1983, p. 619) reported: 'Anyone who is not significantly deteriorated can recall at least three of the five character sets.' This cut-off score (i.e. fewer than nine items reproduced) has often been criticized as too non-specific for persons with true impairment, but other researchers have recommended higher cut-off scores, concluding a cut-off of less than 9 is too insensitive. Frederick (2000b, 2003), and Rogers *et al.* (1993) reviewed many of the issues involved in selecting a cut-off score for the RMT. In general, scores of nine or higher cannot necessarily be construed as indicative of cooperation. Scores below nine are generally meaningful and should lead to further investigation of why the performance is so poor. Malingering and significant neuropsychological impairment remain competing explanations; poor performances in the absence of obvious neuropsychological impairment should lead to pointed consideration of malingering. The RMT is a useful procedure to investigate suspicious presentations, but it does not appear to have the capacity to be used reliably as a primary detection method for malingered cognitive impairment.

Other procedures incorporating a floor effect

One strategy of identifying feigned performances has been to identify a floor for some commonly administered neuropsychological tests. For example, Greiffenstein *et al.* (1994, 1996) compared performances between impaired individuals and probable malingerers on a number of tasks in order to establish the floor for individuals with true memory impairments. Generally, probable malingerers performed below these floor.

Most of the two-alternative forced-choice tests which were designed to identify malingering by below-chance responding have modified their primary detection strategy to a floor effect. The tests can still employ a below-chance strategy, but the current cut-off scores for many of these procedures are above chance, but below the mean score for groups of significantly impaired individuals. For example, as noted above, the cut-off score for the TOMM is less than 90 per cent correct; even most individuals with significant cognitive and memory impairment can correctly identify 90 per cent of the target responses, particularly on a second administration of the test.

Performing below personal floors

Frederick *et al.* (2000) compared performance on a cognitive test to an individual's *own* floor. That is, the highest demonstrated capacity of the individual to consistently respond correctly to test items was construed not as a ceiling, but as the individual's 'floor' (a *personal* floor). Failure of the test-taker to respond perfectly or near-perfectly for test items below their own floor strongly supported a conclusion of inadequate effort. Frederick (2000*a*) extended the application of personal floor to a comparison of performance on word recognition memory tasks (easier) with word recall memory tasks (more difficult). Because recognition memory is typically much stronger than recall memory for most individuals (e.g. see Robinson and Johnson 1996), individuals who are exerting their best effort should easily recognize more words than they are able to recall without prompting. In this construction, performance on the recall task constitutes a personal floor; performance on a recognition task that does not exceed the floor is considered indicative of non-compliance.

The advantage of the personal floor effect is that the floor is established by the individual taking the test and not by a normative group. When performance is below a floor established by a normative group, there exist competing explanations for why the performance is below the floor: severe impairment, bad intentions, or poor effort. But, when individuals have themselves demonstrated a capacity to respond correctly at a certain level, it is difficult to explain how performing below that level on an easier task could be construed as evidence of good intentions and strong effort. Poor performance below a personal floor cannot be properly construed as a result of severe impairment.

Atypical performance

The strategy of 'atypical performance' when applied to testing concerns how closely performance resembles that of genuine patients. For example, Mittenberg *et al.* (1995, 1996) and McKinzey *et al.* (1997) have proposed discriminant function analyses to evaluate performance on neuropsychological test batteries. Test scores are inserted into a lengthy formula, and a value is generated. If this value exceeds a cut-off, the test-taker is classified as a malingerer. Cross-validations of these regression formulas generally result in unduly inflated false positive rates, identifying a high rate of truly impaired individuals as malingerers (e.g. McKinzey and Russell 1997). In an examination of the effectiveness of discriminant function analysis of patient performances on neuropsychological test batteries, Van Gorp *et al.* (1999, p. 249) concluded: '... [clinicians] should rely more heavily on neuropsychological measures which have either been designed to detect malingering or are clinical measures which have been validated for the detection of malingering in making a determination of malingering versus honest responding.' These findings support the recommendations of Pankratz (1988) who concluded the atypical performance strategy was unwise given the prevalence of 'atypical' presentations.

A different approach to the strategy of atypical performance is to measure consistency of performance across two administrations of the same tests. Reitan and Wolfson (1996, 1997, 1998) found notable distinctions in test–retest performance for groups of individuals who were either in litigation or not. Individuals who were not in litigation consistently demonstrated test performance which conformed to expectations of post-injury habilitation. Individuals in litigation (and not necessarily suspected of malingering) consistently demonstrated unreliable test performance. Analysis of the validity of responding on the VIP (Frederick 1997) includes comparison of consistency of response on two equivalent forms of the test imbedded in the total test (e.g. two 50-item equivalent forms in the 100-item non-verbal VIP). Frederick (1997) and Frederick and Crosby (2000) reported three distinct ways to evaluate the consistency of performance when many of the items are too difficult for test-takers to answer correctly without guessing.

Performance curve analysis

Performance curve analysis consists of examining performance on test items across a broad range of difficulty. Essentially, the subject's average performance on test items is compared against average item difficulty with the expectation that response accuracy will decrease as item difficulty increases (see Gudjonsson and Shackleton 1986; McKinzey *et al.* 1999). Frederick and Foster (1991) and Frederick *et al.* (1994) presented large-scale studies demonstrating the effectiveness of a performance curve strategy to identify invalid responding. These initial studies were the basis for publishing the VIP.

Validity Indicator Profile

The VIP (Frederick 1997; see also Frederick 2002*b*) is a measure of response validity which is intended to be administered concurrently within a battery of cognitive tests. The VIP consists of two sub-tests; each can be administered and scored separately. The VIP non-verbal subtest presents 100 picture-matrix problems that require simple matching, complex matching, analogous decision-making, progression, addition, subtraction, and abstraction. The VIP verbal subtest consists of 78 word definition problems. Test-takers are presented with a stimulus word (e.g. *carpet*) and are asked to choose one of two possible answers that is more similar in meaning to the stimulus (e.g. *rug* or *shoe*). For both sub-tests, the items have a hierarchy of difficulty but are presented randomly with respect to item difficulty. Subjects are required to provide a response for each item. Once testing is completed, the items are scored and then re-ordered by difficulty.

As its fundamental analysis of response validity, the items are re-ordered by difficulty, scored (0 = incorrect, 1 = correct), and plotted to generate a performance curve demonstrating the average performance of the test taker across a increasingly difficult range of test items. The plotted points of the performance curve are *running means*, computed by averaging a set of 10 consecutive scored item responses. Responses to items 1–10 are averaged to yield the first plotted running mean, representing the individual's average performance on the 10 easiest items. Responses 2–11 are averaged to compute the second plotted running mean. This process continues until the last (most difficult) item has been included in the plot of the last running mean. The performance curve is then a plot of the running mean on the vertical axis against the plot of its serial position (i.e. 1, 2, 3, and so on) on the horizontal axis.

For compliant test-takers, the two-alternative forced-choice format should result in near-perfect or perfect performance within the test-taker's range of capacity to answer items correctly and

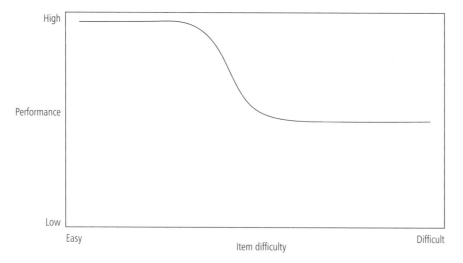

Figure 25.1 Performance curves for compliant test-takers.

random responding once the test-taker has reached his/her ceiling of ability. This means that performance curves for compliant test-takers should be fairly similar in shape regardless of differences in ability. The curves will start and remain at about 100 per cent correct performance, go through a period of transition at the test taker's ceiling of ability, and then remain at about 50 per cent correct performance (i.e. random responding) through the remainder of the curve (see Fig. 25.1). Differences in cognitive capacity should result in differences in the length of the initial and ending segments of the curve, but the shape should remain similar among compliant performers.

Significant deviations from this expected curve have meaning and allow for some reasonable conclusions about the response style of the individual. For example, an individual who performs at 80 per cent throughout most of the test (see Fig. 25.2, line A) may intend to respond correctly but is probably expending insufficient effort (*careless responding* or *inconsistent responding*). It is likely that the test-taker could have performed perfectly on much easier items, given that he/she correctly solved 80 per cent of the moderately difficult items. Another deviation from the expected curve might be for an individual who performs at about 50 per cent throughout the entire test (Fig. 25.2, line B). Such an individual is probably marking answers without regard to item content (*irrelevant responding*). As a final example, consider an individual who demonstrates a consistent increase in correct responding as the test items become more difficult (Fig. 25.2, line C). Such an individual is most likely intentionally choosing the wrong answer despite knowing the correct solution (*malingering* or *suppression*) and responding randomly only when the correct answer is not known.

Frederick (1997) postulated that the shape of performance curves observed on the VIP result from a combination of two test-taking characteristics: *motivtion* and *effort*. Motivation refers to the intention of the test taker to perform well or poorly. Effort refers to the intensity of application of true ability to perform well or poorly (e.g. low effort or high effort). In this scheme, effort and intention are independent constructs.

This cross-classification of motivation and effort results in four response styles: compliant, careless, malingered, and irrelevant (see Fig. 25. 1).[1] *Compliant* responding is characterized by *high*

---

[1] In a revision to the VIP scheduled for release in late 2002, the classifications of 'careless' and 'malingering' will be replaced respectively by 'inconsistent' and 'suppression'.

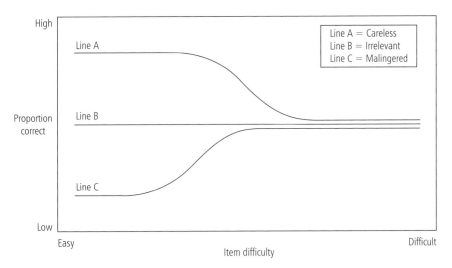

Figure 25.2 Deviation from the expected performance curve.

effort and an *intention to respond correctly*). Compliant test-takers are cooperative with testing procedures, and their performance accurately represents their ability. *Careless* or *inconsistent* test taking is also characterized by the *intention to perform well*. However, it differs from compliant responding in that there is *incomplete effort* to respond correctly. Careless test taking may result from inattention, distraction, or fatigue. *Malingering* or*suppression* is characterized by *high effort when intending to perform poorly*, in which the test-taker strives to feign cognitive deficits in a convincing manner. Finally, *irrelevant* responding is characterized by *token effort when intending to perform poorly*. Irrelevant test-takers may be disengaged from the task of responding correctly, perhaps not caring about the outcome of the assessment. Random responding is included in this category.

Evidence of the construct validity of these sub-classifications was reported in Frederick *et al.* (2000). They examined data for a large sample of criminal defendants who were completing court-ordered examinations of competency and criminal responsibility. Classifications of response style by VIP performance curve characteristics were supported by an analysis of concurrently administered Rey malingering tests when matched on essential VIP measures of test performance to control for potential effects from cognitive capacity. Large to very large effect sizes on malingering test performance were seen for individuals classified as 'motivation to perform well' ('compliant' and 'careless' classifications) when compared to individuals classified as 'motivated to perform poorly' ('irrelevant' and 'malingering'). Moderate to large effect sizes on malingering test performance were seen for differences in motivation even when the effort of subjects was presumed to be low ('irrelevant' versus 'careless' performance curves). There were zero-order effects on malingering test performance when 'compliant' test takers were compared with those classified as 'careless' (i.e. both classes presumed motivated to perform well, but different in effort expended), but defendants classified as 'careless' had significantly higher scores on MMPI-2 (Butcher *et al.* 1989) carelessness indicators when compared to defendants classified as 'compliant'. Furthermore, Frederick *et al.* (2000) hypothesized a mechanism of careless responding and simulated that process by computer for 4000 'compliant' curves. The simulation of careless responding resulted in the predicted changes to the performance curve features which are used to classify responding as 'careless'.

Criterion group contamination in the development of procedures to identify malingering

It is difficult to establish pure criterion groups for research concerning the diagnostic efficiencies of tests that purport to detect malingered cognitive impairment. Rogers (1997*a,b*) has promoted the use of 'known groups' (clinical criterion groups) in malingering research because of the superior generalizability of such designs over the use of 'simulators' (analogue criterion groups in which individuals play roles). Nevertheless, it is only with great optimism that one may speak of a 'known groups' design, given that the nature of malingering research typically precludes one from 'knowing' the true status of clinical participants (Greiffenstein *et al.* 1994, 1995, 1996; Viglione *et al.* 1995). Within simulation designs, researchers can only hope that participants perform as instructed; often it turns out that many did not (Goebel 1983; Frederick *et al.* 1994; Arnett *et al.* 1995). For example, in an article on the validation of the VIP, Frederick and Crosby (2000) noted it was clear that the cross-validation group of 'non-compliant participants' contained a large proportion of individuals who had obviously completed the VIP compliantly. Including them in the computations of test diagnostic efficiency obviously resulted in significant underestimations of VIP sensitivity.

More recent research on the VIP (Frederick *et al.* 2000) has avoided criterion group methodology. Instead, comparison groups have been formed by matching subjects performance curve characteristics suggesting different response sets with respect to the accompanying effect on concurrently administered tests of response style. Additionally, Frederick (2000*b*) demonstrated that, with appropriate methodology and analysis, the problem of criterion group impurity can be overcome by using comparison groups which contain both malingerers and compliant participants. Doing so actually allows for potentially more accurate estimates of sensitivity and specificity. For example, in that paper, Frederick (2000*b*) found that using a differential prevalence design for the RMT resulted in far superior estimates of sensitivity and specificity than reported in the literature on that test. Researchers who wish to develop malingering tests are strongly encouraged to address the limitations of criterion group methodology and to attempt validations of instruments in ways that do not depend on criterion group designs.

Conclusions

Individuals commonly feign neuropsychological impairment to win monetary claims related to putative disability or to persuade judges or juries that they should not be tried or convicted. Failure to include an assessment of feigned impairment in such examinations cannot be justified; clinical judgment alone is an insufficient substitute for available psychological tests and techniques. A large number of tests and techniques exist and can address a wide variety of complaints. In making decisions about which instruments to use, clinicians should consider the reliability and validity of the techniques. In particular, clinicians should question the process by which the procedure was validated, because some estimates of classificatory accuracy for certain tests vary widely. Criterion group contamination ('impaired' or 'control' groups containing individuals unmotivated to do their best or 'malingering' groups containing individuals unmotivated to simulate malingering or patients incorrectly classified as malingerers) should be considered as a primary reason for variability in reports of test sensitivity (true positive rate) and specificity (true negative rate).

References

Arnett, P. A., Hammeke, T. A., and Schwartz, L. (1995). Quantitative and qualitative performance on Rey's 15-Item test in neurological patients and dissimulators. *Clinical Neuropsychologist* **9**, 17–26.

Bernard, L. C., Houston, W., and Natoli, L. (1993). Malingering on neuropsychological memory tests: potential objective indicators. *Journal of Clinical Psychology*, **49**, 45–53.

Binder, L. M. (1990). Malingering following mild head trauma. *Clinical Neuropsychologist*, **4**, 25–36.

Butcher, J. N., Dahlstrom, W. G., Graham, J. R., Tellegen, A., and Kaemmer, B. (1989). *MMPI-2: Manual for administration and scoring*. University of Minnesota Press, Minneapolis, MN.

Denney, R. L. (1996). Symptom validity testing of remote memory in a criminal forensic setting. *Archives of Clinical Neuropsychology*, **11**, 589–603.

Faust, D. and Auckley, M. A. (1998). Did you think it was going to be easy? Some methodological suggestions for the investigation and development of malingering detection techniques. In *Detection of malingering during head injury litigation* (ed. C. R. Reynolds). Plenum, New York, NY.

Faust, D., Hart, K., and Guilmette, T. J. (1988a). Pediatric malingering: capacity of children to fake believable deficits on neuropsychological testing. *Journal of Consulting and Clinical Psychology*, **56**, 578–82.

Faust, D., Hart, K., Guilmette, T. J. and Arkes, H. R. (1988b). Neuropsychologists' capacity to detect adolescent malingerers. *Professional Psychology: Research & Practice*, **19**, 508–15.

Frederick, R. I. (1997). *The Validity Indicator Profile*. NCS Assessments, Minnetonka, MN.

Frederick, R. I. (2000a). A personal floor effect strategy to evaluate the validity of performance on memory tests. *Journal of Clinical and Experimental Neuropsychology*, **22**, 720–30.

Frederick, R. I. (2000b). Mixed group validation: a method to address the limitations of criterion group validation in research on malingering detection. *Behavioral Sciences and the Law*, **18**, 693–718.

Frederick, R. I. (2002a). A review of Rey's strategies for detecting malingered neuropsychological impairment. *Journal of Forensic Neuropsychology*. **2**, 1–25.

Frederick, R. I. (2002b). Review of the Validity Indicator Profile. *Journal of Forensic Neuropsychology*, **2**, 125–45.

Frederick, R. I. and Crosby, R. D. (2000). Development and validation of the Validity Indicator Profile. *Law and Human Behavior*, **24**, 59–82.

Frederick, R. I. and Denney, R. L. (1998). Minding your "*p*s and *q*s" when conducting forced-choice recognition tests. *The Clinical Neuropsychologist*, **12**, 193–205.

Frederick, R. I. and Foster, H. G. (1991). Multiple measures of malingering on a forced-choice test of cognitive ability. *Psychological Assessment*, **3**, 596–602.

Frederick, R. I., Sarfaty, S. D., Johnston, J. D., and Powel, J. (1994). Validation of a detector of response bias on a forced-choice test of nonverbal ability. *Neuropsychology*, **8**, 118–25.

Frederick, R. I., Crosby, R. D., and Wynkoop, T. F. (2000). Performance curve classification of invalid responding on the Validity Indicator Profile. *Archives of Clinical Neuropsychology*, **15**, 281–300.

Frederick, R. I., Carter, M., and Powel, J. (1995). Adapting symptom validity testing to evaluate suspicious complaints of amnesia in medicolegal evaluations. *Bulletin of the American Academy of Psychiatry and the Law*, **23**, 231–7.

Goebel, R. A. (1983). Detection of faking on the Halstead–Reitan neuropsychological test battery. *Journal of Clinical Psychology*, **39**, 731–42.

Goldberg, J. O. and Miller, H. R. (1986). Performance of psychiatric inpatients and intellectually deficient individuals on a task that assesses the validity of memory complaints. *Journal of Clinical Psychology*, **42**, 792–5.

Greiffenstein, M. F., Baker, W. J., and Gola, T. (1994). Validation of malingered amnesia measures in a large clinical sample. *Psychological Assessment*, **6**, 218–24.

Greiffenstein, M. F., Baker, W. J., and Gola, T. (1996). Comparison of multiple scoring methods for Rey's malingered amnesia measures. *Archives of Clinical Neuropsychology*, **11**, 283–93.

Greiffenstein, M. F., Gola, T., and Baker, W. J. (1995). MMPI-2 validity scales versus domain specific measures in detection of factitious traumatic brain injury. *The Clinical Neuropsychologist*, **9**, 230–40.

Gudjonsson, G. H. and Shackleton, H. (1986). The pattern of scores on Raven's Matrices during "faking bad" and "non faking" performances. *British Journal of Clinical Psychology*, **25**, 35–41.

Guilmette, T. J., Hart, K. J., Giuliano, A. J., and Leininger, B. E. (1994). Detecting simulated memory impairment: comparison of the Rey Fifteen-Item Test and the Hiscock Forced-Choice Procedure. *The Clinical Neuropsychologist*, **8**, 283–94.

Hays, J. R., Emmons, J., and Lawson, K. A. (1993). Psychiatric norms for the Rey 15-Item Visual Memory Test. *Perceptual and Motor Skills*, **76**, 1331–4.

Lee, G. P., Loring, D. W., and Martin, R. C. (1992). Rey's 15-Item Visual Memory Test for the detection of malingering: normative observations on patients with neurological disorders. *Psychological Assessment*, **4**, 43–6.

Lezak, M. D. (1983). *Neuropsychological assessment*, 2nd edn. Oxford University Press, New York, NY.

McKinzey, R. K. and Russell, E. W. (1997). A partial cross-validation of a Halstead–Reitan battery malingering formula. *Journal of Clinical and Experimental Neuropsychology*, **19**, 484–8.

McKinzey, R. K., Podd, M. H., Krehbiel, M. A., Mensch, A. J., and Trombka, C. C. (1997). Detection of malingering on the Luria–Nebraska Neuropsychological Battery: an initial and cross-validation. *Archives of Clinical Neuropsychology*, **12**, 505–12.

McKinzey, R. K., Podd, M. H., Krehbiel, M. A., and Raven, J. (1999). Detection of malingering on the Raven's Standard Progressive Matrices: a cross-validation. *British Journal of Clinical Psychology*, **38**, 435–9.

Mittenberg, W., Theroux-Fichera, S., Zielinski, R. E., and Heilbronner, R. L. (1995). Identification of malingered head injury on the Wechsler Adult Intelligence Scale—Revised. *Professional Psychology*, **26**, 491–8.

Mittenberg, W., Rotholc, A., Russell, E., and Heilbronner, R. (1996). Identification of malingered head injury on the Halstead–Reitan Battery. *Archives of Clinical Neuropsychology*, **11**, 271–81.

Pankratz, L. (1979). Symptom validity testing and symptom retraining: procedures for the assessment and treatment of functional sensory deficits. *Journal of Consulting and Clinical Psychology*, **47**, 409–10.

Pankratz, L. (1988). Malingering on intellectual and neuropsychological measures. In *Clinical assessment of malingering and deception* (ed. R. Rogers), pp. 169–92. Guilford, New York, NY.

Pankratz, L., Fausti, S. A., and Peed, S. (1975). A forced-choice technique to evaluate deafness in the hysterical or malingering patient. *Journal of Consulting and Clinical Psychology*, **43**, 421–2.

Reitan, R. and Wolfson, D. (1996). The question of validity of neuropsychological test scoes among head-injured litigants: development of a Dissimulation Index. *Archives of Clinical Neuropsychology*, **11**, 573–80.

Reitan, R. and Wolfson, D. (1997). Consistency of neuropsychological test scores of head-injured subjects involved in litigation compared with head-injured subjects not involved in litigation: development of the Retest Consistency Index. *The Clinical Psychologist*, **11**, 69–76.

Reitan, R. and Wolfson, D. (1998). Detection of malingeringand invalid test results using the Halstead–Reitan Battery. In *Detection of malingering during head injury litigation* (ed. C. R. Reynolds). Plenum, New York, NY.

Rey, A. (1941). L'examen psychologie dans les cas d'encephalopathie traumatique. *Archives de Psychologie*, **28**, 286–340.

Rey, A. (1958). *L'Examen clinique de psychologie*. Presses Universitaires de France, Paris.

Robinson, M. D. and Johnson, J. T. (1996). Recall memory, recognition memory, and the eyewitness confidence-accuracy correlation. *Journal of Applied Psychology*, **81**, 587–94.

Rogers, R. (ed.) (1988). *Clinical assessment of malingering and deception*. Guilford, New York, NY.

Rogers, R. (1990a). Development of a new classificatory model of malingering. *Bulletin of American Academy of Psychiatry and the Law*, **18**, 323–33.

Rogers, R. (1990b). Models of feigned mental illness. *Professional Psychology*, **21**, 182–8.

Rogers, R. (ed.) (1997*a*). *Clinical assessment of malingering and deception*, 2nd edn. Guilford, New York, NY.

Rogers, R. (1997*b*). Researching dissimulation. In *Clinical assessment of malingering and deception* (ed. R. Rogers), 2nd edn, pp. 398–426. Guilford, New York, NY.

Rogers, R., Harrell, E. H., and Liff, C. D. (1993). Feigning neuropsychological impairment: a critical review of methodological and clinical considerations. *Clinical Psychology Review*, **13**, 255–74.

Rogers, R., Sewell, K. W., and Goldstein, A. (1994). Explanatory models of malingering: a prototypical analysis. *Law and Human Behavior*, **18**, 543–52.

Rohling, M. L., Binder, L. M., and Langhinrichsen-Rohling, J. (1995). Money matters: a meta-analytic review of the association between financial compensation and the experience and treatment of chronic pain. *Health Psychology*, **14**, 537–47.

Schretlen, D., Brandt, J., Krafft, L., and van Gorp, W. (1991). Some caveats in using the Rey 15-Item Memory Test to detect malingered amnesia. *Psychological Assessment*, **3**, 667–72.

Siegel, S. (1956). *Nonparametric statistics for the behavioral sciences*. McGraw-Hill, New York, NY.

Slick, D., Hopp, G., Strauss, E., Hunter, M., and Pinch, D. (1994). Detecting dissimulation: profiles of simulated malingerers, traumatic brain-injury patients, and normal controls on a revised version of Hiscock and Hiscock's forced-choice memory test. *Journal of Clinical and Experimental Neuropsychology*, **16**, 472–81.

Tombaugh, T. N. (1997). The Test of Memory Malingering (TOMM): normative data from cognitively intact and cognitively impaired individuals. *Psychological Assessment*, **9**, 260–8.

Van Gorp, W. G., Humphrey, L. A., Kalechstein, A., Brumm, V. L., McMullen, W. J., Stoddard, M., and Pachana, N. A. (1999). How well do standard clinical neuropsychological tests identify malingering? A preliminary analysis. *Journal of Clinical and Experimental Neuropsychology*, **21**, 245–50.

Viglione, D. J., Fals-Stewart, W., and Moxham, Z. (1995). Maximizing internal and external validity in MMPI malingering research: a study of a military population. *Journal of Personality Assessment*, **55**, 280–95.

26 Misrepresentation of pain and facial expression

Kenneth D. Craig and Marilyn Hill

Abstract

A realistic human intuitive expectation that others will endeavour to optimize available opportunities usually leads to careful monitoring of their credibility. Consistent with this general social propensity, clinicians, and others are prepared to question the veracity of patient representations of being in pain. A high incidence of personal experience with pain and opportunities to observe others in pain appears to lead to good training in the role of being in pain when people are motivated to dissimulate pain. Personal, social, and economic pressures can also lead people to suppress evidence of pain, often leading to failure to secure needed medical care. Patients voluntarily faking or suppressing pain displays are generally quite successful in misleading observers. Nevertheless, consistent with theoretical expectations that there would be differences between genuine, faked, and suppressed pain, detailed coding of facial displays during these episodes suggests subtle differences that could be available to highly discerning observers. Investigations of training programmes designed to assist in the detection of deception indicate that corrective feedback is capable of improving detection accuracy.

Introduction

Suspicions concerning the credibility of representations about pain are commonplace in a broad range of clinical, organizational, and informal settings. Clinicians and others with responsibilities for people complaining of pain invariably feel an obligation to identify misrepresentation. This seems to be the case even if the estimate of the real incidence of malingering were low because of a sense of duty to discover deception. Hence, virtually all contacts with people in pain involve at least some form of assessment of the trustworthiness of their reports of symptoms and disability. This appears motivated by the necessity of using indirect evidence to assess the subjective experience of pain. Pain cannot be observed directly, as can physical pathology, and must be inferred through verbal or nonverbal evidence. Contributing to this skepticism is the tenuous relationship between organic pathology and reports of pain (Turk and Melzack 2001). If the person complaining of pain were known to suffer from an injury or painful disease, skepticism would usually be deemed inappropriate. The converse expectation argues that one should be wary if there is a minimal relationship between injury and complaints of pain. Many complaints of pain do not present with physical pathology, for example many forms of headache, abdominal pain, and neuropathic pain.

Evidence has not supported beliefs in a direct correspondence between tissue damage and pain; hence, a complex, multi-faceted model of pain has emerged which features the thoughts and feelings of the person in pain as well as sensory input (Wall and Melzack 1999).

Concern about misrepresentation is expressed most often regarding faked or exaggerated pain complaints, with suppression of pain receiving relatively minimal attention. Malingering is usually defined in accordance with the American Psychiatric Association (2000) interpretation as the intentional production of false or grossly exaggerated symptoms when motivated by external incentives. Suppression concerns efforts to disguise or deny the presence of pain. Documentation of the perceived benefits is less substantial here, but may include efforts to avoid recognition of dangerous illnesses, avoidance of the sick role, or fear of addictive pain medications (Kotarba 1983). Both fraudulent misrepresentation and defensive suppression deserve scrutiny because of their social and personal consequences. The former usually triggers anger, whereas the latter is likely to be ignored, or to lead to pity, with the imbalance perhaps reflecting a preoccupation with betrayal of trust and the perceived costs of the former. A sense of moral indignation does not seem to be provoked by people behaving stoically and the potential losses associated with denial of pain are not so obvious. While the individual would represent less of a demand on the health care system, increased personal risks of morbidity and mortality and long-term costs are a consequence, as denial of pain can be associated with failure to receive early or needed intervention.

Deception in everyday life

The interaction between the person complaining of pain and an interrogator evaluating information concerning the true nature of the person's complaints resembles many interpersonal transactions. Tendencies to be opportunistic can be recognized as commonplace and most people guard against being deceived. Not all ruses involve conscious deliberation or represent exploitation of others. One can conceive of a scale of duplicity ranging from impression management that most often is not conscious or the simplest of 'white lies' to major treachery and abuse of others, with malingered illness varying in terms of where it would fall on the scale. On the one hand, taking advantage of sick days provided in a union contract might be perceived to be of minor significance, if not favourably sanctioned by fellow employees; whereas fraudulent claims of injury designed to bilk insurance companies represent criminal behaviour. It may be possible to identify qualitative variations relating to the consequences of apprehension of lying, as more dramatic lies likely entail greater risks of detection, embarrassment, shame, or punishment.

A capacity for deception emerges early in life (Talwar and Lee 2002a, 2002b). Children learn to confront social demands as problems requiring solutions consistent with their perception of personal best interests. Children's minor deceits are usually treated with humour and patience, but they can be recognized as providing the grounds or even practice for dishonesty later in life. At the same time, children will be socialized in the perception and meaning of somatic experience, as parents seek to understand and control expressions of discomfort and illness behaviour. Socialized display rules come to govern the manner in which pain is expressed. This is dependent upon cognitive development relating to the ability to reason about the causes and effects of emotional displays, the ability to discriminate oneself from others, and the ability to implement knowledge to fit social and other contextual requirements (Zemen and Garber 1996). Frequent, usually minor, painful events are associated inevitably with childhood play and risk-taking (Gilbert-MacLeod *et al.* 2000). These personal experiences, and observation of other children's difficulties, provide opportunities to learn what represents danger, how adults react to minimize threat and provide care, and how to take care of oneself or to engage the help of parents and other adults (Craig 1986).

Young children can often be observed modelling their parents in minor complaints and parents often are suspicious of their children's credibility when avoidance of school or responsibilities seem to provide the motivation for complaints of being ill. It seems likely that the co-emergence of a capacity to deceive others and skill in sick role behaviour would provide the foundation for falsifying pain and illness behaviour later in life.

The ubiquity of at least minor and often unwitting social deceits tends to be paralleled by skepticism and an inherent propensity to carefully screen the credibility of others in virtually all social situations (Cosmides and Tooby 1992), particularly those where there is a likelihood of gain from misrepresentation. Under these latter circumstances there appears to be a potential for conscious intention to exploit others. Some dissemblers do get caught (Rogers 1997). In clinical settings, the process usually entails successive screening of different sources of information, often beginning with insights gained in the course of an initial interview. Thereafter, suspicions can be pursued through structured interviews, careful psychometric appraisal, planned behavioural observation, sometimes undertaken covertly using private surveillance, and evaluation of collateral information from archival sources or significant others (Craig et al. 1999). Various events can initiate an extensive search for evidence confirming malingering. Investigations usually emerge from observations of discrepancies between physical pathology and complaints or disabilities, but doubts about credibility often arise or exceed threshold as a result of observations made during an interview or physical examination.

A theoretical rationale for distinguishing spontaneous and dissembled pain expression

Is it possible that dissembled pain can be discriminated behaviourally from genuine pain? Clinicians often believe they can distinguish between falsified and genuine clinical presentations. The challenge appears considerable, as people are skilled in dissembling pain. Poole and Craig (1992) examined observer judgements of low back pain patients' reactions to a painful movement that was voluntarily intended to exaggerate pain or conceal pain. The judgements were more consistent with the patients' intentions than the actual pain they were suffering. Nevertheless, careful investigation of differences between genuine and voluntarily faked presentations, described below, suggests there are prospects for being able to make the discrimination. There also is a theoretical basis for expecting that misrepresentations of pain, either faked or suppressed, should differ qualitatively from actions instigated by the actual experience or absence of pain. There is reason to believe that behaviour under higher cortical control would differ from reflexive, automatic activity. The following develops these arguments and provides empirical investigations describing their legitimacy.

One can know the presence, severity, and nature of another person's pain only if it is manifest in behaviour, either verbal or nonverbal, and the observer is attuned to this information (Hadjistavropoulos and Craig 2002). Both deserve careful analysis. The use of language is a uniquely human adaptation permitting great control over situational demands. In the case of communications about pain, self-report is often characterized as the gold standard, but this fails to recognize its limitations (Craig 1992). Clinicians usually are enjoined to believe what the patient says (Meinhart and McCaffery 1983). This reflects efforts to rectify long traditions of excessive skepticism and undermanagement of pain (Lander 1990; Chambers et al. 1999). But, self-report is heavily influenced by the individual's perception of the adaptive demands of the immediate social context and will reflect response biases, situational demand factors, and environmental contingencies (Jensen 1997). It is not difficult to mouth the words of a lie and admitting the truth may well be seen as contrary to one's best interests. As well, people are often challenged when confronted with the need to characterize complex, multifaceted experiences using simple language (Melzack and Katz 1999). It becomes clear that self-report of pain is under the control of higher mental processes and usually is the product of complex reasoning concerning perceived best interests. Of course, the usual optimal adjustment to situations in which pain has become paramount would involve as honest and objective a report of personal experience as can be mustered. For that reason, self-report is commonly a good, methodologically convenient first measure. But the trust we have for self-report needs to be recognized as making us vulnerable to exploitation through misrepresentation of pain and illness behaviour.

In contrast, non-verbal behaviour often seems automatic or over-rehearsed and less subject to voluntarily control. Attention is finite and selective; hence, usually focused upon immediate situational demands and problem solving. Under these circumstances, well-rehearsed actions and sub-routines do not seem rigorously monitored or subjected to conscious executive control. Nonverbal actions of this type include paralinguistic qualities of speech, facial expression, and many features of body actions. Their independence of higher mental processes leaves them less subject to conscious distortion (Hadjistavroupoulos and Craig 2002). This is generally appreciated in daily social interactions. Observers often assume that non-verbal behaviour is less amenable to deception (Ekman and Friesen 1969, 1974), and assign greater importance to people's non-verbal behaviour when it is discordant with their verbal self-reports of emotion (DePaulo *et al.* 1978; Craig and Prkachin 1980; Jacox 1980). Pain research indicates that naïve judges and clinicians assign greater weight to nonverbal expression than to patient self-reports when judging the location, nature, and severity of pain experienced (Johnson 1977; Poole and Craig 1992). We have recognized the importance of nonverbal behaviour in identifying and measuring pain in people for whom self-report and higher cognitive functions are not available. For example, non-verbal measures provide valuable approaches to assessing pain in infants and young children, people with intellectual disabilities, brain damage, or dementia, and others (Hadjistavropoulos *et al.* 2001). But they also have potential for helping to identify spontaneous expression of pain when the credibility of self-report is questioned. There is an anatomical basis for the distinction. Voluntary movements appear controlled by cortical/pyramidal systems and involuntary facial movements appear under the control of subcortical/extrapyramidal systems (Rinn 1984). Current brain imaging investigations of the distributed regions of the brain involved during painful events implicate regions involved in motoric control of behaviour (Rainville *et al.* 1997, 2000). These seem to provide the potential of a physiological basis for distinguishing between genuine and deceptive facial expressions of pain.

This distinction between voluntary and involuntary manifestations of pain leads one to question how reasonable it is to characterize pain as an inherently private experience incomprehensible to observers. It may be more reasonable to acknowledge pain as having social dimensions, reflecting the public value of automatic, reflexive manifestations. Pain certainly plays an important internal role in warning of threats to personal safety and survival, enabling the individual to take action and either avoid or escape noxious perils. But overt manifestations in the form of vocalizations and other actions capable of signalling danger and threat to conspecifics would have potential survival value for these others. They then would be in a position either to escape the menace themselves, or, even if the harm to the injured person threatened them, to attend to the needs of that person. The public nature of pain and distress is evident in human infants (Craig and Grunau 1993). Their reactions to distress and pain are dramatic when the totality of the vocalizations and non-vocal behaviour are considered. This probably reflects human infants' protracted substantial dependency upon mothers and other adults in the early years of life. The adaptive functions of signalling distress are evident from the perspective of evolutionary psychology. While humans in hunter/gatherer communities would have been subject to predators, their social systems would have been organized around care for the young. Hence, cry and other expressions of infant distress would not have been as subject to the risk of signalling vulnerability to predators, as would be the case in non-human, less socially adapted species. Thus, the human ancestral environment would have supported overt, spontaneous manifestations of pain as a form of instigating succorance. This characterization of pain as a public display designed to control the social environment is consistent with Fridlund's (1994) account of emotional displays as socially motivated, rather than as expressive of internal states.

Facial expression during genuine, faked, and suppressed pain

A broad range of non-verbal behaviours displayed during painful events is available for observation, including such instrumental activities as limping, guarded movements, protective postures, non-linguistic vocalizations, and facial activity (Keefe and Block 1982; Keefe et al. 1985, 2001). Facial expression has received special attention as it is a rich and complex source of information, serves as a visual focus during social interactions, and is identified by others as a key source of information (Craig et al. 1999). The study of facial expression was advanced substantially by development of the Facial Action Coding system (Ekman and Friesen 1978), which allows one to identify from a comprehensive, exhaustive set of 44 anatomically defined facial actions those that are associated with specific events.

Various studies have identified 'core' facial actions related to acute clinical pain (e.g. Lilley et al. 1997), exacerbations of chronic pain (Hadjistavropoulos and Craig 1994), and experimentally induced pain (Craig and Patrick 1985). These comprise: a lowered brow, raised cheeks, tightened eye lids, a raised upper lip or opened mouth, and closed eyes (Prkachin and Mercer 1989; Craig et al. 1991; Prkachin 1992b). Research has less consistently identified horizontal or vertical stretching of the lips, a wrinkled nose, deepening of the nasolabial fold, and drooping eyelids as pain-related actions. These inconsistencies across studies may reflect methodological variations, such as the type of pain experienced (LeResche 1982; Prkachin and Mercer 1989), pain severity (Patrick et al. 1986; Prkachin and Mercer 1989), situational factors (Prkachin et al. 1983; Prkachin and Craig 1985; Hill 1996), and individual difference variables (Craig 1992). But, generally, there is consistency in the facial display across sources of pain (Prkachin 1992b).

Detailed studies of the genuine pain expression examining acute procedural pain and exacerbation of chronic pain, for example, when patients with persistent low back pain are subjected to painful range of motion activities, confirm its clinical utility. The magnitude of facial activity increases with the intensity of noxious stimulation (Prkachin et al. 1983) and it correlates with self-reports of pain severity (Patrick et al. 1986; Prkachin and Mercer 1989) and unpleasantness (LeResche and Dworkin 1988; Prkachin and Mercer 1989). The pain expression can be differentiated from expressions of disgust, fear, anger, and sadness (LeResche 1982; Hale and Hadjistavropoulos 1997; LeResche and Dworkin 1988), and is unrelated to measures of anxiety and depression (LeResche and Dworkin 1988), despite consistent findings of a correlation between anxiety, depression, and verbal pain reports (Craig 1999).

Naïve observers can discriminate facial expressions of pain from various emotional states, and are sensitive to quantitatively graded information (Prkachin et al. 1983; Prkachin and Craig 1985; Patrick et al. 1986; Prkachin and Mercer 1989; Prkachin 1992a) as they identify the degree of suffering based on facial information (Boucher 1969; von Baeyer et al. 1984; Prkachin and Craig 1985). Observers rely on specific pain-related facial cues (primarily brow lowering, upper lip raise, cheek raise) to judge pain levels, as these variables account for 74 per cent of the variance in pain judgements (Patrick et al. 1986). Finally, pain judgements based upon self-report appear to tap different aspects of the pain experience than those based on non-verbal behaviour. We have observed that social models, representing themselves as either tolerant or intolerant of pain to people receiving experimental pain, had a substantially more potent influence on self-report measures and a lesser, more inconsistent impact on nonverbal pain displays (Prkachin *et al.* 1983; Patrick *et al.* 1986). Self-report appears more plastic and responsive to contextual variables and may best represent the individual's conscious understanding of best interests.

While facial expressions of pain appear less amenable to conscious deception than verbalizations (Craig and Prkachin 1983), even these manifestations of pain cannot be considered simply innate or reflexive responses to tissue insult. Affect and cognition do substantially moderate the experience of pain (Turk *et al.* 1983). As well, facial expressions of pain do change consistent with the social context. People tend to moderate their behavioural pain reactions when in the presence of others (Kleck *et al.* 1976; Badali 2000). As well, the social modelling influences described above provoke behaviour in the tolerant or intolerant direction, albeit inconsistently, and people can readily follow instruction to represent themselves in non-verbal behaviour as either tolerant or intolerant of the pain, again imperfectly as our detailed research indicates. Facial expressions, therefore, do not represent a direct measure of pain intensity, and are amenable to personal distortion. Nevertheless, useful information in facial expressions is available to the clinician and others when assessing the credibility of self-report.

Empirical discrimination of genuine and deceptive pain expressions

Faked pain expressions differ from genuine pain expressions in the increased frequency and intensity of pain-related and non pain-related facial actions (Craig *et al.* 1991; Hadjistavropoulos and Craig 1994), as well as in the timing and temporal contiguity of component facial actions (Hill and Craig 2003). In contrast, the masked pain expression tends to be a diminished display, somewhat intermediate to baseline, non-pain expressions and the genuine pain expression. The residual, uninhibited display appears to be a 'micro-expression' which 'leaks out' when there is an attempt to neutralize the genuine facial display (Ekman and Friesen 1969). These differences are subtle and would be difficult for observers to distinguish.

Judge's ability to discriminate genuine and deceptive pain displays

Given evidence of qualitative and quantitative variations among genuine, faked, and suppressed facial displays, it is of interest to know whether judges, trained and untrained, can discriminate the displays, how effectively they can understand the nature of pain being experienced, and the types of information they use or fail to use when making such judgements. Poole and Craig (1992) used videotaped facial expressions to have judges rate the severity of pain being experienced by patients voluntarily exhibiting faked pain, masked pain, genuine pain, and neutral expressions. In general, naïve judges were fooled by the deceptive pain expressions, as their ratings of the severity of pain being experienced corresponded with the intended effects rather than the actual levels of pain being experienced. Alerting the judges to the possibility of deception did not increase their ability to accurately estimate the pain being experienced. Rather, it reduced the observer's willingness to attribute pain to patients in any of the conditions. They were more conservative in their judgements, irrespective of whether genuine, faked, or suppressed pain was being represented. This finding is consistent with earlier investigations indicating that increasing the base rate expectation of deception has little impact on success in detecting deception (Faust *et al.* 1988).

Nevertheless, the discrimination appears possible (Prkachin 1992*a*). Hadjistavropoulos *et al.* (1996) used a forced choice design to evaluate whether naïve judges could accurately categorize videotaped images of baseline, genuine, suppressed, and exaggerated facial expressions of pain. There was 53 per cent success in discriminating the spontaneous and deliberate facial displays, an outcome substantially greater than the 25 per cent accuracy expected by chance. The forced choice format would have maximized judgement accuracy; nevertheless, the findings indicated that there is information available to make the discriminations. In general, the findings indicate that faking pain or its absence can be successful, but there are qualitative variations between genuine states of pain or its absence and faked pain or suppressed pain. It is conceivable that a solid training programme may facilitate accurate discrimination of faked and genuine states.

Variables influencing the detection of deception

Deception research confirms that people do not do well at 'lie detection' when judgements are based on observations of behaviour alone. Accuracy in the binary distinction of lying/not lying rarely exceed 60 per cent, only modestly exceeding the chance expectation of 50 per cent (Ekman and O'Sullivan 1991). Ekman and O'Sullivan's preliminary research using professionals thought to be experienced at detecting deception (police, customs officials, federal law enforcement agents) did not show advanced skills in detection accuracy. This supports the position of others that there is little utility in training to detect deception (Kraut and Poe 1980; Zuckerman *et al.* 1985; DePaulo and Pfeifer 1986; Kohnken 1987). However, these early studies rarely were able to provide judges with specific information on the distinction between genuine and faked displays. For example, Ekman and O'Sullivan (1991) attributed the lack of success in these studies to a lack of information concerning videotaped deceptive behaviours.

In contrast, Ekman and O'Sullivan (1991) used videotaped samples of behaviour which could correctly classify 86 per cent of the participants as truthful or lying, based on an empirical analysis of facial actions and vocalizations (Ekman *et al.* 1991). Secret Services agents showed detection accuracies significantly above chance levels and better than the performance of college students, other untrained adults, and various professionals with experience in lie detection. Furthermore, 53 per cent of the Secret Service agents scored above 70 per cent accuracy and 29 per cent were above 80 per cent accuracy. The Ekman and O'Sullivan (1991) findings denote individual differences in detection accuracy and imply that detection accuracy may be improved with training.

To date, efforts to train deception detection in interviews have been only marginally successful (Zuckerman *et al.* 1984; Kohnken 1987); however, 'training' usually has been limited to provision of corrective feedback, based on the assumption that subjects who are made aware of their errors will look for alternative strategies to improve their performance. Failures to improve detection indicate that participants simply do not see, or do not use, the facial cues which distinguish deceptive and truthful communications. There is some evidence that training in discriminating facial actions improves the accuracy of distinguishing truthful from deceptive facial behaviour (Ekman and Friesen 1974), but there was no training on facial cues likely to facilitate the distinction. Gallin and Thorn (1993) reported that corrective feedback and information-based training modestly improved judges' accuracies in identifying genuine cold-pressor induced pain, masked pain, posed pain, and no pain.

In a recent investigation of efforts to improve training to detect pain deception, Hill and Craig (submitted for publication) evaluated the accuracy of participants who judged the credibility of the facial behaviour of physiotherapy patients who engaged in faking while undertaking potentially painful range of motion exercises. The patients voluntarily cooperated with experimental instructions by either dissembling faked pain or by attempting to suppress pain reactions. In another condition, the spontaneous or 'genuine' pain, they were allowed to react without instructions. These were contrasted against a baseline condition in which ongoing pain was not exacerbated with movement. The participant judges were assigned to groups receiving: (a) corrective feedback following trials; (b) specific training in deception detection; (c) both corrective feedback and training; and (d) neither corrective feedback nor training deception, as a baseline control condition.

The training manual provided written descriptions of facial activity during genuine, faked, and suppressed pain, as identified in the studies reviewed above, accounts of the cues that distinguished the types of displays, and example photographs of the genuine pain expression. These included differences in the frequency and intensity of the pain-related facial actions, the timing of the facial expressions, and cues possibly specific to deception (Hill and Craig 2002).

Only corrective feedback improved judgemental accuracy across the several types of pain display. The training programme did not improve accuracy relative to the control condition, nor did it improve accuracy beyond that found for the corrective feedback alone. The feedback condition appeared to make cues useful in accurate discrimination available, whereas the training program did not appear to provide this specific, useful information. It was possible that the feedback training made whatever differences were conspicuous, such that an additive effect of the information training had little significance.

Individual differences in deception detection

A variety of factors have been postulated to influence one's ability to detect deception.

Cue utilization and decision-making confidence

More skilled judges use different cues during the judgement process (Ekman and O'Sullivan 1991). Accurate judges listed more varied behaviours as being useful, emphasized non-verbal behaviours more than verbal behaviours, and were better at recognizing 'micro-expressions'. In pain research, judges indicate that movements of the eyes, eyebrows, eyelids, and mouth were the most important sources of information (Prkachin *et al.* 1983). However, this represents only a beginning in understanding the specific cues that are used or could be used when judging the veracity of another's pain representations. Studies have reported that retrospective ratings of high levels of confidence in one's judgements of deception were not related to improved judgement accuracy (DePaulo and Pfeifer 1986; Kohnken 1987). However, these studies did not examine the relationship between accuracy on individual cases and rated confidence in these decisions, an approach that may yield better relationships.

Sex differences

The deception literature has not found consistent gender differerences in detection abilities. Hurd and Noller (1988), in the most comprehensive investigation to date, found that females used more cues, had a longer latency to response time, and appeared less confident during the decision making process. Females appear to use a slower, cue-based or analytical approach, while males made quicker, confident decisions which were more intuitive and less reliant on cues. None of these decision-making variables were related to accuracy, but low accuracy levels in general and a lack of variability may have influenced these findings. The findings contradict Buck's (1984) conclusion that females use a perception-based decoding strategy whereas males use an analytic, cognitively based decoding strategy

Empathy

The relationship between empathy and the ability to detect deception has not been investigated. Empathy is likely best described as multi-faceted, being comprised of several interrelated and overlapping processes (Moore 1990). Current definitions of empathy stress both an increased social acuity, which may be related to accuracy in judging characteristics of others, and an emotional identification with others, which may be more highly related to the probability of helping others (Chlopan *et al.* 1985).

Summary and conclusions

Skepticism concerning the credibility of pain complaints and pain-related disabilities is common-place, particulary when organic pathology cannot be identified as responsible for the symptoms. The doubts seem inevitable, even appropriate, in human society where social conventions necessitate varying degrees of impression management in daily social intercourse. This is matched by constant vigilance concerning the possibility of being cheated or exploited. Various social factors can lead to misrepresentations about pain. On the one hand, there are financial and social incentives for consciously pretending to be in pain when this is not the case. Less attention is paid to the personal, social and financial factors that lead to denial or suppression of pain. The theoretical argument was advanced that people would have difficulty matching the spontaneous expression of pain when voluntarily attempting to fake pain and that they would have difficulty over-riding the involuntary expression of pain when in pain. Self-report measures of pain appear more vulnerable to dissembling because they are the product of higher level, cognitive functions. In contrast, the reflexive, automatic nature of non-verbal expression would be more difficult to dissimulate or suppress. Fine-grained analyses of facial activity during genuine, faked, and suppressed pain confirmed expectations. Reliable distinctions can be made among spontaneous, faked, and suppressed pain. However, these differences are decidedly subtle and people acting roles of pain or suppressed pain tend to be convincing. There are prospects for improving people's abilities to make the discrimination through training, particularly corrective feedback. However, the task is difficult, as rates of judgemental accuracy are not high and there are many false positives and negatives. Nevertheless, the findings are consistent with continued efforts to use behavioural data to improve clinical assessment and identification of misrepresented illness.

References

American Psychiatric Association (2000). *Diagnostic and Statistical Manual of Mental Disorders*, 4th edn, Text Revision. American Psychiatric Association, Washington, DC.

Badali, M. A. (2000). Expressive and intentional parameters of pain behaviour: audience effects. Unpublished Master's Thesis, University of British Columbia, Vancouver, BC.

Boucher, J. D. (1969). Facial displays of fear, sadness and pain. *Perceptual and Motor Skills*, **28**, 239–42.

Buck, R. (1984). *The communication of emotion*. Guilford Press, New York, NY.

Chambers, C. T., Reid, G. J., Craig, K. D., McGrath, P. J., and Finley, G. A. (1999). Agreement between child and parent reports of pain. *Clinical Journal of Pain*, **14**, 336–42.

Chlopan, B. E., McCain, M. L., Carbonell, J. L., and Hagen, R. L. (1985). Empathy—review of available measures. *Journal of Personality and Social Psychology*, **48**, 635–53.

Cosmides, L. and Tooby, J. (1992). Cognitive adaptations for social exchange. In *The adapted mind: evolutionary psychology and the generation of culture* (eds J. H. Barkow, L. Cosmides, and J. Tooby). Oxford University Press, New York, NY.

Craig, K. D. (1983). A social learning perspective on pain experience. In *Perspectives on behavior therapy in the eighties* (eds M. Rosenbaum, C.M. Franks and Y. Jaffe), pp. 311–27. Springer, New York, NY.

Craig, K. D. (1986). Social modeling influences: pain in context. In *Psychology of pain* 2nd edn. (ed. R.A. Sternback), pp. 67–96. Raven Press, New York, NY.

Craig, K. D. (1992). The facial expression of pain: better than a thousand words? *American Pain Society Journal*, **1**, 153–62.

Craig, K. D. (1999). Emotions and psychobiology. In *Textbook of pain* 4th edn. (eds P.D. Wall and R. Melzack), pp. 103–22. Churchill Livingstone, Edinburgh.

Craig, K. D. and Grunau, R. V. E. (1993). Neonatal pain perception and behavioral masurement. In *Neonatal pain and distress: Pain research and clinical management* (eds K.J.S. Anand and P.J. McGrath), Vol. 4, pp. 67–105. Elsevier Science, Amsterdam.

Craig, K. D., Hill, M. L., and McMurtry, B. (1999). Detecting deception and malingering. In *Handbook of chronic pain syndromes: biopsychosocial perspectives* (eds A.R. Block, E.F. Kramer and E. Fernandez). Lawrence Erlbaum, New York, NY.

Craig, K. D., Hyde, S. A., and Patrick, C. J. (1991). Genuine, suppressed, and faked facial behavior during exacerbation of chronic low back pain. *Pain*, **46**, 161–72.

Craig, K. D. and Patrick, C. J. (1985). Facial expression during induced pain. *Journal of Personality and Social Psychology*, **48**, 1080–91.

Craig, K. D. and Prkachin, K. M. (1980). Social influences on public and private components of pain. In *Stress and anxiety* (eds I.G. Sarason and C. Spielberger), Vol. 7, pp. 57–72. Hemisphere, New York, NY.

Craig, K. D. and Prkachin, K. M. (1983). Nonverbal measures of pain. In *Pain measurement and assessment* (ed. R. Helzack) , Raven Press, New York, NY.

Craig, K. D., Prkachin, K. M., and Grunau, R. V. E. (2001). The facial expression of pain. In *Handbook of pain assessment* 2nd edn. (eds D.C. Turk and R. Melzack). Guilford Press, New York, NY.

DePaulo, B. M. and Pfeifer, R. L. (1986). On the job experience and skill at detecting deception. *Journal of Applied Social Psychology*, **16**, 249–67.

DePaulo, B. M., Rosenthal, R., Eisenstat, R. A., Rogers, P. C., and Finkelstein, S. (1978). Decoding discrepant nonverbal cues. *Journal of Personality and Social Psychology*, **36**, 313–23.

Ekman, P. and Friesen, W. V. (1969). Nonverbal leakage and clues to deception. *Psychiatry*, **32**, 88–105.

Ekman, P. and Friesen, W. V. (1974). Detecting deception from the body or face. *Journal of Personality and Social Psychology*, **29**, 288–98.

Ekman, P. and Friesen, W. V. (1978). *Facial action coding system: a technique for the measurement of facial movement*. Consulting Psychologists Press, Palo Alto, CA.

Ekman, P., Friesen, W. V., O'Sullivan, M., and Scherer, K. (1991). Face, voice and body in detecting deceit. *Journal of Nonverbal Behavior*, **15**, 125–35.

Ekman, P. and O'Sullivan, (1991). Who can catch a liar? *American Psychologist*, **46**, 913–20.

Faust, D., Hart, K. J., Guilmette, T. J., and Arkes, H. R. (1988). Neuropsychologists' capacity to detect adolescent malingerers. *Professional Psychology: Research and Practice*, **19**, 508–15.

Fridlund, A. J. (1994). *Human facial expression: an evolutionary view*. Academic Press, San Diego, CA.

Galin, K. E. and Thorn, B. E. (1993). Unmasking pain: detection of deception in facial expressions. *Journal of Social and Clinical Psychology*, **12**, 182–97.

Gilbert-MacLeod, C. A., Craig, K. D., Rocha, E. M., and Mathias, M. D. (2000). Everyday pain responses in children with and without developmental delays. *Journal of Pediatric Psychology*, **25**, 301–8.

Hadjistavropoulos, H. D. and Craig, K. D. (1994). Acute and chronic low back pain: Cognitive, affective and behavioral dimensions. *Journal of Consulting and Clinical Psychology*, **62**, 341–9.

Hadjistavropoulos, H. D. and Craig, K. D. (2002). A theoretical fraework for understanding self-report and observational measures of pain: a communication model. *Behaviour Research and Therapy*, **40**, 551–70.

Hadjistavropoulos, H. D., Craig, K. D., Hadjistavropoulos, T., and Poole, G. D. (1996). Subjective judgments of deception in pain expression: accuracy and errors. *Pain*, **65**, 247–54.

Hadjistavropoulos, H. D., von Baeyer, C., and Craig, K. D. (2001). In *Handbook of pain assessment* 2nd edn. (eds D.C. Turk and R. Melzack), Guilford, New York, NY.

Hale, C. and Hadjistavropoulos, T. (1997). Emotional components of pain. *Pain Research and Management*, **2**, 217–25.

Hill, M. (1996). Deception in facial expressions of pain: strategies to improve detection. Unpublished doctoral dissertation. University of British Columbia, Vancouver, BC.

Hill, M. L. and Craig, K. D. (2002). Detecting deception in pain expressions: the structure of genuine and deceptive pain displays. *Pain*, **96**, 135–44.

Hurd, K. and Noller, P. (1988). Decoding deception: a look at the process. *Journal of Nonverbal Behavior*, **12**, 217–33.

Jacox, A. K. (1980). The assessment of pain. In *Pain, meaning and management* (eds L. Smith, H. Merskey, and S. Grass). Spectrum, New York, NY.

Jensen, M. P. (1997). Validity of self-report and observation measures. In *Proceedings of the 8th World Congress on Pain. Progress in Pain Research and Management*, (eds T.S. Jensen, J.A. Turner, and Z. Wiesenfeld-Hallin), Vol. 8, IASP Press, Seattle, WA.

Johnson, M. (1977). Assessment of clinical pain. In *Pain: a sourcebook for nurses and other health professionals* (ed. A.K. Jacox). Little, Brown, Boston, MA.

Keefe, F. J. and Block, A. R. (1982). Development of an observational method for assessing pain behavior in chronic low back pain patients. *Behavior Therapy*, **13**, 363–75.

Keefe, F. J., Brantley, A., Manuel, G., and Crisson, J. E. (1985). Behavioral assessment of head and neck cancer pain. *Pain*, **23**, 327–36.

Keefe, F. J., Williams, D. A., and Smith, S. J. (2001). Assessment of pain behaviors. In *Handbook of pain assessment* (eds D.C. Turk and R. Melzack) 2nd edn, pp. 170–87. Guilford, New York, NY.

Kleck, R. E., Vaughan, R. C., Cartwright-Smith, J., Vaughan, K. B., Colby, C. Z., and Lanzetta, J. T. (1976). Effects of being observed on expressive, subjective, and physiological responses to painful stimuli. *Journal of Personality and Social Psychology* **34**, 1211–18.

Kohnken, G. (1987). Training police officers to detect deceptive eyewitness statements: does it work? *Social Behaviour*, **2**, 1–17.

Kotarba, J. A. (1983). *Chronic pain: its social dimensions*. Sage Publications, Beverley Hills, CA.

Kraut, R. E. and Poe, D. (1980). On the line: the deception judgements of customs inspectors and laymen. *Journal of Personality and Social Psychology*, **39**, 784–98.

Lander, J. (1990). Clinical judgements in pain management. *Pain*, **42**, 15–22.

LeResche, L. (1982). Facial expression in pain: a study of candid photographs. *Journal of Nonverbal Behavior*, **7**, 46–56.

LeResche, L. and Dworkin, S. (1988). Facial expressions of pain and emotion in chronic TMD patients. *Pain*, **35**, 71–8.

Lilley, C. M., Craig, K. D., and Grunau, R. V. E. (1997). The expression of pain in infants and toddlers: developmental changes in facial activity. *Pain*, **72**, 161–70.

Meinhart, N. T. and McCaffrey, M. (1983). *Pain: a nursing approach to assessment and analysis*. Appleton-Century-Crofts, Norwalk, CT.

Melzack, R. and Katz, J. (1999). Pain measurement in persons in pain. In *Textbook of pain* 4th edn. (eds P.D. Wall and R. Melzack), pp. 409–26. Churchill Livingstone, Edinburgh.

Patrick, C. J., Craig, K. D., and Prkachin, K. M. (1986). Observer judgments of acute pain: facial action determinants. *Journal of Personality and Social Psychology*, **50**, 1291–8.

Poole, C. D. and Craig, K. D. (1992). Judgments of genuine, suppressed and faked facial expressions of pain. *Journal of Personality and Social Psychology*, **63**, 797–805.

Prkachin, K. M. (1992a). Dissociating spontaneous and deliberate expressions of pain: signal detection analyses. *Pain*, **51**, 57–65.

Prkachin, K. M. (1992b). The consistency of facial expressions of pain: a comparison across modalities. *Pain*, **51**, 297–306.

Prkachin, K. M. and Craig, K. D. (1985). Influencing nonverbal expressions of pain: signal detection theory analyses. *Pain*, **21**, 399–409.

Prkachin, K. M., Currie, N. A., and Craig, K. D. (1983). Influencing non-verbal expressions of pain. *Canadian Journal of Behavioural Science*, **15**, 409–21.

Prkachin, K. M. and Mercer, S. R. (1989). Pain expression in patients with shoulder pathology: validity, properties and relationship to sickness impact. *Pain*, **39**, 257–65.

Rainville, P., Bushnell, M. C., and Duncan, G. H. (2000). PET studies of the subjective experience of pain. In *Pain imaging. Progress in pain research and management* (eds K.L. Casey and M.C. Bushnell), Vol. 18, pp. 123–56. IASP Press, Seattle, WA.

Rainville, P., Duncan, G. H., Price, D. D., Carrier, B., and Bushnell, M. C. (1997). Pain affect encoded in human anterior cingulate but not somatosensory cortex. *Science*, **277**, 968–71.

Rinn, W. E. (1984). The neuropsychology of facial expression: a review of the neurological and psychological mechanisms for producing facial expressions. *Psychological Bulletin*, **95**, 52–77.

Rogers, R. (ed.) (1997). *Clinical assessment of malingering and deception*, 2nd edn. Guilford, New York, NY.

Talwar, V. and Lee, K. I. (2002*a*). Emergence of white lie telling in children between 3 and 7 years. *Merrill-Palmer Quarterly*, **48**, 160–81.

Talwar, V. and Lee, K. I. (2002*b*). Development of lying to conceal a transgression: children's control of expressive behavior during verbal deception. *International Journal of Behavioral Development*.

Turk, D. C., Meichenbaum, D. H., and Genest, M. (1983). Pain and behavioural medicine: theory, research and clinical guide. Guilford, New York, NY.

Turk, D. C. and Melzack, R. (eds) (2001). *Handbook of pain assessment*, 2nd edn. Guilford, New York, NY.

von Baeyer, C. L., Johnson, M. E., and McMillan, M. J. (1984). Consequences of nonverbal expressions of pain: patient distress and observer concern. *Social Sciences and Medicine*, **19**, 1319–24.

Wall, P.D. and Melzack, R. (eds.) (1999). *Textbook of pain, 4th edn*. Churchill Livingstone, Edinburgh.

Zemen, J. and Garber, J. (1996). Display rules for anger, sadness and pain: it depends who is watching. *Child Development*, **67**, 957–73.

Zuckerman, M., Koestner, R., and Alton, A. O. (1984). Learning to detect deception. *Journal of Personality and Social Psychology*, **46**, 519–28.

Zuckerman, M., Koestner, R., and Colella, M. J. (1985). Learning to communicate deception from three communication channels. *Journal of Nonverbal Behavior*, **9**, 188–94.

27 Deceptive responses and detecting deceit

Aldert Vrij and Samantha Mann

Abstract

This chapter discusses (i) the relationship between deception, non-verbal behaviour, and speech content; and (ii) people's ability to detect deceit. Although there is not a clear giveaway cue such as Pinocchio's growing nose, some non-verbal and verbal cues are, to some extent, related to deception. We will discuss these cues and reasons why they differentiate between liars and truth tellers. Research has demonstrated that people, including professional lie catchers such as police officers, are generally not good at detecting deceit. We discuss explanations for this poor ability as well as guidelines which might help those who want to improve at this task.

Introduction

There are three different ways to detect lies: (i) by observing people's non-verbal behaviour (the movements they make, whether or not they show gaze aversion, their vocal pitch, whether or not they stutter, and so on); (ii) by analysing what is being said (speech content); and (iii) by examining physiological responses (blood pressure, heart rate, palmar sweating, and so on). This chapter discusses the relationship between lying (throughout this chapter the terms 'lying' and 'deception' will be used interchangeably), non-verbal behaviour and speech content. Are there systematic differences between liars and truth tellers in their non-verbal and verbal responses? Are people able to detect lies while paying attention to these aspects? This chapter answers both questions by reviewing the relevant deception research. Although some responses are more likely to occur during deception than others, neither laypersons nor professional lie catchers are generally good at detecting lies. This chapter will provide some reasons why, and will give guidelines which might enhance lie detection.

Theoretical reasons for differences between liars and truth tellers

For many years, researchers have shown great interest in examining people's verbal and non-verbal responses during deceit. DePaulo et al. (2003) recently reviewed more than 110 studies investigating these issues. In particular, one finding emerged: typical deceptive speech content and non-verbal behaviour does not exist. In other words, nothing like Pinocchio's growing nose exists.

The mere fact that someone lies will not affect his or her verbal or non-verbal response. However, liars may experience three different processes during deception, called *emotional, content complexity* and *attempted control* processes (Zuckerman *et al.* 1981; DePaulo *et al.* 1985; Vrij 2000*a*), and each of these processes may influence a liar's verbal and non-verbal behaviour. Each process emphasizes a different aspect of deception, and lies may well feature all three aspects. Therefore, the three processes should not be considered as opposing camps.

The *emotional process* proposes that deception can produce different emotions in the deceiver. The three most common types of emotion associated with deceit are guilt, fear, and excitement (Ekman 1992). A liar might feel *guilty* because he/she is lying, might be *afraid* of getting caught, or might be *excited* about having the opportunity to fool someone. Guilt might result in gaze aversion because the liar does not dare to look the target straight in the eye (Keltner and Harker 1998). Fear and excitement might result in signs of stress, such as an increase in hand and body movements, an increase in speech fillers (e.g. ah-filled pauses) and stutters (e.g. repetition of words), or a higher pitched voice (Ekman *et al.* 1976; DePaulo *et al.* 2003).

The *content complexity process* emphasizes that lying can be a cognitively complex task (Burgoon *et al.* 1989 (see Chapter 20)). Liars have to think of plausible answers, should not contradict themselves, should tell a lie that is consistent with everything which the observer knows or might find out, and should not give their lies away by making slips of the tongue. Moreover, they have to remember what they have said so that they can remain consistent when someone asks them to repeat their story. People engaged in cognitively complex tasks make more speech fillers and stutters and wait longer before giving an answer (Goldman-Eisler 1968). Cognitive complexity also leads to fewer illustrators (hand and arm movements designed to modify and/or supplement what is being said verbally) and to more gaze aversion. The decrease in illustrators is a consequence of a greater cognitive load resulting in a neglect of body language, reducing overall animation (Ekman and Friesen 1972). Gaze aversion (usually to a motionless point) occurs because looking at the conversation partner distracts from thinking too much. It is easy to examine the impact of content complexity on movements and gaze aversion. Ask people what they ate 3 days ago, and observe their behaviour while they try to remember what they have eaten. Most people will look away and will sit still while thinking about the answer.

Verbal differences might emerge as well due to content complexity (Steller 1989). For example, sometimes truth tellers, especially when they are upset, might tell a story in an unstructured, non-chronological order. For example, they may start by explaining the essential facts of the event ('We had a near-fatal accident, and I haven't been in a car since'), may then describe the beginning ('We were on the brow of a hill'), may then give information about subsequent events ('The car filled with smoke'), and then go back to the beginning ('I saw the glare of headlights . . .'). However, fabricated stories typically follow a structured, coherent and chronological order.

Truth tellers might also tend to include more details than liars, for example more details which are unusual but meaningful in the context ('The tall man had a stutter'); might include more contextual embeddings, that is, more information about time ('I heard that noise outside while I was watching the news') and location ('Her bag was on the counter when the man took it and disappeared'); might report more descriptions of interactions between the interviewee and others involved in the event ('The policeman said we should stay in the car, but my husband refused and got out'); and might report more reproductions of speech (spoken words apparently reported in their original form: 'I said: "am I going to die?" ' fulfils this criterion but 'Then I asked whether it was serious' would not).[1]

---

[1] Several of these verbal differences can also be predicted on the basis of reality monitoring (Johnson and Raye 1981, 1998). See Vrij (2000*a,b*) for a discussion about reality monitoring and deception.

Liars may respond intentionally in order to avoid getting caught. This is emphasized in the *attempted control process*. Most people lie less frequently than they tell the truth. DePaulo *et al.* (1996) found that people lie in one quarter of interactions with others, whereby an interaction was defined as an exchange with another person that lasted for 10 min or longer. This makes lying a more special event which merits special attention. While lying, people may worry about the impression they make on others and may be particularly keen on making an honest impression, perhaps even more so than when they are telling the truth. Someone who tries to smuggle something is probably more keen on making an honest impression on customs officers than someone who is not smuggling, because the stakes of getting stopped and searched are much higher for the smuggler than for the non-smuggler. It will not harm the non-smuggler much when a customs officer asks her to open her suitcase. She might be annoyed about the time it takes and the delay it causes, but, other than that, there are no negative consequences. The smuggler, however, will be in trouble when a customs officer wants to check his luggage. In summary, the attempted control process suggests that liars will put more effort into behaving 'normally' or in making an honest and convincing impression than will truth tellers. But this is not easy. They should suppress their nerves effectively, should not only mask evidence that they are having to think hard, but also know how they normally behave in order to behave naturally, as well as know how to make an honest and convincing impression and be able to show the behaviour they want to show.

Hocking and Leathers (1980) argued that liars' attempts to control their behaviour will focus on those behaviours that fit the cultural stereotype of liars. There is a widespread belief, at least amongst Caucasian people, that liars look away, increase their movements, and stutter (Akehurst *et al.* 1996; Vrij and Semin 1996; Taylor and Vrij 2000; Vrij and Taylor 2003).

Eye contact should be easier to control than movements and speech disturbances (Ekman and Friesen 1974). The face is important in the exchange of information. For example, via facial expressions people can demonstrate whether they are interested in someone's conversation, and whether they feel happy or sad (Ekman 1992). The great communicative potential of the face means that people are practised at using and therefore controlling it.

By contrast, the body may not be salient in communication and is less often attended to and reacted to by others. We are therefore less practised at controlling the body. It may well be the case that, when controlling their behaviour, liars exhibit a pattern of body language that will appear planned, rehearsed, and lacking in spontaneity (DePaulo and Kirkendol 1989). For example, liars may believe that frequent movements will give their lies away, and will therefore move very deliberately and tend to avoid any movements which are not strictly essential. This will result in an unusual degree of rigidity and inhibition, because most people normally make movements which are not essential.

Like most movements, speech hesitations and speech errors are usually made unintentionally and are not generally important in the exchange of information. We therefore may assume that people do not often practise controlling these behaviours, and are not very good at controlling them. It is likely that liars will think that the use of speech hesitations and speech errors sound suspect. Therefore, they will try to avoid making such non-fluencies. This, however, may result in a speech pattern which sounds unusually smooth, as it is normal for most people to make some errors in speech.

Another possible cue as a result of inadequate control of behaviour is that performances may look flat due to a lack of involvement. An artist who applies for a job as salesperson because he needs the money may not look enthusiastic enough during the selection interview. A mother who punishes her child for wrongdoing might not look sincere enough if she, in fact, was amused by the trick played on her.

Verbal differences might emerge as well. Liars will try to construct a report which they believe will give a credible impression to others, and will leave out information which, in their view, will damage their appearance of being a sincere person (Köhnken 1999). For example, liars might make less spontaneous corrections (spontaneously admitting that the previous description was incorrect and modifying that description).

Before discussing which responses liars typically show, three comments are important. First, the approaches only suggest that the presence of signs of emotions, content complexity and overcontrol *may* be indicative of deception. None of these approaches claim that the presence of these signs *necessarily* indicates deception. Some truth tellers might experience exactly the same processes. For example, innocent (truthful) people might also be afraid that they will not be believed (Ofshe and Leo 1997). Because of that fear, they may show the same nervous behaviours as guilty liars who are afraid of being caught (Bond and Fahey 1987). This puts the lie detector in a difficult position: how to interpret the signs of fear, as a sign of guilt or as a sign of innocence? The behaviour does not provide the answer. Ekman (1992) labelled this phenomenon the *Othello error*, after Shakespeare's play. Othello falsely accuses his wife, Desdemona, of infidelity. He tells her to confess since he is going to kill her for her treachery. Desdemona asks Cassio (her alleged lover) to be called so that he can testify her innocence. Othello tells her that he has already murdered Cassio. Realizing that she cannot prove her innocence, Desdemona reacts with an emotional outburst. Othello, however, misinterprets this outburst as a sign of her infidelity.

Second, signs of emotion, content complexity, and attempted control may only become apparent if a liar experiences one of the three processes. That is, if a liar does not experience any fear, guilt, or excitement (or any other emotion), if the lie is not difficult to fabricate, and if the liar does not try to control himself, cues to deception are unlikely to occur. Most lies in everyday life fall in this category (DePaulo *et al.* 1996).

Third, the three processes are hypothetical and are typically introduced *post hoc* to explain verbal and non-verbal differences between liars and truth tellers (Zuckerman *et al.* 1981; DePaulo *et al.* 1985; Miller and Stiff 1993). However, there is evidence that liars actually experience the three processes when they lie. In Vrij *et al.* (1996) experiment, participants were asked either to lie or to tell the truth. Afterwards they were asked to what extent they had experienced the three processes. Results showed that liars experienced all three processes significantly more than truth tellers. Vrij *et al* (2001c) found individual differences in experiencing these processes. For example, a negative correlation was found between being good at acting and having to think hard while lying.[2] Although these studies were correlational studies, the relationship between the three processes and lying is more likely to be causal: They are the consequence of being engaged in lying.

Non-verbal and verbal characteristics of lying

In studies of actual indicators of deception, participants are typically instructed to give either true or deceptive reports on certain issues. Their responses are then analysed with particular coding systems and the average frequencies of occurrence of certain responses during truthful and deceptive messages are compared. DePaulo *et al.* (2003) and Vrij (2000a) have provided reviews of such deception studies. The outcomes are summarized in Table 27.1 (first column). Definitions of the cues are given in Table 27.2.

Table 27.1 reveals some cues to deception. Liars tend to have a higher pitched voice than truth tellers, which is in line with the emotional approach, probably caused by stress (Ekman *et al.* 1976). The results concerning speech errors and speech hesitations show a conflicting pattern. In some studies an increase in such errors and hesitations has been found during deception, whereas other studies have revealed the opposite pattern. There is some evidence that variations of lie

---

[2] One might wonder whether psychopaths experience the three processes during deception to the same extent as non-psychopaths. This has never been investigated.

Table 27.1 Actual indicators of deception (column 1), the behaviour of 13 male suspects in police interviews (column 2), and subjective indicators of deception (column 3)

	1 Actual indicators[a]	2 Behaviour of 13 male suspects[a]	3 Subjective indicators[b]
Vocal characteristics			
High-pitched voice	>	*	>
Speech hesitations	</>	—	>
Speech errors	</>	—	>
Slow speech	—	*	—
Latency period	—	*	>
Non-vocal characteristics			
Gaze aversion	—	—	>
Smiling	—	—	>
Illustrators	<	<[c]	>
Self-manipulations	—	<[c]	>
Hand/finger	<	<[c]	>
Leg/foot	—	*	>
Head	—	—	—
Trunk	—	—	>
Shifting positions	—	*	>
Verbal characteristics			
Unstructured reproduction	<	*	
Number of details	<	*	
Unusual details	<	*	
Contextual embedding	<	*	
Description of interactions	<	*	
Reproduction of speech	<	*	
Spontaneous corrections	<	*	

[a] Explanations of the signs: > = increase during deception; < = decrease during deception; – = no relationship with deception; * = relationship was not investigated.

[b] Explanation of the signs: > = observers associate an increase in the behaviour with deception; < = observers associate a decrease in the behaviour with deception; – = observers do not associate the behaviour with deception; * = relationship was not investigated.

[c] Illustrators, self manipulations, and hand/finger movements combined.

complexity are responsible for these conflicting findings (Vrij and Heaven 1999). Lies that for various reasons are 'difficult to tell' result in an increase in speech errors and speech hesitations (in line with the content complexity approach), whereas lies that are 'easy to tell' result in a decrease in speech hesitations and speech errors (in line with the attempted control approach).

Moreover, liars tend to make fewer illustrators and fewer hand and finger movements than truth tellers. The decrease in these movements might be the result of both lie complexity and attempted control.

Contrary to popular beliefs, gaze aversion is not specifically related to deception. In fact, Table 27.1 suggests that the face does not reveal information about deception. However, as Ekman's (1992) work has shown this is not true. Lies may result in fraudulent facial emotional expressions, so-called 'micro-expressions'. These are facial expressions that are displayed for only a fraction of a second, but clearly reveal the liar's true feelings before being quickly covered with a false expression. Ekman also argues that fake facial expressions, such as fake smiles, differ from genuine expressions, such as felt smiles (Ekman et al. 1988).

With regard to the verbal characteristics, liars' statements are more likely to be presented in a chronological order and include fewer details, fewer unusual details, fewer contextual embeddings, fewer descriptions of interactions, and fewer reproductions of speech. Liars also make fewer

Table 27.2 Overview and descriptions of the non-verbal behaviours

Vocal Characteristics
 Speech hesitations: use of speech fillers such as 'ah', 'um', 'er' and so on
 Speech errors: word and/or sentence repetition, sentence change, sentence incompletions, slips of the
  tongue and so forth
 Pitch of voice: changes in pitch of voice, such as rise in pitch or fall in pitch
 Speech rate: number of spoken words in a certain period of time
 Latency period: period of silence between question and answer

Facial Characteristics
 Gaze: looking at the face of the conversation partner
 Smile: smiling and laughing

Movements
 Self manipulations: scratching the head, wrists, and so forth
 Illustrators: hand and arm movements designed to modify and/or supplement what is being said
  verbally
 Hand and finger movements: non-functional movements of hands or fingers without moving the
  arms
 Leg and foot movements: movements of feet and legs
 Head movements: head nods and head shakes
 Trunk movements: movements of the trunk (usually accompanied with head movements)
 Shifting position: movements made to change the sitting position (usually accompanied with trunk and
  foot/leg movements)

Verbal Characteristics
 unstructured production: information which is scattered throughout the statement rather than presented
  in a chronological order
 number of details: specific descriptions of place, time, people, objects, and events
 unusual details: details which are unusual but meaningful in the context
 contextual embeddings: details that place the event within its temporal and spatial context
 descriptions of interactions: information about interactions involving at least the interviewee and one
  other person
 reproduction of speech: reporting speech in its original form
 spontaneous corrections: correcting one's own statement without any prompts to do so

spontaneous corrections. The latter finding might be the result of attempted control, whereas the other findings might be caused by content complexity.

Perhaps a striking finding is that liars do not seem to show clear patterns of nervous behaviours (gaze aversion, fidgeting, and so on). However, this might be the result of an artefact. Deception research has almost exclusively been conducted in the laboratory where people tell the truth and lie for the sake of the experiment. Perhaps in experimental laboratory studies, the stakes (the positive and negative consequences of getting caught) are not high enough for the liar to exhibit clear deceptive cues to deception (Miller and Stiff 1993).

In order to raise the stakes in laboratory experiments, participants have been offered money if they successfully get away with their lies (Vrij 1995). In other studies, participants are told that they will be observed by a peer who will judge their sincerity (DePaulo *et al.* 1985). In an attempt to raise the stakes even further, participants in Frank and Ekman's (1997) study were given the opportunity to 'steal' US$50. If they could convince the interviewer that they had not taken the money, they could keep all of it. If they took the money and the interviewer judged them as lying, they had to give the US$50 back and also lost their US$10 per hour participation fee. Moreover, some participants faced an additional punishment if they were found to be lying. They were told that they would have to sit on a cold, metal chair inside a cramped, darkened room ominously labelled XXX, where they would have to endure anything from 10 to 40 randomly sequenced 110-decibel starting blasts of white noise over the course of 1 h.

A study like this should raise ethical concerns. Also, one might argue that the stakes in such a study are still not comparable with the stakes in some real-life situations, such as during police interviews. Laboratory studies are not suitable for examining the responses in high-stake situations as raising the stakes to a comparable extent is not usually possible due to ethical reasons. Therefore, the only way to investigate how liars behave in high-stake real-life situations is to examine their behavioural responses in such situations. This has proven to be difficult. Researchers face three problems in particular (Vrij 2002): (i) obtaining video footage of the truths and lies (for scoring the frequency of occurrence of verbal and non-verbal behaviours, the high-stakes interviews need to be videotaped and the researcher needs permission to use these tapes for further coding); (ii) establishing the ground truth, that is, to obtain conclusive evidence that the person is lying or telling the truth; and (iii) obtaining deceptive and truthful fragments which are comparable (this will be further discussed in the 'guidelines to detect deceit' section). As a result, behavioural and verbal examinations of real-life high-stake situations are virtually non-existent.

In the most comprehensive study of real-life high-stakes lies to date, Mann (2001) examined the behaviour displayed by 13 male suspects during their police interviews. The suspects were all being interviewed with regard to serious crimes such as murder, rape, and arson. Clips of video footage were selected where other sources (reliable witness statements and forensic evidence) provided evidence that the suspect lied or told the truth. Truthful and deceptive behaviours were compared (for each suspect both truthful and deceptive fragments were available). The results are summarized in Table 27.1, column 2 (see Mann 2001; Mann *et al.* 2002, for further details about this study). The suspects in these high-stakes situations did not demonstrate clear nervous behaviour either. In fact, they showed a decrease in movements which is more in agreement with the content complexity and attempted control approaches than with the emotional approach. The strongest evidence that content complexity has affected suspects' behaviour more than nervousness was the finding regarding eyeblinks (not reported in Table 27.2). Suspects made fewer blinks when they lied. Research has shown that nervousness results in an increase in blinking (Harrigan and O'Connell 1996), whereas increased cognitive load results in a decrease in eye blinking (Wallbott and Scherer 1991). Many suspects had had frequent contact with the police. In that respect they were probably familiar with police interviews which might have decreased their nervousness during those interviews. However, suspects in police interviews are frequently of below average intelligence (Gudjonsson 1992). There is evidence that less intelligent people will have difficulties in inventing convincing stories (Ekman and Frank 1993).

People's ability to detect lies

In scientific studies concerning detection of deception, observers are typically given videotaped or audiotaped statements of a number of people who are either lying or telling the truth. After each statement observers are asked to judge whether the statement is truthful or false. Vrij (2000*a*) calculated the percentages of lie detection (the 'accuracy rate'), derived from a review of 39 studies. Included were studies in which judges were college students who tried to detect lies and truths told by people they were not familiar with. The total accuracy rate was 56.6 per cent, which is a low score as 50 per cent accuracy would be expected by chance alone. (Guessing whether someone is lying or not gives a 50 per cent chance of being correct.) If accuracy at detecting lies is computed separately from accuracy at detecting truth, results show a *truth-bias*, that is, judges are more likely to consider that messages are truthful than deceptive and, as a result, truthful messages are identified with more accuracy than deceptive ones. Vrij's (2000*a*) review shows that observers are

Table 27.3 Accuracy scores of professional lie catchers

References	Accuracy Rates (%)		
	Truth	Lie	Total
DePaulo and Pfeifer (1986) (federal law enforcement)	64[a]	42[a]	53
Ekman and O'Sullivan (1991) (Secret Service)			64
Ekman and O'Sullivan (1991) (federal polygraphers)			56
Ekman and O'Sullivan (1991) (police officers)			56
Ekman et al. (1999) (CIA)	66	80	73
Ekman et al. (1999) (sheriffs)	56	78	67
Ekman et al. (1999) (law enforcement)	54	48	51
Köhnken (1987) (police officers)	58	31	45
Porter et al. (2000) (parole officers)	20	60	40
Vrij (1993) (police detectives)	51	46	49
Vrij and Graham (1997) (police officers)			54
Vrij and Mann (2001a) (police officers)	70	57	64
Vrij and Mann (2001b) (police officers)		51	

[a] Experienced and unexperienced officers together.

reasonably good at detecting truths (correctly judging that someone is telling the truth: 67 per cent accuracy rate) but particularly poor at detecting lies (correctly judging that someone is lying: 44 per cent accuracy rate). In fact, 44 per cent is below the level of chance, and people would be more accurate at detecting lies if they simply guessed! One explanation for the truth-bias is that in daily life people are more often confronted with truthful than with deceptive statements (DePaulo *et al.* 1996), so people are therefore more inclined to assume that the behaviour they observe is honest (the so-called *availability heuristic*; O'Sullivan *et al.* 1988).

It could be argued that college students are not habitually called upon to detect deception. Perhaps professional lie catchers, such as police officers or customs officers, would obtain higher accuracy rates than laypersons. Indeed, trained experts who analyse written transcripts in order to detect deceit are better than laypeople (Tye *et al.* 1999). In several other studies, professional lie catchers were exposed to videotaped footage of liars and truth tellers and their ability to detect lies was tested. The findings of these studies are summarized in Table 27.3.

Three findings emerged from these studies. First, most accuracy rates were similar to the accuracy rates found in studies with college students as observers, and most fall in the 45–60 per cent range. Second, some groups seem to be better than others. Ekman's research has shown that members of the Secret Service, CIA, and Sheriffs were better lie detectors than others. Third, the truth-bias, consistently found in studies with students as observers, is much less profound or perhaps even lacking in studies with professional lie catchers. Perhaps their job makes them more suspicious.[3]

However, how realistic are these findings of scientific lie detection studies? Clearly, there are many differences between lie detection in scientific deception studies and lie detection in real-life. For example, in deception studies observers watch videotapes of liars and truth tellers, whereas in real-life they often actually interview people. However, it is doubtful whether having the opportunity to interview the potential liar improves detection accuracy. Some studies, in which the accuracy scores of observers who actually interviewed potential liars were compared with those who observed the interviews but did not interview the potential liars themselves have found

---

[3] Given the fact that police detectives overwhelmingly believe that the suspects they interview are guilty, for example, in their analysis of real-life police interviews, Moston *et al.* (1992) found that in 73% of the cases police detectives were 'sure' of the suspect's guilt before they interviewed the suspect, a lie-bias (an inclination that the person is lying) could be expected in these studies. One might argue that the absence of a lie bias in studies with professional lie catchers could be seen as a truth-bias.

that observers were more accurate in detecting truths and lies than were interviewers (Feeley and deTurck 1997; Granhag and Strömwall 2001). These findings suggest that actually interviewing someone is a disadvantage, and not an advantage in detecting deceit. Both studies found a strong truth-bias amongst interviewers. In other words, interviewers are reluctant to accept that some people are convincing liars and are able to fool them. Their reluctance to believe that others might be able to fool them will hamper lie detection.

There are at least three reasons why people are poor at detecting deceit. First, differences between liars and truth tellers are usually very small (Vrij 1994), due to the fact that they may experience the same processes. Also, truth tellers might be nervous, might have to think hard, and might try to control their behaviour.

Second, perhaps in these laboratory studies the stakes were not high enough for the liar to elicit clear cues to deception (Miller and Stiff 1993), which makes the lie detection task difficult. In a series of experiments in which the stakes were manipulated (although the stakes were never really high), it was found that such 'high stake' lies were easier to detect than low stake lies (DePaulo et al. 1983, 1988, 1991; Feeley and deTurck 1998; Heinrich and Borkenau 1998; Bond and Atoum, 2000; Forrest and Feldman 2000; Vrij 2000b).

Third, people have poor insight into how liars respond. Table 27.1 (column 3) summarizes Vrij's (2000a) review of research about how people think liars behave. This review showed that laypersons and professional catchers have similar views, although these views are often incorrect. Basically, observers expect liars to behave nervously although liars often do not show such responses. There are four reasons why people have incorrect views. First, probably everybody has come across examples of people who did show nervous behaviour when they lied. This will support their views that liars show nervous behaviour. Second, people are not aware of how they behave themselves when they lie and incorrectly believe that they themselves show nervous behaviours such as gaze aversion and fidgeting (Vrij et al. 1996, 2001). In other words, they are looking in others for cues they incorrectly believe they themselves show when they lie. Third, people are taught the wrong cues. In their influential manual about police interviewing— *Criminal interrogation and confessions*—Inbau et al. (1986) describe in detail how, in their view, liars behave. This includes showing gaze aversion, displaying unnatural posture changes, exhibiting self manipulations, and placing hands over the mouth or eyes when speaking. None of these behaviours have been found to be reliably related to deception in deception research. Not surprisingly, when in their detection of deception study, Kassin and Fong (1999) trained half of their participants to look at the cues Inbau and colleagues claim to be related to deception, these trained observers actually performed worse than naive observers who did not receive any information about deceptive behaviour. Fourth, observers do not take individual differences into account. Non-verbal behaviours are culturally determined and do differ across cultures. For example, looking into the eyes of the conversation partner is regarded as polite in Western cultures but is considered to be rude in several other cultures (Vrij and Winkel 1991). Therefore, Afro-American people display more gaze aversion than white Americans, and people from Turkey and Morocco who are living in the Netherlands show more gaze aversion than native Dutch people (Vrij 2000a). However, white observers are often not aware of these culturally defined behaviours and sometimes tend to interpret these behaviours (such as gaze aversion) as indications of deceit (Vrij and Winkel 1992, 1994).

These reasons imply that lie detectors commonly make mistakes, and that they might become better if they are trained to detect lies. Indeed, some training programmes have revealed promising results. Porter et al. (2000) published results of a two-day training programme of parole officers. The training consisted of 'myth dissolution' (e.g. Pinocchio's growing nose, such as liars look away and fidget, does not exist), 'information provision' (they were given a detailed overview of verbal and non-verbal cues to deception), and 'practice judgements' (videotaped clips of liars and truth tellers were shown and discussed). Although the officers were particularly poor at detecting truths and lies at the beginning of the programme (they only obtained an accuracy rate of 40 per cent), they considerably improved and obtained an accuracy rate of 77 per cent after 2 days of training.[4]

As mentioned before, some people are better lie detectors than others. Perhaps we can learn from the good lie detectors. Obviously, we can only learn from them if we know their strategies. The ability to detect lies is not correlated with gender, age or experience in interviewing suspects (Ekman and O'Sullivan 1991; Porter *et al.* 2000; Vrij and Mann 2001*a*).[5] Ekman and O'Sullivan's (1991) preliminary results showed that good lie detectors use different cues when observing different people (for instance, they mention speech-related cues when detecting a lie in one person, voice-related cues for a second person, and body movement-related cues for a third person), whereas inaccurate lie detectors seem to use a 'rule of thumb' strategy, using the same cues in order to detect lies in different people. Vrij and Mann (2001*a*) also found that good lie detectors rely less on stereotypical beliefs such as 'liars look away' and 'liars fidget' than poor lie detectors. A stereotypical rule of thumb strategy is doomed to fail because different people show different behaviours when lying. Ekman and colleagues found that observers' ability to detect facial micro-expressions of emotions (as measured with a special micro-expression test) was positively correlated with their ability to detect deceit in the lie detection task (Ekman and O'Sullivan 1991; Frank and Ekman 1997). In other words, good lie detectors are good at noticing facial micro-expressions of emotions.

Guidelines to detecting deceit

The following guidelines might help those who want to detect deceit.

(1)   Lies may only be detectable if the liar experiences fear, guilt, or excitement (or any other emotion), when the lie is difficult to fabricate, or when the liar attempts to make a credible impression.

(2)   There are large individual differences in people's non-verbal behaviour and speech. One person talks more than another person, one person makes more movements than another person, one persons speaks faster than another person, etc. Suppose there are two people, one person who naturally moves a lot (e.g. fidgets or gesticulates) and one person who naturally sits still. It is possible that in both persons lying is associated with a small decrease in movements. In that case, however, the more fidgety person who lies will probably still make more movements than the restless person who is telling the truth. Comparing the movements different people make *per se* is therefore not particularly useful in detecting deceit. A more accurate judgement could be made by comparing the same person's response under investigation with the person's natural truthful response. A deviation from the latter response might indicate that a person is lying. However, keep the Othello-error in mind and do not disregard other explanations for deviations in responses. This so-called baseline method (comparing the response under investigation with someone's natural truthful response (baseline response) could only work if the method is applied correctly. Crucial in the use of the baseline technique is that the correct parts of the interview are compared. One should not compare apples with oranges. Unfortunately, that happens often in police interviews (Moston and Engelberg 1993). Small talk at the beginning of the interview is used to establish a baseline, which is then compared with the behaviour shown in the actual interview. This is an incorrect way of employing the technique as small talk and the actual investigation part of

---

[4]   Both in the training session and in the actual lie detection test, police officers were exposed to videotapes of participants who told truths or lies for the sake of the experiment. It is therefore possible that the improvement in accuracy was obtained because parole officers became more experienced in judging these types of lie. If this is true, it implies that they not necessarily will be better when they judge more forensically relevant material.

[5]   Although recent research (Mann 2001) suggests that there is a positive relationship between accuracy and experience, depending on how experience is measured.

the police interview are totally different situations. Not surprisingly, both guilty and innocent people tend to change their behaviour the moment the actual interview starts (Vrij 1995).

We have employed this so-called *baseline method* several times (Vrij 1998; Vrij and Mann 2001*a,b*), including in the following murder case. During a videotaped real-life police interview, a man was asked to describe his activities during a particular day (Vrij and Mann 2001*a*). The murder suspect gave descriptions of his activities during the morning, afternoon, and evening. Detailed analyses of the videotape revealed a sudden change in his behaviour as soon as he started to describe his activities during the afternoon and evening. One possible reason for this may have been that he was lying. Evidence supported this view. Police investigations could confirm his story about his morning activities, but revealed that his statement about the afternoon and evening were fabricated. In reality, he met the victim and killed her later on that day. In the case of the murderer, we were able to make a good comparison. There seemed no other reasons why different behaviours would emerge while describing the morning or the afternoon and evening. Interestingly, the question on which we based the baseline method 'What did you do that particular day?' could be asked in many police interviews.

(3) The judgement of untruthfulness should only be made when all other possible explanations are negated.

(4) A person suspected of deception should be encouraged to talk. This is necessary to negate the alternative options regarding somebody's behaviour. Moreover, the more a liar talks, the more likely it is that he or she (finally) will give their lies away via verbal and/or non-verbal cues (as they continuously have to pay attention to both speech content and non-verbal behaviour).

Inbau *et al.* (1986) claim that sometimes during police interviews police detectives confront suspects with pieces of evidence they have already gathered. They hereby try to show suspects that it is meaningless to remain silent and that it might be better for them to talk. This interview style will hamper lie detection. One of the difficulties for liars is that they do not know what the observer knows. They therefore do not know what they could tell without running the risk of getting caught out. By disclosing to suspects the facts they know, police officers reduce the uncertainty for lying suspects and make it easier for them to lie.

Another unfortunate strategy is if police detectives accuse suspects of lying by referring to their behaviour, for example, 'You are lying, I can see it in your eyes!' (Inbau *et al.* 1986).[6] This gives suspects the ideal opportunity to 'escape' from the interview situation. They might tell police detectives that they no longer want to continue co-operating with the investigation, and give a 'no comment' interview, as further interviewing does not make sense given the fact that the police detectives do not believe them (the suspect) anyway. Also keep in mind that accusing someone in itself might elicit response changes (Othello error).

(5) There are stereotypical ideas about cues to deception (such as gaze aversion, fidgeting and so on), which research has shown to be unreliable indicators of deception. More accurate cues are listed in Table 27.1. These can be a guide, but keep in mind that not everyone will exhibit these cues during deception.

(6) There is evidence that people are better lie detectors when they are asked indirectly whether they think someone is lying (DePaulo 1994). In some studies, after watching a truthful or deceptive story, participants were asked to detect deception both in a direct way (i.e. 'Is the person lying?') and in an indirect way (i.e. 'Does the speaker sincerely like the person (s)he just described?'). These studies found greater accuracy in the indirect measures (see Vrij *et al.* 2001*b*). It might be the result of conversation rules which regulate politeness. Observers are often unsure as

---

[6] Sometimes professional lie catchers tell us that they believe that eye movements are associated with deception. They then typically refer to the neurolinguistic programming (NLP) model. However, not a single scientific study has demonstrated that eye movements are related to deception in the way described in the NLP model (Vrij and Lochun 1997). NLP teachers who claim the opposite therefore are engaged in deceiving their pupils.

to whether someone is lying to them. In these cases it would be impolite or for other reasons undesirable to accuse someone of being a liar (e.g. 'I do not believe you'), but it might be possible to challenge the words of a speaker more subtly (e.g. 'Do you really like that person so much?'). Alternatively, people might look at different cues when detecting lies than when applying an indirect method. In Vrij *et al.*'s (2001*b*) study, police officers could distinguish between truths and lies, only by using an indirect method (by judging whether truth tellers and liars had to think hard instead of by judging whether they were lying). Moreover, only in the indirect method they did pay attention to the cues which actually discriminated between the truth tellers and liars, such as a decrease in hand movements.

Conclusions

Research has indicated that both laypersons and professional lie catchers are commonly mistaken when they try to detect deceit. However, the picture is not entirely gloomy. Some people seem to be capable of detecting lies and perhaps the poor lie detectors can learn from them. Also, some training programmes aimed at enhancing detecting deceit have obtained promising results. Both this chapter and publications cited in this chapter provide a variety of tips which could be used by those who would like to become better lie detectors. There is evidence that lie detection skills can be easily improved. Disregarding reliance on popular cues such as gaze aversion and fidgeting is a step in the right direction in becoming a better lie detector.

References

Akehurst, L., Köhnken, G., Vrij, A., and Bull, R. (1996). Lay persons' and police officers' beliefs regarding deceptive behaviour. *Applied Cognitive Psychology*, **10**, 461–73.

Bond, C. F. and Atoum, A. O. (2000). International deception. *Personality and Social Psychology Bulletin*, **26**, 285–395.

Bond, C. F. and Fahey, W. E. (1987). False suspicion and the misperception of deceit. *British Journal of Social Psychology*, **26**, 41–6.

Burgoon, J. K., Kelly, D. L., Newton, D. A., and Keely-Dyreson, M. P. (1989). The nature of arousal and non-verbal indices. *Human Communication Research*, **16**, 217–55.

DePaulo, B. M. (1994). Spotting lies: can humans learn to do better? *Current Directions in Psychological Science*, **3**, 83–6.

DePaulo, B. M., Kashy, D. A., Kirkendol, S. E., Wyer, M. M., and Epstein, J. A. (1996). Lying in everyday life. *Journal of Personality and Social Psychology*, **70**, 979–95.

DePaulo, B. M. and Kirkendol, S. E. (1989). The motivational impairment effect in the communication of deception. In *Credibility assessment* (ed. J. C. Yuille), pp. 51–70. Kluwer, Dordrecht.

DePaulo, B. M., Kirkendol, S. E., Tang, J., and O'Brien, T. P. (1988). The motivational impairment effect in the communication of deception: replications and extensions. *Journal of Non-verbal Behavior*, **12**, 177–201.

DePaulo, B. M., Lanier, K., and Davis, T. (1983). Detecting the deceit of the motivated liar. *Journal of Personality and Social Psychology*, **45**, 1096–103.

DePaulo, B. M., LeMay, C. S., and Epstein, J. A. (1991). Effects of importance of success and expectations for success on effectiveness at deceiving. *Personality and Social Psychology Bulletin*, **17**, 14–24.

DePaulo, B. M., Lindsay, J. J., Malone, B. E., Muhlenbruck, L., Charlton, K., and Cooper, H. (2003). Cues to deception. *Psychological Bulletin*, **129**, 74–118.

DePaulo, B. M. and Pfeifer, R. L. (1986). On-the-job experience and skill at detecting deception. *Journal of Applied Social Psychology*, **16**, 249–67.

DePaulo, B. M., Stone, J. L., and Lassiter, G. D. (1985). Deceiving and detecting deceit. In *The self and social life* (ed. B. R. Schenkler), pp. 323–70. McGraw-Hill, New York, NY.

Ekman, P. (1992). *Telling lies*. W. W. Norton, New York, NY.

Ekman, P. and Frank, M. G. (1993). Lies that fail. In *Lying and deception in everyday life* (eds M. Lewis and C. Saarni), pp. 184–201. Guildford Press, New York, NY.

Ekman, P. and Friesen, W. V. (1972). Hand movements. *Journal of Communication*, **22**, 353–74.

Ekman, P. and O'Sullivan, M. (1991). Who can catch a liar? *American Psychologist*, **46**, 913–20.

Ekman, P., O'Sullivan, M. and Frank, M. G. (1999). A few can catch a liar. *Psychological Science*, **10**, 263–66.

Ekman, P., O'Sullivan, M., and O'Sullivan, M. (1988). Smiles when lying. *Journal of Personality and Social Psychology*, **54**, 414–20.

Ekman, P., O'Sullivan, M., and Scherer, K. R. (1976). Body movement and voice pitch in deceptive interaction. *Semiotica*, **16**, 23–7.

Feeley, T. H. and deTurck, M. A. (1997). Perceptions of communication as seen by the actor and as seen by the observer: the case of lie detection. Paper presented at the International Communication Association Annual Conference. Montreal, Canada.

Feeley, T. H. and deTurck, M. A. (1998). The behavioral correlates of sanctioned and unsanctioned deceptive communication. *Journal of Non-verbal Behavior*, **22**, 189–204.

Forrest, J. A., and Feldman, R. S. (2000). Detecting deception and judge's involvement: Lower task involvement leads to better lie detection. *Personality and Social Psychology Bulletin*, **26**, 118–25.

Frank, M. G. and Ekman, P. (1997). The ability to detect deceit generalizes across different types of high-stake lies. *Journal of Personality and Social Psychology*, **72**, 1429–439.

Goldman-Eisler, F. (1968). *Psycholinguistics: experiments in spontaneous speech*. Doubleday, New York, NY.

Granhag, P. A. and Strömwall, L. A. (2001). Detection deception based on repeated interrogations. *Legal and Criminological Psychology*, **6**, 85–101.

Gudjonsson, G. H. (1992). *The psychology of interrogations, confessions and testimony*. Wiley and Sons, Chichester.

Harrigan, J. A. and O'Connell, D. M. (1996). Facial movements during anxiety states. *Personality and Individual Differences*, **21**, 205–12.

Heinrich, C. A. and Borkenau, P. (1998). Deception and deception detection: the role of cross-modal inconsistency. *Journal of Personality*, **66**, 687–712.

Hocking, J. E. and Leathers, D. G. (1980). Non-verbal indicators of deception: a new theoretical perspective. *Communication Monographs*, **47**, 119–31.

Inbau, F. E., Reid, J. E., and Buckley, J. P. (1986). *Criminal interrogation and confessions*. Williams and Wilkins, Baltimore, MD.

Johnson, M. K. and Raye, C. L. (1981). Reality monitoring. *Psychological Bulletin*, **88**, 67–85.

Johnson, M. K. and Raye, C. L. (1998). False memories and confabulation. *Trends in Cognitive Sciences*, **2**, 137–45.

Kassin, S. M. and Fong, C. T. (1999). 'I'm innocent!': effects of training on judgments of truth and deception in the interrogation room. *Law and Human Behavior*, **23**, 499–516.

Keltner, D. and Harker, L. A. (1998). Forms and functions of the non-verbal signal of shame. In *Interpersonal approaches to shame* (eds P. Gilbert and B. Andrews), pp. 78–98. Oxford University Press, Oxford.

Köhnken, G. (1987). Training police officers to detect deceptive eyewitness statements. Does it work? *Social Behaviour*, **2**, 1–17.

Köhnken, G. (1999). Statement Validity Assessment. Paper presented at the pre-conference programme of applied courses 'Assessing credibility' organized by the European Association of Psychology and Law. Dublin, Ireland.

Mann, S. (2001). Suspects, lies and videotape: an investigation into telling and detecting lies in police/suspect interviews. PhD thesis. University of Portsmouth, Psychology Department, Portsmouth, England.

Mann, S., Vrij, A., and Bull, R. (2002). Suspects, lies and videotape: an analysis of authentic high-stakes liars. *Law and Human Behavior*, **26**, 365–76.

Miller, G. R. and Stiff, J. B. (1993). *Deceptive communication*. Sage Publications, Newbury Park, CA.

Moston, S. J. and Engelberg, T. (1993). Police questioning techniques in tape recorded interviews with criminal suspects. *Policing and Society*, **3**, 223–37.

Moston, S. J., Stephenson, G. M., and Williamson, T. M. (1992). The effects of case characteristics on suspect behaviour during police questioning. *British Journal of Criminology*, **32**, 23–39.

Ofshe, R. J. and Leo, R. A. (1997). The decision to confess falsely: rational choice and irrational action. *Denver University Law Review*, **74**, 979–1112.

O'Sullivan, M., Ekman, P., and Friesen, W. V. (1988). The effect of comparisons on detecting deceit. *Journal of Non-verbal Behavior*, **12**, 203–16.

Porter, S., Woodworth, M., and Birt, A. R. (2000). Truth, lies, and videotape: an investigation of the ability of federal parole officers to detect deception. *Law and Human Behavior*, **24**, 643–58.

Steller, M. (1989). Recent developments in statement analysis. In *Credibility assessment* (ed. J. C. Yuille), pp. 135–54. Kluwer, Deventer.

Taylor, R. and Vrij, A. (2000). The effects of varying stake and cognitive complexity on beliefs about the cues to deception. *International Journal of Police Science and Management*, **3**, 111–24.

Tye, M. C., Amato, S. L., Honts, C. R., Kevitt, M. K., and Peters, D. (1999). The willingness of children to lie and the assessment of credibility in an ecologically relevant laboratory setting. *Applied Developmental Science*, **3**, 92–109.

Vrij, A. (1993). Credibility judgments of detectives: the impact of non-verbal behavior, social skills and physical characteristics on impression formation. *Journal of Social Psychology*, **133**, 601–11.

Vrij, A. (1994). The impact of information and setting on detection of deception by police detectives. *Journal of Non-verbal Behavior*, **18**, 117–37.

Vrij, A. (1995). Behavioral correlates of deception in a simulated police interview. *Journal of Psychology: Interdisciplinary and Applied*, **129**, 15–29.

Vrij, A. (1998). To lie or not to lie. *Psychologie*, **17**, 22–5.

Vrij, A. (2000a). *Detecting lies and deceit: the psychology of lying and the implications for professional practice*. Wiley and Sons, Chichester UK.

Vrij, A. (2000b). Telling and detecting lies as a function of raising the stakes. In *New trends in criminal investigation and evidence II* (eds C. M. Breur, M. M. Kommer, J. F. Nijboer, and J. M. Reintjes), pp. 699–709. Intersentia, Antwerp.

Vrij, A. (2002). The camera never lies: investigating and detecting the lies of murderers and thieves during police interviews. Inaugural Lecture, University of Portsmouth.

Vrij, A. and Heaven, S. (1999). Vocal and verbal indicators of deception as a function of lie complexity. *Psychology, Crime, and Law*, **4**, 401–13.

Vrij, A., Edward, K., and Bull, R. (2001). People's insight into their own behaviour and speech content while lying. *British Journal of Psychology*, **92**, 373–89.

Vrij, A. and Lochun, S. (1997). Neuro-linguistic programming and the police: worthwhile or not? *Journal of Police and Criminal Psychology*, **12**, 25–31.

Vrij, A. and Mann, S. (2001a). Telling and detecting lies in a high-stake situation: the case of a convicted murderer. *Applied Cognitive Psychology*, **15**, 187–203.

Vrij, A. and Mann, S. (2001b). Who killed my relative? Police officers' ability to detect real-life high-stake lies. *Psychology, Crime, and Law*, **7**, 119–32.

Vrij, A. and Semin, G. R. (1996). Lie experts' beliefs about non-verbal indicators of deception. *Journal of Non-verbal Behavior*, **20**, 65–81.

Vrij, A., Semin, G. R., and Bull, R. (1996). Insight in behavior displayed during deception. *Human Communication Research*, **22**, 544–62.

Vrij, A., Semin, G. R., and Bull, R. (2001a). Stereotypical verbal and non-verbal responses while deceiving others. *Personality and Social Psychology Bulletin*, **27**, 899–909.

Vrij, A., Semin, G. R., and Bull, R. (2001b). Police officers' ability to detect deceit: the benefit of indirect deception measures. *Legal and Criminological Psychology*, **6**, 185–96.

Vrij, A. and Suaham, S. (1997). Individual differences between and the ability to detect lies. *Expert Guidance*, **5**, 144–8.

Vrij, A. and Taylor, R. (2003). Police officers' and students' beliefs about telling and detecting little and serious lies. *International Journal of Police Science and Management*.

Vrij, A. and Winkel, F. W. (1991). Cultural patterns in Dutch and Surinam non-verbal behavior: an analysis of simulated police/citizen encounters. *Journal of Non-verbal Behavior*, **15**, 169–84.

Vrij, A. and Winkel, F. W. (1992). Crosscultural police–citizen interactions: the influence of race, beliefs and non-verbal communication on impression formation. *Journal of Applied Social Psychology*, **22**, 1546–559.

Vrij, A. and Winkel, F. W. (1994). Perceptual distortions in crosscultural interrogations: the impact of skin color, accent, speech style and spoken fluency on impression formation. *Journal of Cross-Cultural Psychology*, **25**, 284–96.

Wallbott, H. G. and Scherer, K. R. (1991). Stress specifics: differential effects of coping style, gender, and type of stressor on automatic arousal, facial expression, and subjective feeling. *Journal of Personality and Social Psychology*, **61**, 147–56.

Zuckerman, M., DePaulo, B. M., and Rosenthal, R. (1981). Verbal and non-verbal communication of deception. In *Advances in experimental social psychology*, (ed. L. Berkowitz), Vol. 14, pp. 1–57. Academic Press, New York, NY.

Index